E. JAMES POTCHEN, M.D., *Consulting Editor*

Professor and Chairman
Department of Radiology
Michigan State University
East Lansing, Michigan

Published

Volume 10 in the Series
SAUNDERS
MONOGRAPHS
IN CLINICAL
RADIOLOGY

Forthcoming Monographs

RADIOLOGIC DIAGNOSIS OF RENAL PARENCHYMAL DISEASE
Alan J. Davidson, M.D.

RADIOLOGY OF THE GALLBLADDER AND BILE DUCTS
Robert N. Berk, M.D., and Arthur R. Clemett, M.D.

THE RADIOLOGY OF VERTEBRAL TRAUMA
John A. Gehweiler, Jr., M.D., Raymond L. Osborne, Jr., M.D., and R. Frederick Becker, Ph.D.

ARTHROGRAPHY: PRINCIPLES AND TECHNIQUES
Tom W. Staple, M.D.

CLINICAL PEDIATRIC AND ADOLESCENT UROGRAPHY
Richard C. Pfister, M.D., and Alfred L. Weber, M.D.

RADIOLOGY OF THE LIVER
James McNulty, M.B., F.F.R.

PEDIATRIC ORTHOPEDIC RADIOLOGY
Michael B. Ozonoff, M.D.

XEROMAMMOGRAPHIC PATHOLOGY
Michael D. Lagios, M.D., H. Joachim Burhenne, M.D., and F. Margolin, M.D.

With a chapter on

Formation and Development of the Alimentary Tract

by

DAVID F. MERTEN, M.D.

Assistant Professor of Radiology and Pediatrics
University of California, Davis
School of Medicine
Davis, California

RADIOLOGY
OF THE
ALIMENTARY TRACT
IN INFANTS
AND CHILDREN

Second Edition

EDWARD B. SINGLETON, M.D.

Director of Radiology, St. Luke's Episcopal Hospital,
Texas Children's Hospital, and the Texas Heart Institute;
Clinical Professor of Radiology,
Baylor College of Medicine and the
University of Texas Medical School,
Houston, Texas

MILTON L. WAGNER, M.D.

Associate Radiologist, St. Luke's Episcopal Hospital,
Texas Children's Hospital, and the Texas Heart Institute;
Clinical Associate Professor of Radiology,
Baylor College of Medicine,
Houston, Texas

ROBERT V. DUTTON, M.D.

Associate Radiologist, St. Luke's Episcopal Hospital,
Texas Children's Hospital, and the Texas Heart Institute;
Clinical Assistant Professor of Radiology and
Clinical Assistant Professor of Pediatrics,
Baylor College of Medicine,
Houston, Texas

1977

W. B. SAUNDERS COMPANY • Philadelphia • London • Toronto

W. B. Saunders Company: West Washington Square
Philadelphia, PA 19105

1 St. Anne's Rd.
Eastbourne, East Sussex BN21 3UN, England

833 Oxford Street
Toronto, Ontario M8Z 5T9, Canada

Radiology of the Alimentary Tract in Infants and Children, 2nd ed.   ISBN   0-7216-8314-2

Last digit is the print number: 9   8   7   6   5   4   3   2   1

FOREWORD

Children are not simply micro-adults, but have their own specific problems.

Béla Schick, 1877–1967

Nowhere is the above aphorism more true than in the field of gastrointestinal radiology. Ever since Cannon's publication of *The Mechanisms of Digestion* in 1911, numerous books and reviews have been devoted to analysis and appreciation of the role of radiology in the diagnosis and management of gastrointestinal disorders. However, until this past decade few publications discussed the important problems that can occur in the alimentary tract of children.

Recently the role of the upper gastrointestinal radiologic examination in the evaluation of dyspepsia has been brought into question because of the availability of alternative diagnostic techniques, such as endoscopy. However, radiology, especially fluoroscopy, remains a vital means for examining the pediatric patient with a gastrointestinal problem.

In adults the efficacy of contrast examination of the colon is limited to relatively few disease entities. On the other hand, in pediatrics the gastrointestinal tract represents a myriad of issues, variations, and complexities that are all too infrequently appreciated by the general clinician whose primary interest has been adult radiology. While reading through this book, I have come to realize the spectrum of disorders and the subtleties of variation that can be revealed by contrast examination in children in whom early diagnosis can clearly yield a significant improvement. This volume is an excellent resource for the radiologist, gastroenterologist, pediatrician, and pediatric surgeon and, in my view, is superior to all other existing publications on the subject.

Edward B. Singleton, the senior author of this completely revised work, is a man well known for his warmth, charm, and sense of humor as well as his important contributions to pediatric radiology. He has been joined by two colleagues at Texas Children's Hospital, Milton L. Wagner and Robert V. Dutton, who are both outstanding pediatric radiologists. This book manifestly represents an accumulation of considerable judgment, experience, and knowledge and sets a new hallmark for future developments in the field.

It is indeed a pleasure to welcome *Radiology of the Alimentary Tract in Infants and Children* to Saunders Monographs in Clinical Radiology.

E. JAMES POTCHEN, M.D.

PREFACE

The first edition of *X-Ray Diagnosis of the Alimentary Tract in Infants and Children* was published in 1959. In the subsequent years, additional experience in the x-ray evaluation of alimentary tract disorders in this age group has demonstrated the necessity for a new edition. During the past ten years there has been an increase in the number of articles pertaining to pediatric radiology, and many of the major pediatric and radiology journals allocate sections for pediatric radiology. Also, a journal specifically devoted to pediatric radiology is now available, and the many seminars on this subject attest to the importance of this relatively young specialty.

The improvement of fluoroscopic equipment and image amplification during the past decade has greatly enhanced the radiologist's diagnostic accuracy in detecting gastrointestinal tract abnormalities. Even more important, the low milliamperage of image amplification has reduced considerably the amount of radiation exposure to these patients during fluoroscopy. This aspect of pediatric radiography is particularly appreciated by those of us who recall the "old days" of dark adaptation followed by prolonged fluoroscopic studies, waiting for the duodenal bulb to fill in a child who was frightened not only by the procedure but also by the dark environment. Of equal importance, especially in the evaluation of tracheoesophageal fistula and swallowing dysfunctions, is the availability of rapid spot film facilities and videotape equipment. Although 16- and 35-mm cine recording devices have been developed, videotape recording is preferable because of the reduced radiation delivered to the patient. These devices, again made possible through the development of image intensification, have provided a much more accurate method of examining physiologic and anatomic abnormalities of the pharynx and esophagus. Unfortunately, because of the size of the fluoroscopic carriage and the addition of television cameras and sophisticated spot film devices, the radiologist frequently is unable to be close enough to the patient for adequate palpation of the stomach and duodenum. However, this is less important in the pediatric patient, since most of the procedures are done with the patient recumbent, and the disadvantage is more than compensated by the improved image. Despite the decline in the "art of fluoroscopy," so well performed by the preamplification radiologists, fluoroscopy remains an indispensable part of the alimentary tract examination of the pediatric patient, as it does in the adult.

More recent introduction of ultrasound studies of abdominal organs is especially important in children because it offers a method of study without using ionizing radiation. The value of computerized tomography of the abdominal organs in the pediatric patient is yet to be determined, but the revolutionary and rapid development of these newer modalities will undoubtedly provide safer and more accurate diagnosis in pediatric as well as adult patients.

There has been an increasing interest and awareness of alimentary tract problems of children, not only by radiologists but also by many pediatricians and surgeons who have developed the subspecialty of pediatric gastroenterology. Endoscopy of the intestinal tract, especially the colon, is now commonly performed and offers reliable methods of diagnosis and, at times, treatment. The interest of the pediatric radiologist in a more accurate radiologic diagnosis and localization of accessible lesions has been helpful in the development of endoscopy.

Malabsorption syndromes have been recognized with increased frequency in the past ten years in all age groups. This is particularly true in infants and children, and although the radiographic findings are frequently nonspecific, the radiologist should have a knowledge of the variety of causes of malabsorption.

Hydrostatic reduction of intussusception has become a recognized method of treatment in many selected cases and is hopefully no longer considered as a competitive approach to the surgical treatment. Advances in pediatric surgery, particularly in both congenital and acquired obstructive lesions of the esophagus, have permitted fluoroscopic observations and videotape recordings of physiologic alterations following the surgical procedures.

The role of hypoxia in the etiology of ischemic bowel disease now seems clearly established. This relationship was first described as noninfectious enterocolitis in the first edition of this book. A spectrum of ischemic bowel disease related to hypoxia and stress is now recognized in both the fetus and young infant.

Since the last edition there has been an increasing awareness of newer concepts in pathogenesis of congenital obstructive lesions. Earlier theories of failure of embryonic canalization of the alimentary tube are now considered to be rare causes of congenital obstruction, intrauterine anoxic or stress insults to the fetus with resulting vascular insult to the bowel and subsequent necrosis and scarring being a more logical consideration. Important experimental investigations have established the etiologic role of ischemic changes in the bowel in obstructive lesions as well as in necrotizing enterocolitis. Additional considerations in the radiologic examination and diagnosis and occasionally treatment of congenital colonic obstructions, including imperforate anus and meconium ileus, are now being applied differently than the older methods. Water-soluble iodide contrast medium had a brief period of popularity but because of its hypertonic qualities has been, for the most part, discarded except for occasional therapeutic use in meconium plug obstructions and some anorectal anomalies.

The importance of hyperalimentation feeding in the treatment of many debilitating gastrointestinal problems in young infants and the utilization of catheter placement under fluoroscopy has become an important procedure in maintaining the nutrition of many of these infants.

Because a knowledge of embryology is imperative in the appreciation of congenital defects, a chapter describing normal embryologic development of the alimentary tract has been written by David F. Merten, M.D. We are very grateful for the dedicated effort he gave to this subject. In addition, for the sake of completeness, a section on abnormalities of the gallbladder, liver, and pancreas is included. These additional chapters will enhance the value of this book for both pediatricians and radiologists.

Many of these considerations, as well as a new look and approach at alimentary tract radiology in the pediatric age group, are presented in this new edition.

Acknowledgment of the cooperation of our secretary Mrs. Vivian Spears, the x-ray technologists of Texas Children's Hospital, and the photography departments of St. Luke's Epsicopal Hospital, Texas Children's Hospital, and the Texas Heart Institute is gratefully given.

The friendly and constructive efforts of Mr. John Hanley, Mr. Herbert Powell, and the staff of the W. B. Saunders Company are also respectfully acknowledged.

EDWARD B. SINGLETON
MILTON L. WAGNER
ROBERT V. DUTTON

CONTENTS

Chapter 1

INDICATIONS FOR RADIOLOGIC EXAMINATION

Although the indications for radiologic examination of the alimentary tract are dependent upon the judgment of the patient's attending physician, the radiologist is frequently consulted regarding the advisability of the examination and the order in which it should be conducted, i.e., upper or lower bowel examination. For this reason, the radiologist should be cognizant of the indications for the examination, as well as the symptomatology of the many disorders of the child's alimentary tract. Only with this knowledge can he assess his radiologic results in an accurate and logical manner. The radiologist's responsibility consists not only of the interpretation of the fluoroscopic and radiographic findings but especially the correlation of these findings with the clinical information.

In general, there are certain major symptoms which influence the pediatrician to refer his patient to the radiologist for an alimentary tract examination. These indications are vomiting, abdominal pain, abdominal mass, abdominal distention, constipation or diarrhea, and rectal bleeding. Each symptom may have a different connotation, depending upon the patient's age, the combination of symptoms, or the characteristics of each symptom. Correlation of the radiologic impression with the symptomatology is especially important in the evaluation of obstructive lesions in the infant age group. At this age, the variability of the intestinal gas pattern is such that errors in judgment may easily occur unless the clinical evidence is closely correlated with the radiologic impression. The most accurate

radiologic diagnoses will be made by the radiologist who is aware of the significance of the child's symptoms, and who is therefore better qualified to demonstrate the causative lesion radiologically. It should be remembered, however, that the typical symptoms of a specific abnormality may not be present or may be masked by another condition. This further emphasizes the value of the radiologic examination.

VOMITING

Vomiting is the most common symptom requiring radiologic evaluation in the young infant and, unlike the problem of abdominal pain, the radiologic studies are usually informative in demonstrating both anatomic and physiologic disorders.

In the neonatal period severe vomiting is usually indicative of a congenital obstructive lesion. Vomiting accompanied by excessive mucus or by strangling during the first feeding attempts is suggestive of esophageal atresia, with or without tracheoesophageal fistula. Vomiting which occurs shortly after the first feeding is more characteristic of high intestinal obstruction. This obstruction may be due to volvulus of the midgut, duodenal atresia or stenosis, peritoneal band, or annular pancreas. Bile in the vomitus is evidence that the obstruction is below the ampulla of Vater.

Persistent regurgitation of feedings after the neonatal period should arouse suspicions of gastroesophageal incompetence, the result either of chalasia or, less likely,

1

achalasia. Hematemesis in the newborn suggests consumptive coagulopathy or anoxic ulceration of the esophagus or stomach. In either case radiologic studies are usually uninformative. Hematemesis after the neonatal period may be a sign of esophagitis secondary to reflux of gastric juices into the esophagus, or of peptic ulceration in the esophagus, stomach, or duodenum. Absence of a demonstrable cause for vomiting in infancy suggests that the parents are overly concerned about the normal "spitting up" of their baby or that the infant may have some unexplained milk intolerance, requiring a milk substitute. Unexplained vomiting in young infants may also be secondary to sepsis or an intracranial lesion.

Projectile vomiting in infants 3 to 7 weeks old, accompanied by a palpable mass in the pyloric region, is characteristic of hypertrophic pyloric stenosis. The sudden onset of vomiting accompanied by abdominal pain in the older infant should arouse the suspicion of intussusception, whether or not blood is present in the stool. Emesis accompanying dysphagia in older infants or in children is often indicative of esophageal stenosis or compression on the esophagus by an extrinsic lesion. Vomiting past infancy is usually the result of an acquired disease, although the possibility of a latent congenital lesion, such as volvulus secondary to malrotation of the midgut or duplication anomalies with pressure on the adjacent bowel, should be considered. Hematemesis in this age group suggests gastric or duodenal ulceration or esphageal varices.

ABDOMINAL PAIN

Most gastrointestinal tract examinations in children past infancy are made in an effort to locate the cause of abdominal pain. In infants, this symptom alone is difficult to evaluate. However, an infant who persistently cries for no apparent reason, and who maintains the thighs flexed on the abdomen or a knee-chest position, should be suspected of having abdominal pain, probably secondary to abnormality of the gastrointestinal tract. Persistence of the discomfort excludes colic, and localized tenderness should raise the question of mesenteric adenitis or appendicitis, the lat-

ter being less common in this age group. If the pain is accompanied by vomiting, an obstructive lesion should be suspected, and if a palpable abdominal mass or rectal bleeding is present, intussusception is the most likely etiology.

There is no explanation for the cause of most "stomach aches" in children past infancy. Periumbilical pain in a child 5 to 12 years old is an especially common complaint. The discomfort usually is present only during the day and is often accompanied by anorexia. A relationship between this type of pain and associated allergies has not been convincingly correlated. Urinary tract abnormalities in this age group are more commonly responsible for abdominal pain than recognizable gastrointestinal tract disease. Consequently, excretory pyelography should precede radiologic investigation of the intestinal tract. Electroencephalographic findings may suggest "abdominal epilepsy" and a clinical trial of Dilantin medication may be confirmative. Emotional factors undoubtedly play a part in the production of abdominal pain in this age group.

Recurrent small bowel intussusception may well be a more common cause of unexplained abdominal pain in children than is suspected, but it will not be demonstrated during gastrointestinal tract examination unless the study is performed during an episode of pain. Epigastric pain, particularly at night and on awakening in the morning, should arouse suspicions of peptic ulcer or abdominal epilepsy. The possibility of parasitic infestation also should be considered in the presence of ill-defined abdominal pain in children. Although appendicitis is uncommon in young children, it should not be discounted as improbable, particularly if there are pain and tenderness in the right lower quadrant accompanied by leukocytosis. Similar tenderness in the right midabdomen and right upper quadrant in an infant should still warrant the consideration of appendicitis because of the high location of the cecum common at this age. Similar symptoms with or without blood in the stool may be produced by Meckel's diverticulitis. Chronic discomfort in the lower abdomen, most often on the right side, accompanied by loss of weight and anemia, may be due to lymphoma or pelvic neoplasms.

ABDOMINAL DISTENTION

Generalized abdominal distention in the neonatal age occurs in all cases of low small bowel and colon obstructions, such as congenital bowel atresias and stenoses, meconium ileus, peritoneal bands, imperforate anus, incarcerated hernias, aganglionosis of small bowel or colon, and pressure from adjacent masses. The obstruction is ordinarily accompanied by vomiting, abdominal pain, and constipation. Pneumoperitoneum resulting from necrotizing enterocolitis and perforation of the gastrointestinal tract is another cause of abdominal distention in this age group. Abdominal distention of the newborn may also result from failure of passage of a meconium plug.

In the infant and young child, distention accompanied by bulky and foul-smelling stools suggests one of the malabsorption syndromes. Distention unaccompanied by other symptoms may result from the ingestion of large quantities of air. Intestinal obstruction in infants and older children will also cause generalized abdominal distention if the obstructive lesion is in the colon or low small bowel. In older children vomiting is usually less conspicuous than in infants. Although mild or moderate abdominal distention may occur in the habit type of constipation, it reaches tremendous proportions in untreated Hirschsprung's disease.

Generalized distention accompanied by signs of peritoneal irritation in either infants or children usually indicates peritonitis, either primary or following perforation of the bowel.

ABDOMINAL MASS

Most abdominal masses (hydronephrosis, renal cystic disease, Wilms' tumor, neuroblastoma, etc.) encountered in infancy or childhood are retroperitoneal and do not produce symptoms of gastrointestinal tract disease. An exception is the diarrhea occasionally produced by the catecholamine-excreting tumors, best exemplified by the neuroblastomas. Usually, pyelographic studies disclose their location and intestinal tract examination is unnecessary. Intra-abdominal cysts occurring at any age may, by encroachment on adjacent bowel, produce an obstruction and accompanying symptoms of abdominal pain and vomiting. The mere presence of these cysts, unaccompanied by symptoms, is sufficient reason for alimentary tract studies in order to ascertain their location and extent as accurately as possible before surgery. Enterogenous cysts and mesenteric lymphangiomas are the commonest of these cysts, and are usually impossible to differentiate radiologically unless the enterogenous cyst communicates with the adjacent bowel. Furthermore, mesenteric cysts are less likely to produce obstruction. Other cystic conditions to be considered are omphalomesenteric cysts, omental cysts (lymphangiomas), pancreatic cysts, choledochal cysts, urachal cysts, ovarian cysts, and hydrometrocolpos.

The presence of an abdominal mass along the passageway of the colon in an infant having abdominal pain, especially if there is also hematochezia, is practically pathognomonic of intussusception.

A palpable epigastric mass in a child, particularly a girl, should raise the suspicion of trichobezoar. A right upper quadrant mass accompanied by jaundice and abdominal pain may be a choledochal cyst. Palpable fecal masses are invariably present in the child who has either organic or functional type of constipation.

OBSTIPATION, CONSTIPATION, AND DIARRHEA

Obstipation may be present in the neonatal period as a result of any of the many types of congenital obstruction of the intestinal tract. However, except for imperforate anus, there is frequently passage of at least one meconium stool. Additional signs of obstruction, namely vomiting and abdominal distention, are present.

Constipation alone in infancy usually has a dietary basis but may be the result of rectal stenosis or Hirschsprung's disease. In children past the bowel-training age, chronic constipation is the most common reason for radiologic examination of the colon. Organic causes should be considered, but most cases represent a functional, habit type of constipation.

Diarrhea, at any age, usually is the result of acute enteritis or accompanies acute parenteral infection and does not warrant radiologic investigation. Chronic diarrhea in infancy is rare but may be due to chronic ulcerative colitis or colitis resulting from a specific infectious agent. In children past infancy, granulomatous or chronic ulcerative colitis is a more common cause of chronic diarrhea. Episodes of diarrhea may also occur in Hirschsprung's disease, and diarrhea is an invariable accompaniment of necrotizing colitis.

RECTAL BLEEDING

In the evaluation of rectal bleeding, consideration must be given to whether the blood is bright or dark, whether on the stool or intermixed with it, and whether or not there is accompanying pain. If pain accompanies passage of the stool and the blood is on the surface of the stool, a low rectal lesion is present, usually an anal fissure. Passage of a bloody stool unaccompanied by pain suggests a colonic polyp. Bleeding Meckel's diverticulum also should be considered when there is rectal bleeding, but in such cases abdominal pain and tenderness are often present, and the blood is usually darker and more intimately mixed with the stool than in colonic polyposis. Bright rectal bleeding is common with any type of severe colitis. The higher the bleeding site, the darker the blood, although with severe bleeding from the upper portions of the alimentary tract, hematochezia may occur. Melena may occur in infancy and childhood and be the result of a number of conditions, including trauma, peptic ulcer, purpura, esophageal varices, small bowel polyps, intestinal lymphosarcoma, and hemangioma.

Table 1–1 illustrates the large number and variety of causes of gastrointestinal bleeding encountered in infants and children in a ten-year period at the Texas Children's Hospital. Unfortunately, relatively few of these can be demonstrated radiologically.

The type of radiologic examination, whether an upper gastrointestinal series or a colon examination, and the order in which these examinations are conducted, depend upon the symptomatology and the suspected site of the lesion. Scout films of the abdomen, both upright and supine, are invaluable in determining the location, and should precede all radiologic examinations. This simple examination frequently precludes any further radiographic procedure. This is particularly true in cases of congenital obstruction of the proximal portions of the intestinal tract. In cases of lower obstruction, where the level of the obstruction cannot be definitely localized, the feeding of barium is contraindicated because it may have serious consequences. In such cases, and in all cases of intestinal obstruction in which the site of obstruction, i.e., small bowel or colon, cannot be determined by radiographs of the abdomen, barium enema studies are indicated. If the colon is demonstrated to be normal, the obstruction may be assumed to be in the terminal small bowel, and the surgeon so advised. Colon examinations should also be performed first in infants and children who have rectal bleeding, since most lesions producing this sign are found in the colon. Failure to demonstrate the source of the bleeding necessitates examination of the upper gastrointestinal tract. In cases of melena, the reverse order applies. Obviously, in cases of constipation or chronic diarrhea, the colon should be examined first.

Infants and children whose predominant symptom is vomiting during or after feeding and who consequently are suspected of having an esophageal or gastric lesion should, of course, have these structures examined radiologically. Preliminary scout films of the abdomen and chest should be obtained in these cases as well, not only to gain information concerning the nature of the lesion, but as a precaution against giving barium by mouth to a patient with large bowel obstruction.

In the localization of abdominal masses excretory pyelograms and upper gastrointestinal tract examinations with interval films to follow the contrast material into the colon will usually suffice. A barium enema may provide additional information concerning the size and location of the mass.

It should be remembered that the preceding discussion serves only to exemplify the significance of those symptoms which influence the pediatrician to refer his patient to the radiologist. A more detailed account of symptomatology and radiologic procedures is included in the following chapters.

TABLE 1–1. Causes of Gastrointestinal Bleeding

CHART I—DARK BLOOD	CHART II—DARK AND/OR BRIGHT BLOOD	CHART III—BRIGHT BLOOD
Swallowed blood	*Hepatobiliary disease*	*Tumors*
Maternal	Hematobilia	Colonic polyps
Bleeding in utero	Hepatitis	Inflammatory
Bleeding nipples	Posttraumatic	Adenomatous
Oral blood	Cholelithiasis	Familial
Respiratory bleeding	Hypoprothrombinemia	Intestinal polyps
		Peutz-Jeghers syndrome
Mucosal ulceration	*Aberrant gastric and pancreatic tissue*	(melanin spots)
Stress	Duplications	Carcinoma
Anoxia	Meckel's diverticulum	Lymphosarcoma
Trauma		Neuroblastoma
Head injury	*Volvulus*	Teratoma
Burns	Mesenteric thrombosis	Sacrococcygeal
Endocrine lesion		Ovarian
Adrenal	*Intussusception*	Gastric
Pheochromocytoma	Acute	Rhabdomyosarcoma
Corticoma	Chronic	
Cushing tumor	Postoperative	*Enterocolitis*
Aldosteroma	Rectal	Infectious
Parathyroidoma		Specific
Pancreatic	*Systemic disease*	Pseudomembranous
Hypothalamic—pituitary	Allergy	Granulomatous
Peptic ulcers	Milk	Ulcerative
Esophagitis	Schönlein-Henoch purpura	Idiopathic
Gastroduodenal	Glomerulonephritis	Amebic
Marginal	(purpuras)	Renal insufficiency
Obstructive	Necrotizing enterocolopathy	
Esophageal		*Anorectal*
Pyloric	*Trauma*	Proctitis
Intestinal	External	Fissures
Drugs	Blunt	Fistula
Aspirin	Penetrating	Hemorrhoids
Antibiotics	Internal	Impactions
Steroids	Gastrointestinal suction	Stercorium ulcers
Nitrogen mustard	Swallow—foreign body	
Numerous poisons	Suppositories	
	Anal—foreign body	
Varices		
Gastric	*Tumors*	
Esophageal	Hemangioma	
Intestinal	Telangiectasia	

In Chart I, a "Pain" bracket spans Peptic ulcers through Marginal.
In Chart II, a "Pain" bracket spans Duplications through Rectal.
In Chart III, a "Pain at some stage of disease" bracket spans Carcinoma through Rhabdomyosarcoma, and a "Pain" bracket spans Enterocolitis through Stercorium ulcers.

REFERENCES

Apley, H. *The Child with Abdominal Pains* (Springfield, Ill.: Charles C Thomas, 1959).

Astley, R. *Radiology of the Alimentary Tract in Infancy* (London: Edward Arnold, Publishers, 1956).

Eklof, O. Abdominal plain film diagnosis in infants and children, *Progr. Pediatr. Radiol.*, 2:3, 1969.

Gross, R. E. *The Surgery of Infancy and Childhood* (Philadelphia: W. B. Saunders Co., 1953).

Mustard, W. T., Ravitch, M. M., Snyder, W. H., Welch, K. J., and Benson, C. D., editors, *Pediatric Surgery* (2nd ed.; Chicago: Year Book Medical Publishers, 1969).

Schaffer, A. J., and Avery, M. E. *Diseases of the Newborn*, Chapter 28 (3rd ed.; Philadelphia: W. B. Saunders Co., 1971).

Chapter 2

TECHNIC OF EXAMINATION OF UPPER GASTROINTESTINAL TRACT

In the radiologic examination of children, regardless of which portion of the anatomy is under investigation, foremost attention should be directed to the problem of radiation protection. The fluoroscopic exposure should be held to a minimum, and performed only by those well-trained in the technics of fluoroscopy. The use of image amplifiers is of inestimable value, particularly in the examination of the pediatric patient, not only because of the enhancement of diagnostic accuracy but also because of the marked reduction in radiation. Radiation exposure, both in fluoroscopy and radiography, should cover only the portion under examination and whenever possible the gonadal area should be protected by lead shielding or equivalent material.

The preparation for upper gastrointestinal tract studies in our institution is as follows. Nothing is given by mouth after midnight if the exam is scheduled in the morning. However, babies accustomed to scheduled feedings may have a bottle as late as five hours before the study, which is normally done by 9 A.M.

The problems of examination of the upper gastrointestinal tract are primarily concerned with the reluctance of the young patient to ingest the contrast media. In this regard, four age groups should be considered. The neonate and very young infant readily take unflavored barium, and consequently these patients are easily examined. Water-soluble iodide contrast materials have no place in the examination of the

stomach and small intestine. The unpalatable taste of these materials is obviously unpleasant to even the youngest patient but, in addition, the hypertonic characteristics of the water-soluble materials produce diarrhea and have, on occasions, resulted in severe hypovolemia and death. Barium, on the other hand, is much more palatable and safer to use.

There is some disagreement regarding a method of introducing contrast media into the stomach of the young infant. A number of pediatric radiologists prefer routinely to pass a nasogastric tube into the stomach and inject barium directly, whereas others prefer to administer barium through a nursing bottle. The latter method is, in our opinion, far preferable and allows the fluoroscopist to evaluate not only esophageal motility but also the suck reflex and swallowing movement (Fig. 2–1). If the opening in the nipple is made slightly larger than in the ordinary nursing nipple, the examination may be carried out rapidly without any more fluoroscopic time than that used by injecting through a catheter. The insertion of a feeding tube just beyond the opening in the nipple also offers a convenient way of administering barium and simultaneously gratifies the infant (Fig. 2–2). Rubber nipples connected to barium containers are now commercially available. Only small amounts of contrast media are necessary, it being unnecessary to distend the stomach with barium in order to examine it.

Examination of the young infant and

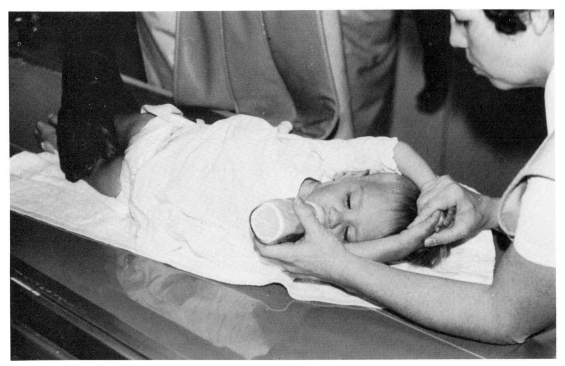

Figure 2-1. Position of administering barium in a nursing bottle to a young infant.

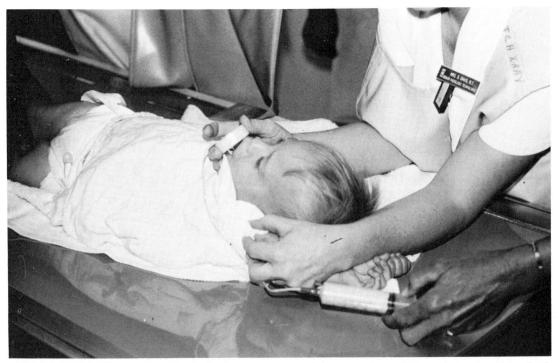

Figure 2-2. Additional method of administering oral barium through a nasogastric tube which has passed just beyond the opening of a rubber nipple.

child is naturally carried out with the patient in the supine position. The contrast media should be administered through a nursing bottle with the infant turned to the right anterior oblique position in relation to the fluoroscopic screen, and with the technician holding the infant's right arm against its head and with the left hand holding the nursing bottle. This allows the pharynx and esophagus to be adequately studied during deglutition, and allows the contrast media to pool in the gastric fundus, prohibiting premature fill of the distal stomach and duodenum. The infant is then turned to the right into the prone position, with the infant's left side elevated, while the fluoroscopist observes the fill of the stomach and waits for gastric peristalsis to fill the duodenum. Because of the normally high transverse position of the infant's stomach and the posterior direction of the first portion of the duodenum, the antrum and lesser curvature of the stomach overlap the pyloric canal and duodenum, making their identification more difficult than in the older patient. But, as the infant is turned to a right lateral and right anterior oblique position in relation to the radiographic table, they can be identified. Forceful palpation and resultant fill of the duodenum is performed with great difficulty, and one must rely mainly on gastric peristalsis to accomplish filling.

Because of the necessity of turning the infant from a supine to a prone position during fluoroscopy, a brat-board is impractical for immobilization. Instead we utilize one of the parents or, preferably, a hospital attendant to restrain the child. Each attendant wears a protective x-ray apron and a film badge. By utilizing the services of many attendants, there is no danger of any one individual receiving an undue amount of exposure.

The older infant and young child, usually between the ages of one and three, is, without question, the most difficult age group to examine because of reluctance to drink the barium voluntarily even when it is flavored. This age group is frequently frightened and at the same time too young to coerce into drinking the necessary contrast material. Rather than forcing a nasogastric tube on this age patient, we prefer to have the infant sit in the fluoroscopist's lap while he forcefully feeds the infant

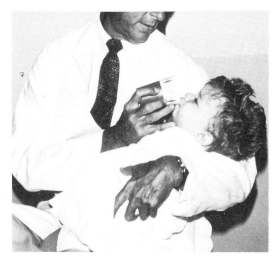

Figure 2–3. Force-feeding of barium through a cup in an older infant.

through a cup (Fig. 2–3). This is sometimes referred to in our department as the swallow or drown technique but, after many years of experience, it has proven successful in the examination of the stomach and small bowel. Although the esophagus is not seen at the time of deglutition, it may be examined by putting the patient in the supine position and giving thick barium in a spoon or using a nursing bottle with a large hole in the nipple to accomplish deglutition. The patient is turned onto the right side for examination of the duodenum in the same method as used for the infant.

The older child is usually agreeable to the examination, particularly if the contrast media is flavored. In our department we prefer chocolate as the flavoring agent, but other agents such as Kool-aid and various forms of flavoring may be utilized satisfactorily. If the child is old enough to stand and cooperate, the examination is carried out with the patient in the upright position and the same technique is used as for the adult (Fig. 2–4).

As the mixture is ingested, its passage down the esophagus into the stomach is carefully observed, with the child being turned to right and left oblique positions in order to determine the configuration and width of the esophagus, its distensibility, patency of the gastroesophageal junction, deviation of the esophagus in the retrocar-

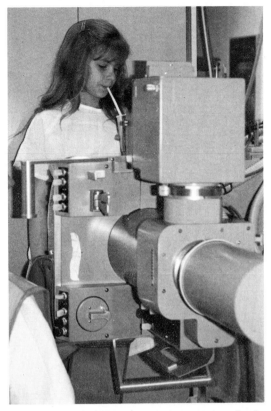

Figure 2-4. Upright examination of the upper gastrointestinal tract in an older child.

diac area, and the location of the aortic arch. Following this, the tumbler is taken from the child and the mucosal pattern of the stomach examined by palpation with the gloved hand. The lateral, anterior, and posterior contours of the stomach are carefully examined by rotating the child into oblique and lateral positions. Then, with the patient in both right and left anterior oblique positions, barium is forced into the duodenum by pressure directed toward the pylorus, and the duodenum is carefully observed for alteration in contour and configuration, and spot films are obtained in both views. Fill of the bulb is frequently facilitated by timing the palpation with gastric peristalsis, which usually begins a few minutes after barium has collected in the stomach. Occasionally, transitory pylorospasm is encountered, necessitating delay in the examination. This is especially prevalent in apprehensive children, and it may be necessary to place the child in the prone position on his right side for a few minutes

before the pylorus relaxes sufficiently to allow barium to pass through it.

After a satisfactory view of the stomach and duodenum has been obtained, the child is placed in a supine position and the fundus of the stomach and its relation to the left hemidiaphragm is studied. Spot films of the duodenum, with the child supine and with the right side slightly elevated, are often of value in obtaining air contrast studies of the pylorus and duodenum, the ingested air rising to fill these structures with the patient in this position. The child is then turned to a prone position and again the stomach and duodenum are briefly visualized. Following this, fluoroscopy is discontinued and PA, AP, and right anterior oblique radiographs of the stomach area are obtained.

Although image amplification has undoubtedly enhanced fluoroscopic accuracy, it has to some extent, because of its size, interfered with the ability to palpate the stomach satisfactorily and manually distend the duodenal bulb. Consequently, the "art of fluoroscopy," as known with the older smaller fluoroscopic screens, is rapidly dying and these young patients are probably examined just as accurately in the recumbent position. Barium is administered through a straw with the patient supine and the right side elevated. This allows the esophagus to be clear of the spine, and barium collects in the fundus of the stomach. After appropriate spot films of the esophagus and gastroesophageal junction are obtained, the stomach is observed fluoroscopically while the patient turns to his right into the prone position with the left side elevated. Adequate visualization and films of the duodenum can then be obtained.

The technic of examination varies, depending upon the suspected type of abnormality. The procedure already described applies to the vast majority of conditions affecting the esophagus, stomach, and duodenum. However, if a lesion of the lower portion of the small intestine is suspected, delayed or interval films concomitant with internal fluoroscopic examination are necessary in order to examine the small bowel completely. The obligation of the radiologist to examine the intestinal tract thoroughly in such cases is no less than that of the surgeon in his examination at the

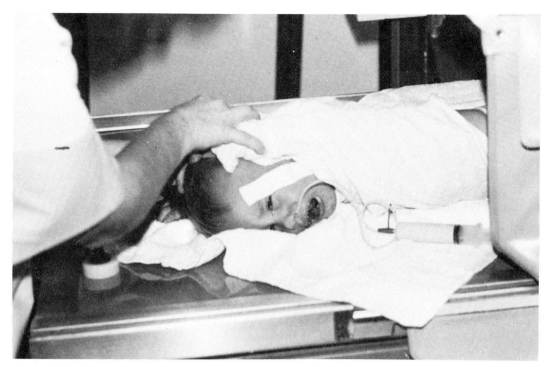

Figure 2–5. Examination for tracheoesophageal fistula. The tip of the catheter has been placed in the upper esophagus and the infant is in a semiprone Trendelenburg position.

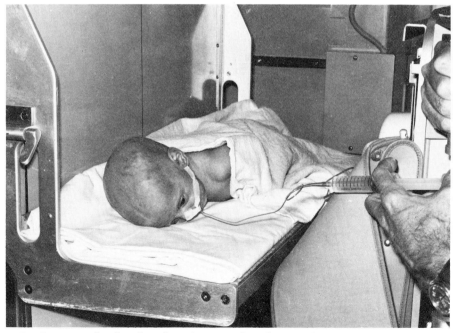

Figure 2–6. Position of infant for identification of tracheoesophageal fistula. The x-ray table is in an upright position, and the infant lies prone on the elevated footboard.

time of laparotomy for unknown intestinal tract disorders.

If a congenital lesion of the esophagus is suspected, particularly esophageal atresia with or without tracheoesophageal fistula, a catheter should be passed through the nose down the esophagus to the level of obstruction and then, under fluoroscopic control, contrast medium injected. The application of a notched plastic strip to hold the catheter avoids the unpleasantness of adhesive tape applied to the infant's nose (Fig. 2–5).

Examination of the infant in the prone and Trendelenburg positions should always be carried out if tracheoesophageal fistula is suspected so as to identify these communications which pass cephalad from the esophagus to the trachea. The method of examination in such conditions is discussed in greater detail under the headings of the individual abnormalities. Placing the infant in the prone position on an elevated footboard or table in front of the upright x-ray table permits excellent lateral fluoroscopic viewing of the neck (Fig. 2–6).

Except in cases of esophageal atresia or tracheoesophageal fistula, barium is the contrast medium of choice, since it is inexpensive and easily swallowed. Iodized oil is difficult for the infant to swallow; consequently, aspiration occurs frequently, acting as an irritant to the pulmonary tissue and often leading to a misdiagnosis of tracheoesophageal fistula.

The value of fluoroscopy in examining the alimentary tract of infants and children is no less than in the examination of the adult patient. The obviously greater difficulties encountered in examining young children and their frequent failure to cooperate should not provide an excuse for indifference or neglect of the fluoroscopic part of the examination. An attitude of patience rather than indifference is vital to the radiologist in his examination of the pediatric patient, and for him to compromise the ideal essentials of the fluoroscopic counterpart and rely solely on radiographic evidence is negligent.

For details regarding the factors of kilovoltage, milliamperage, and time of exposure in obtaining radiographs of the highest diagnostic quality, the reader is referred to the bibliography. It will suffice here to emphasize that only equipment having high milliamperage rating and short exposure times will provide satisfactory radiographs.

REFERENCES

Becker, M. H., and Genieser, N. B. A new device for feeding infants during fluoroscopy, *J. Pediatr.* 80:291, 1972.

Darling, D. B. *Radiography Of Infants And Children* (2nd ed.; Springfield, Ill.: Charles C Thomas, 1971).

Giedion, A. Pacifier nipple (dummy) in pediatric radiology: a remote control pacifier for radiographic studies, *Ann. Radiol.* (Paris), 516:437, 1968.

Gwinn, J. L. Tracheoesophageal fistula with and without esophageal atresia, *Progr. Pediatr. Radiol.*, 2:170, 1969.

Harris, P. D., Neuhauser, E. B. D., and Gerth, R. L. The osmotic effect of water soluble contrast media on circulating plasma volume, *Am. J. Roentgenol. Radium Ther. Nucl. Med.*, 91:694–698, 1964.

Kuhns, L. R., and Poznanski, A. K. A device for control of esophageal tubes in infants, *Radiology*, 102:438, 1972.

Nelson, S. W., Christofordis, A. J., and Roenigk, W. J. Dangers and fallibilities of iodinated radiopaque mediums in obstruction of small bowel, *Am. J. Surg.*, 109:546, 1965.

Poznanski, A. K. *Practical Approaches to Pediatric Radiology.* Chicago: Year Book Medical Publishers, 1976.

Sauvegrain, J. The technique of upper gastro-intestinal investigation in infants and children, *Progr. Pediatr. Radiol.*, 2:26, 1969.

Shurtleff, F. E. *Children's Radiologic Technic* (2nd ed.; Philadelphia: Lea & Febiger, 1962).

Chapter 3

THE FORMATION AND DEVELOPMENT OF THE ALIMENTARY TRACT

Because many alimentary tract abnormalities are the result of abnormal embryogenesis, an understanding of the normal development of the alimentary tract is necessary for an appreciation and clarification of anomalous development. Although in the subsequent chapters a brief description of the embryonic defect as it relates to specific anomalies will be given, this chapter will serve as a reference in understanding the pathogenesis of anomalous development as related to normal development.

The fully developed alimentary tract of the newborn infant is a complex organ system derived from a simple digestive tube through a complicated but orderly series of events that span a period from very early embryonic life to birth.

In order to simplify the presentation of this process, we shall for the most part consider the growth and development of the various segments of the primitive gut individually. It is, however, most important to keep in mind that the end result of the growth process is the sum total of the development of the individual members of this complex organ system, appearing at different points in embryonic life and developing at different rates. Reference to errors in the normal process of alimentary tract

development will be described in the following chapters.

DETERMINATION AND SEGMENTATION OF THE PRIMITIVE ALIMENTARY CANAL

The first evidence of a developing digestive system is found in the embryo of only several weeks of age, and consists of the incorporation of the gut-entoderm into the arching embryonic disc, forming a pouch-like-extension of the vitelline or yolk sac. As the embryo rapidly elongates, the head and tail folds are formed, containing cephalic and caudal extensions of the yolk sac. These blind tubes are the first step in the segmentation of the alimentary canal and are termed the *foregut* and *hindgut* (Fig. 3–1A). The intervening open portion of the primitive gut, the *midgut*, is gradually separated from the yolk sac by constriction of its ventral connection with the yolk sac. This vitelline duct, which attaches at the midportion of the midgut, is completely closed by the end of the fifth week. The resultant tubular alimentary canal can be further divided into the mouth and pharynx (cephalic foregut) and the digestive tube (caudal foregut, midgut, and hindgut) (Fig. 3–1B).

All segments of the primitive gut consist of a lining of entoderm and surrounding mesoderm. The endoderm gives rise to the

This chapter was prepared and written by Dr. David F. Merten, Assistant Professor of Radiology and Pediatrics, University of California Medical Branch, Davis, California.

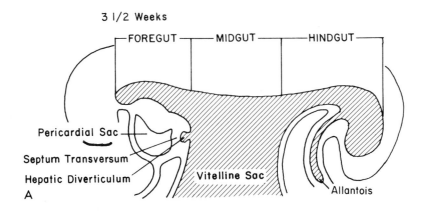

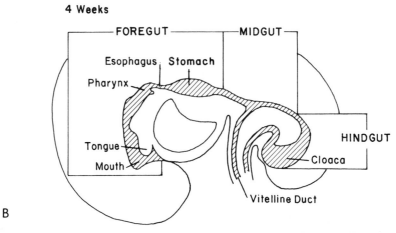

Figure 3–1. Segmentation of the primitive alimentary tract (adapted from Allan). *A*, 3½ weeks. *B*, 4 weeks.

epithelial lining of the alimentary canal and its diverticula, from which the parenchyma of the secretory glands are derived. The mesoderm gives rise to the muscular and mesenteric tissue components of the gut, as well as to the peritoneal lining of the celomic cavity.

THE ESOPHAGUS AND LOWER RESPIRATORY TRACT

In the embryo of four weeks gestation, the esophagus consists of a short section of foregut that extends from the level of the last pharyngeal arch to the cephalic border of the yolk stalk (see Fig. 3–1*B*). From the ventral floor of the most caudal portion of the pharynx a midline cleft is formed, called the *laryngotracheal groove*. This

evagination rapidly elongates along with the esophagus and from its caudal extent paired lateral *lung buds* appear that will become the mainstem bronchi and associated structures (Fig. 3–2). The lumen of the combined esophageal-tracheal tube gradually assumes a narrow vertical configuration, and is soon divided in a caudal to cephalic progression by the folding in and fusion of the lateral walls of the thoracic foregut. The respiratory and alimentary tubes thus formed are soon completely separated by degeneration of the fused area, to be joined only at the level of the larynx.

With further growth of the cardiac and pulmonary structures, the esophagus elongates rapidly and its caudal extent is soon delineated by the developing diaphragm and stomach. No esophageal mesentery, as such, develops.

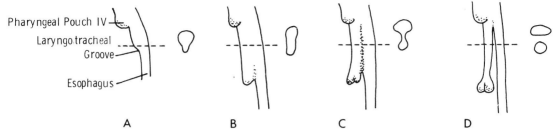

Pharyngeal Pouch IV

Laryngotracheal Groove

Esophagus

A   B   C   D

Figure 3–2. Separation of esophagus and tracheobronchial tree (from Bremer).

THE FORMATION OF THE BODY CAVITIES AND DIAPHRAGM

The formation of the body cavity, or *celom*, begins in the latter part of the second week as bilateral clefts in the mesoderm lateral to the primitive gut. These expand rapidly in a cephalocaudal progression, forming first the single pericardial cavity and the paired pleural canals. The primitive peritoneal cavity is a caudal extension of the pleural canals, remaining for the most part as a single cavity divided dorsally by the mesentery and ventrally only at its superior extent by the septum transversum.

The formation of the ventral abdominal wall by continued elongation and folding of the embryo gradually separates the primitive peritoneal cavity from the extraembryonic celom; the point of final closure is at the umbilical cord.

Division of the celom into the thoracic and abdominal cavities begins at five weeks with the formation of paired lateral pleuroperitoneal folds which ultimately fuse with the midline septum transversum to form the primitive diaphragm (Fig. 3–3). At the beginning of the eighth week, the pleuroperitoneal canals are obliterated by fusion of the pleuroperitoneal folds with the mesoesophagus and by the end of this week, the definitive diaphragm has been formed by the addition of muscular elements derived from mesoderm split from the thoracic wall by the expanding lungs. The central tendon of the diaphragm develops from the septum transversum (Fig. 3–4).

GROWTH AND ROTATION OF THE ABDOMINAL DIGESTIVE TRACT

Below the developing diaphragm, the stomach, proximal duodenum, liver, and pancreas are derived from the foregut, the distal duodenum, small intestine, and large bowel to the distal transverse colon from the midgut, and the distal colon and rectum from the hindgut. The digestive tube has by the beginning of the sixth week become a continuous tubular structure which includes the proximal gastric dilatation and extends caudally to the cloaca. The entire tube is attached to the posterior wall of the abdomen by a midline reflection of connective tissue, the *dorsal mesentery,* through which course the nervous and vascular elements of the developing gut. In addition to this dorsal connection, a short ventral mesentery is derived from the septum transversum and extends from the liver to the stomach and proximal duodenum.

Figure 3–3. Formation of diaphragm and division of abdominal and thoracic cavities.

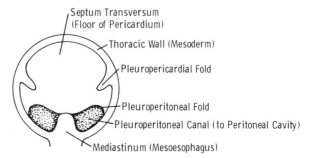

Septum Transversum (Floor of Pericardium)

Thoracic Wall (Mesoderm)

Pleuropericardial Fold

Pleuroperitoneal Fold

Pleuroperitoneal Canal (to Peritoneal Cavity)

Mediastinum (Mesoesophagus)

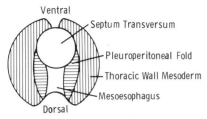

Figure 3–4. The embryonic components of the diaphragm.

The ventral arteries of the abdominal aorta coalesce into three major arteries to the intra-abdominal gut segments. The proximal *celiac artery* supplies the foregut structures, the *superior mesenteric artery* extends to the midgut, and the *inferior mesenteric artery* to the colonic portion of the hindgut. The cloaca and its derivatives derive their vascular supply from the *iliac arteries* and their branches (Fig. 3–5).

The neural elements of the alimentary tract are derived from the autonomic nervous system. Of particular interest to the pediatric radiologist is the development of the intestinal neural plexuses. No intramural ganglion cells are present in the intestinal tract until five weeks gestation. In the ensuing seven weeks, neuroblasts appear in the intermuscular layer, beginning in the proximal portion of the alimentary canal and following a cephalocaudal migration. By the twelfth week of gestation, the neuroblasts are found in the rectum. The neuroblasts migrate from these myenteric plexuses into the submucosa to form the submucosal plexuses. The maturation of the neuroblasts follows the same cephalocaudal progression, with the ratio of mature to immature ganglion cells being greater in the proximal portions of the gut. The maturation process continues on into postnatal life and throughout childhood.

Growth and development of the subdiaphragmatic gut follows a cephalic to caudal progression, showing a continuous zone of growth that advances down the primitive digestive tube in relatively orderly fashion. Thus, the development of the foregut is advanced over that of the mid- and hindgut. This growth pattern is important in the ultimate configuration of the abdominal contents and, according to Lauge-Hansen, is responsible for the rotation of the midgut into its final intra-abdominal position. The rotation of the midgut is an integral part of the normal expansion and elongation of the subdiaphrag-

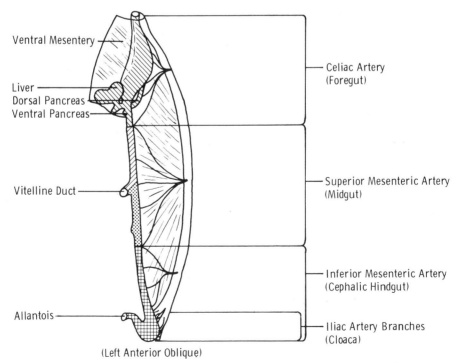

(Left Anterior Oblique)

Figure 3–5. Segmentation and vascular supply of the abdominal gut.

matic alimentary canal. In order to facilitate the understanding of this complex process, it will be considered as a function of the normal growth habit of the gut and not as a separate phenomenon.

The spindle-shaped dilatation of the foregut begins during the fourth week, and thereafter there is rapid asymmetrical expansion and displacement to the left, presumably secondary to the growing liver mass. At the same time the duodenal portion of the foregut grows to the right and forms a slight junction curve with the midgut. By the sixth week the midgut describes an arc or loop toward the ventral abdominal wall, with its apex at the site of the vitelline duct remnant. The superior mesenteric artery with its midpoint at the site of the vitelline duct divides the midgut into *pre- and postarterial* subsegments, and serves as the axis around which the midgut will rotate. During this phase, the midgut mesentery is oriented in a midsagittal plane (Fig. 3–6A). The cecum, which may be found as a distinct bulge in the postarterial midgut by the sixth week, will be used as the reference point in the rotation process. The midgut and hindgut form another small loop at their juncture.

At about this same time, the sudden rapid growth of the alimentary canal is heralded by an increase in numbers of epithelial cells resulting in narrowing and even occlusion of the primitive gut lumen. This is thought to involve the entire gut, although not simultaneously or completely. Obliteration of the lumen may pass as a wave of solidification, or, more probably, according to Bremer, only in certain, variable regions does complete occlusion occur. Following this solid stage, vacuoles appear in the epithelial mass. With continued development of the intestinal tract, intervening epithelial cells are carried away to cover the mucosal surface of the elongating intestinal tract, and the vacuoles expand, coalesce, and are incorporated into the continuous gut lumen.

During the seventh week, the stomach has grown to a point where it is approaching its final shape and orientation. The duodenal foregut has also increased greatly in size and length, forming the first portion of the duodenal loop and forcing the junction loop with the midgut posteriorly (dorsally) and toward the left. The midgut has

elongated rapidly so that the pre- and postarterial subsegments come to lie side by side in the interlobar hepatic fissure, with the apex of the loop pointing at the umbilicus. Soon the elongating midgut loop outstrips the confines of the abdominal cavity and herniates into the umbilical cord (Fig. 3–6B).

During this phase of rapid elongation of the prearterial midgut, the ventral surface of the duodenum, by virtue of its asymmetric expansion and elongation, has rotated to the right. This rotation carries the plane of the midgut mesentery into a horizontal or frontal orientation. The postarterial midgut and cecum have therefore rotated 90° to the left in a counterclockwise direction around the arterial axis (Fig. 3–6B).

Because of the cephalocaudal progression of the zone of rapid growth, the prearterial midgut becomes longer than the postarterial segment, forming multiple loops and shifting the original arterial midpoint caudally. Both the midgut and hindgut colon remain relatively straight but elongate somewhat, so that the junction loop is shifted cephalad and to the left.

Between the eighth and ninth weeks, both the foregut and midgut portions of the duodenal loop continue to grow, pushing the forming duodeno-jejunal junction loop to the left of the midline, dorsal (posterior) to the superior mesenteric artery. Additional loops form in the umbilical hernia and the intra-abdominal prearterial midgut continues to elongate, forming the jejunal loops in the left upper part of the celom. This mass of jejunal loops forces the postarterial proximal colon ventrally and to the right and, at the same time, along with the expanding greater curvature of the stomach, pushes the hindgut colon laterally, thereby elongating the transverse colon. The cecum thus traverses another 90° rotation around the arterial axis, and the midgut mesentery again comes to lie in a sagittal plane (Fig. 3–6C).

As the wave of accelerated growth sweeps caudally during the ninth week, more and more intraumbilical prearterial midgut coils begin to pass into the abdomen dorsal (posterior) to the superior mesenteric artery, first filling the left side of the celom and then forming the ileal loops to the right. The transverse colon and midgut-hindgut juncture are forced farther dorsally and then laterally up into the posterior left abdominal cavity. By this continuous process, the slowly lengthening postarterial midgut and cecum which lag behind the growth of the prearterial segment are gradually lifted toward the umbilical ring and by the tenth week the cecum has regained an intra-abdominal position, leaving several loops of terminal ileum in the umbilical sac. At this point in development, the right colon passes in a curve ventral (anterior) to the returning loops of small intestine lying in the right side of the abdominal cavity.

At about eleven weeks, the last coils of small intestine leave the umbilical sac and the latter is obliterated. The pre- and postarterial coils of small intestine that were the last to enter the cavity, and lie dorsal (posterior) to the right colon, increase in size, forcing the right colon and cecum to the right dorsolateral aspect of the celom. During this period the cecum completes its final 90° of rotation around the arterial axis.

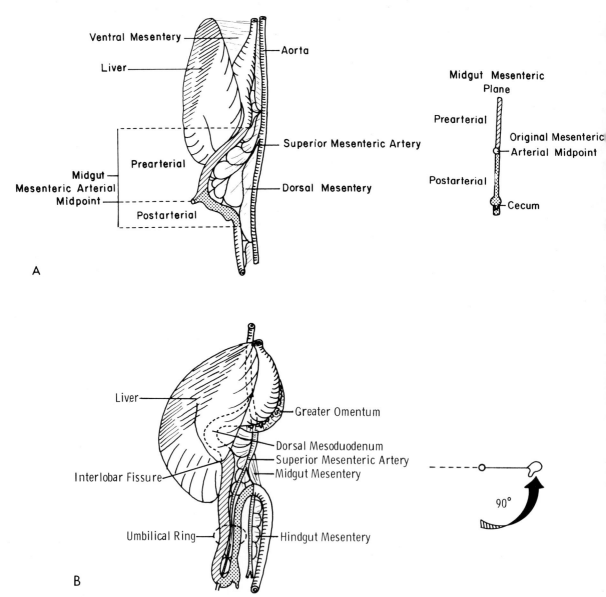

Figure 3-6. Rotation process of the alimentary tract. A, 0° rotation (lateral view). B, 90° rotation (frontal view).

Illustration continued on the opposite page.

The ileocecal valve, which at the beginning of rotation pointed ventrally, has traversed a 270° counterclockwise rotation, coming to point to the left, and the midgut mesentery again lies in a frontal plane (Fig. 3–6D).

The final development of the colon extends from the twelfth week through the rest of gestation. At the third month, the diameter of the colon has increased very little and remains smaller than the proximal bowel. By the fourth month, the slowly elongating colon comes to overlie the descending duodenum and fusion of their mesenteries occurs, anchoring the mobile colon at this point in the right upper abdomen. The right colon continues to elongate and the cecum gradually "descends" into the right lower abdomen. The expansion of the colon, moving caudally from right to left, reaches a point during the fifth month where its diameter is equal to the small bowel and the ascending colon can be identified. The transverse colon, followed by the descending and sigmoid portions, gradually attain their final size and configuration as the mesenteric fixation is established. Continued dilation of the colon to its normal size at birth is dependent upon the intrauterine transit of meconium into its lumen. Meconium is first noted within the intestinal lumen at the third month. It is a thick greenish mixture of swallowed amniotic fluid and its contents (lanugo hairs and vernix caseosa) as well as gastrointestinal secretions and cells.

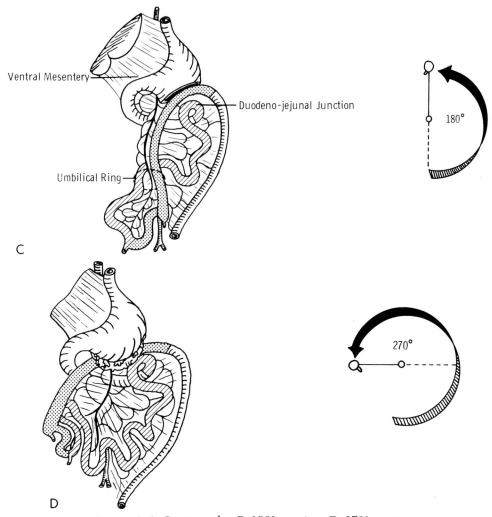

Figure 3–6. Continued. C, 180° rotation. D, 270° rotation.

The dorsal mesentery of the foregut forms the *mesogastrium* and *mesoduodenum*. As the stomach expands and rotates, its dorsal mesentery also expands rapidly into a purse-like structure, the greater omentum. The posterior wall of this sac contains the dorsal pancreas and the spleen.

The greater omentum ends at about the pylorus, and the dorsal mesentery continues onto the duodenum as the mesoduodenum. As the duodenum elongates and expands asymmetrically to the right, forming the duodenal loop, its dorsal mesentery containing the head of the dorsal pancreas fans out, extending caudally to the developing duodeno-jejunal loop (Fig. 3–6B).

The midgut continuation of the dorsal mesentery initially arises from a relatively long stretch of the dorsal abdominal wall; however, as the midgut elongates, forming multiple loops, the peripheral connection of the mesentery becomes greatly increased in length while the dorsal abdominal base remains relatively short (Fig. 3–6B). The midgut mesentery rotates around this relatively narrow mesenteric root, with the superior mesenteric arterial axis as described in the preceding section (Fig. 3–6D).

The hindgut mesentery, originally very short, elongates with the descending colon, experiencing only slight rotation and being carried up into the left abdomen with the developing splenic fissure.

By the end of the third month of gestation, the digestive tube and its mesenteries are mobile, while exhibiting the relationships found in the fully mature fetus. The dorsal mesentery has maintained a more or less straight mid-dorsal line of attachment despite the complex growth and rotation of the bowel (Fig. 3–7A). During the fourth month certain segments of the dorsal mesentery begin to agglutinate with the posterior abdominal wall and some opposing mesenteric surfaces. The series of fusions that follow ultimately fix the bowel into a more or less permanent position. First, the posterior wall of the greater omentum begins to fuse with the dorsal abdominal wall, beginning at its esophageal origin, and progressively agglutinates to form a new line of mesenteric connection running from left to right. The dorsal mesentery of the duodenal loop fuses with the posterior abdominal wall as far as the duodeno-jejunal junction, where the plane of fixation stops at the future level of the ligament of Treitz (Fig. 3–7A).

The lesser omentum, running from the

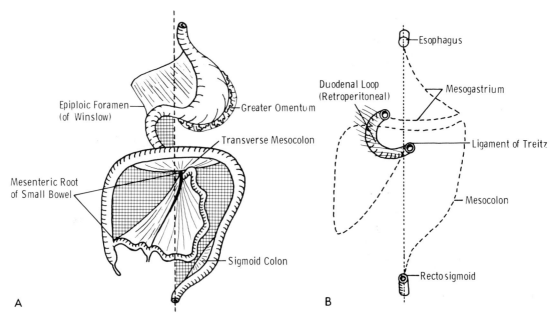

Figure 3–7. Normal postrotation position of the gastrointestinal tract with mesenteric attachments and retroperitoneal fixation.

lesser curvature of the stomach to the post-bulbar portion of the duodenum, remains free with the exception of its distal extent, containing the ventral pancreas and distal common bile duct which is incorporated into the retroperitoneal space by fusion with the dorsal duodenal mesentery. The free edge of the lesser omentum contains the more proximal common bile duct and the various vascular structures going to the liver. It forms the anterior extent of the epiploic foramen of Winslow into the lesser sac and omental bursa.

The midgut mesentery to the small intestine remains relatively free, but at the fourth month the colonic mesenteries agglutinate with the posterior abdominal wall, fixing the ascending and descending colon. The mesentery of the transverse colon fuses with the greater omentum, retaining a small apron of free mesentery. The hindgut mesocolon agglutinates with the posterior wall to the level of the sigmoid colon, where a free mesentery is again found attaching to the sigmoid loop. This ends at the rectosigmoid junction (Fig. 3–7A).

The incorporation of the mesocolon into the posterior abdominal wall results in a new line of mesenteric attachment for the small bowel, running obliquely across the abodmen from the ligment of Treitz to the right lower quadrant and cecum (Fig. 3–7A). By the fifth month the mesenteric connections are completed, forming an erratic line of attachment differing markedly from the primitive mid-dorsal mesenteric origin (Fig. 3–7B). The digestive tube with the exception of the stomach, small bowel, and portions of the colon has either become retroperitoneal in position or firmly fixed to the posterior abdominal wall.

THE CLOACA AND DERIVATIVES

The primitive alimentary canal terminates caudally in a dilatation called the cloaca. This primitive sac receives the hindgut dorsally, the allantoic stalk ventrally, the ducts of the developing upper urinary tract laterally, and the tailgut, which obliterates early, distally. The endodermal lining of the cloaca comes in contact with the embryonic ectoderm, forming the midline cloacal membrane between the allantoic stalk and the tailfold (Fig. 3–8A).

Beginning at the sixth week, the cloaca begins to divide into separate ventral genitourinary and rectal compartments. This division is thought to be accomplished (according to Stephens) by the combined craniocaudal descent of a crescentic fold originating between the allantois and the hindgut, as well as by the formation and midline fusion of the lateral folds (Fig. 3–8B). By the end of the seventh week, division is completed and the urorectal septum fuses with the cloacal membrane, forming the primitive *perineum*. Dorsal (posterior) to this structure is the *anal membrane* which lies in a surface indentation, the *anal pit*. The rectum and anal pit are quickly brought into continuity by the breakdown of the anal membrane during the eighth week. The ectodermal wall of the anal pit, together with the caudal endoderm of the rectum, form the *anal canal* (Fig. 3–8C).

THE LIVER AND PANCREAS

The liver first appears in the 3½-week embryo as a ventral evagination of the foregut at its junction with the yolk sac

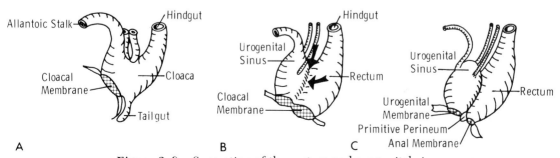

Figure 3–8. Separation of the rectum and urogenital sinus.

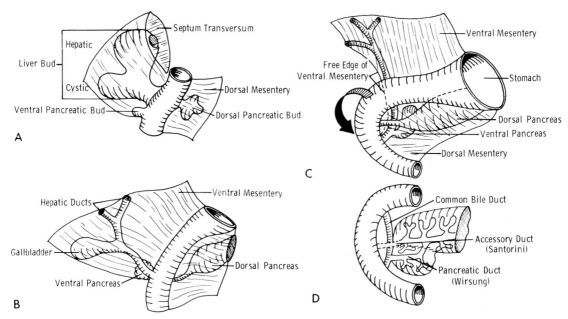

Figure 3-9. Development of the liver and pancreas. *A*, Lateral view. *B*, Anteroposterior view. *C*, Anteroposterior view. *D*, Pancreatic and bile duct formation.

(Fig. 3–1*A*). The bud rapidly expands into the septum transversum, dividing into an hepatic segment that becomes the glandular structures and ducts of the liver, and a cystic portion that forms the gall bladder and cystic duct (Fig. 3–9*A*). The hepatic portion elongates and soon divides into the right and left lobes of the liver. The connective tissue framework and vascular structures of the liver, as well as the mesenteric connections and biliary structures, are derived from the mesoderm of the septum transversum and vitelline veins.

The hepatic mass expands rapidly, so that by the fifth week the liver occupies almost the entire abdominal cavity. The original area of contact with the septum transversum becomes the base area of the liver in contact with the diaphragm, and the reflections of the ventral mesentery become the coronary and triangular ligaments of the liver. The falciform ligament is the ventral mesenteric remnant extending from the interlobar fissure to the abdominal wall, carrying the umbilical veins.

The liver remains large in relation to the rest of the alimentary tract until about the ninth week, when the expanding stomach and loops of midgut returning from the umbilical hernia force the liver into its final size and position.

The cystic portion of the primitive hepatic diverticulum elongates into the gallbladder and cystic duct, which drain into the main biliary duct (Fig. 3–9*B*). The lumen of the biliary duct system is established by the seventh week and bile is secreted by the twelfth week.

The pancreas develops from two separate foregut buds appearing at the fourth week. The ventral pancreatic bud arises from the wall of the duodenal foregut at a point marking the most caudal extent of the ventral mesentery, while the dorsal pancreas arises from the opposite wall at a point somewhat more cephalic than the ventral bud (Fig. 3–9*A*).

The dorsal pancreatic bud, which will form the major part of the pancreas, grows into the dorsal duodenal mesentery, extending ultimately into the gastric mesentery as far as the developing spleen. With the asymmetric growth and rotation of the stomach, the dorsal pancreas comes to lie along the dorsal (posterior) abdominal wall in the dorsal mesogastrium, and is progressively incorporated into a retroperitoneal position by fusion of the mesentery with the abdominal wall (Fig. 3–9*C*).

The ventral pancreatic bud is rapidly incorporated into the hepatic bud as the gut wall between them is absorbed. It is carried away from the duodenum within the ventral mesentery by the elongating common bile duct (Fig. 3–9B). As the duodenum elongates and rotates, the ventral mesentery and its contents rotate 270° to the right in a counterclockwise direction around the duodenum, and are carried somewhat caudally, coming to be posterior to the first and descending portions of the duodenum. The bile duct and ventral pancreas are then posterior to the dorsal pancreas which, being relatively fixed, has only rotated about 90° (Fig. 3–9C). The two pancreatic primordia then fuse, the ventral mass joining with the right side of the dorsal pancreas. The short ventral duct fuses with the dorsal duct which then usually atrophies, leaving the single pancreatic duct emptying into the common bile duct,

although persistence of the dorsal connection as the accessory duct is not unusual (Fig. 3–9D).

REFERENCES

Allan, F. D. *Essentials of Human Embryology* (New York: Oxford University Press, 1969).

Arey, L. B. *Developmental Anatomy* (5th ed., Philadelphia: W. B. Saunders, 1950).

Bremer, J. L. *Congenital Anomalies of the Viscera* (Cambridge, Mass.: Harvard University Press, 1957).

Hamilton, W. J., Boyd, J. D., and Massman, H. W. *Human Embryology* (Baltimore: Williams & Williams, 1962).

Lauge-Hansen, N. *The Developmental and The Embryonic Anatomy of the Human Gastrointestinal Tract* (Eindhoven: Centrex Publishing Co., 1960).

Stephens, F. D., and Smith, E. D. *Ano-rectal Malformation in Children* (Chicago: Year Book Medical Publishers, 1971).

Chapter 4

THE NORMAL ESOPHAGUS

ROENTGENOLOGIC ANATOMY. The normal infantile esophagus extends from the fourth or fifth cervical vertebra to its junction with the stomach at about the level of the ninth thoracic vertebra, which is one vertebral level higher at both upper and lower extremities than in the older child and adult. The identification of air in the esophagus is frequently a normal finding (Fig. 4–1), but its persistence suggests abnormality of the lower esophageal segment (chalasia or achalasia) or tracheoesophageal fistula. When the esophagus of the newborn is demonstrated radiologically, either fluoroscopically or on radiographs, it is seen as a straight or slightly fusiform tube, slightly wider in its inferior portion. Because of the excessive redundancy of the retropharyngeal soft tissues in infancy, the pharynx and upper esophagus often appear to be displaced anteriorly and to the right, especially if the x-ray examination is made in less than full inspiration. Unless this is appreciated the tracheal displacement may be mistaken for a retropharyngeal mass. It should be recognized that this buckled ap-

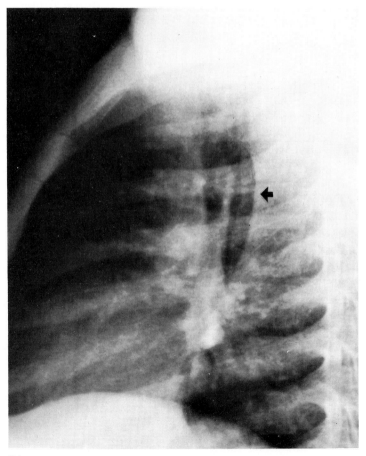

Figure 4–1. Lateral chest radiograph of normal 18-month-old infant. Air is identified in the midportion of the esophagus (arrow) as well as in the trachea and bronchi anterior to this.

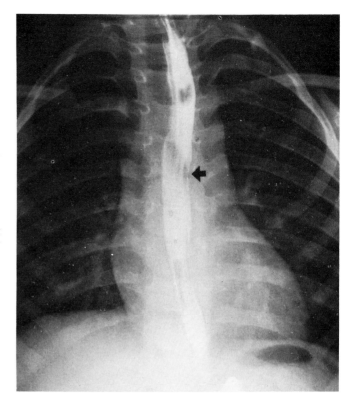

Figure 4–2. Normal esophagus in a 3-year-old child. The esophagus is deviated normally to the left in the lower cervical area and slightly to the right in the lower thoracic area. These deviations are increased during expiration. Indentation produced by left main stem bronchus is indicated by arrow.

pearance of the pharyngotracheal airway is a normal finding. If the infant is having respiratory distress, the lungs are frequently hyperinflated, the diaphragm depressed, and the tracheal air column straight.

The deviations and compressions produced by adjacent normal structures are not as prominent as in the older infant or child. The superior segment in the upper thoracic region is slightly convex to the left, forming the left flexure of the esophagus. The middle portion deviates to the right, often projecting slightly past the midline, and the lower segment, known as the right esophageal flexure, passes to the left, entering the diaphragmatic hiatus at approximately the superior border of the ninth dorsal vertebra (Fig. 4–2). This level varies considerably in different children and in the same child at different examinations, depending upon the phase of respiration. The transverse portion of the aorta crosses the esophagus anteriorly and produces a normal indentation on the left anterior border of the esophagus at about the level of the fourth dorsal vertebra. This aortic impression is nearly always identifiable, even in the neonatal infant, and is seen to

best advantage fluoroscopically with the infant in the supine and right anterior oblique position. A similar but less prominent indentation, frequently noted at a slightly lower level, is produced by the left main stem bronchus as it passes across the anterior surface of the esophagus (Fig. 4–3). This occasionally appears as an oblique filling defect in the barium column, particularly on films exposed with the infant supine (Fig. 4–2). In this position, the weight of the bronchus, thymus, and other mediastinal structures increases the pressure defect of the left bronchus on the esophagus. A similar configuration may be produced by an ectopic right subclavian artery, but lateral or oblique views demonstrate the anterior position of the bronchial indentation and the posterior location of the retroesophageal subclavian artery. The normal indentations made by the aorta and bronchus become more prominent with growth of the child, and beyond infancy are identified with greater clarity. This is especially true of the aortic impression, which increases in prominence with the age of the individual and with the resulting elongation of the aorta. The retrocardiac portion

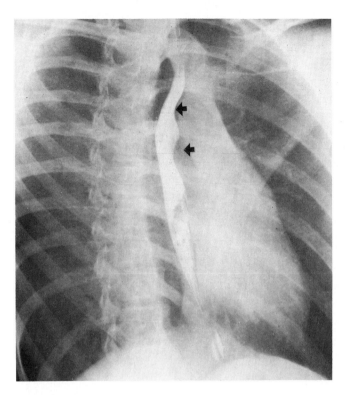

Figure 4-3. Right anterior oblique view showing normal indentations on esophagus produced by aortic arch (upper arrow) and left bronchus (lower arrow).

of the esophagus is in direct contact with the left atrium. Consequently, enlargement of this chamber leads to posterior displacement of the esophagus, which is readily identified when the esophagus is outlined by barium. However, in many normal infants, because of the short vertical dimension of the chest and the relatively broad mediastinum, the esophagus becomes posteriorly displaced in the retrocardiac region during the expiratory phase of respiration. Recognition of this will enable the radiologist to avoid a misdiagnosis of left atrial enlargement (Fig. 4-4).

The esophagus enters the anteromedial wall of the stomach at an oblique angle (the angle of His), which probably aids in preventing reflux of stomach contents into the esophagus. Although the exact site of transition between the esophageal squamous epithelium and the columnar epithelium of the stomach is impossible to detect roentgenologically, the radiographic appearance of the mucosa of the two structures aids in locating the transition zone, the mucosal pattern of the esophagus consisting of fine longitudinal striations and the mucosa of the stomach containing larger, irregularly distributed folds. Although differentiation of these types of mucosal markings is more difficult in infants than in older children, they may frequently be visualized even in young infants. The identification of the junction between gastric and esophageal mucosa is subject to many inaccuracies, as discussed in the section on the gastroesophageal junction. Nevertheless, it is often the only roentgenologic means of determining the presence of hiatus hernia.

ROENTGENOLOGIC PHYSIOLOGY. The normal process of deglutition consists of the nursing infant putting the tongue upward and forward against the nipple and moving it back against the palate so that the material entering the mouth is passed posteriorly over the lower dorsal surface of the tongue into the oral pharynx (Fig. 4-5). This is accompanied by elevation of the velum palatinum and apposition with the contracted posterior pharyngeal muscles, thereby closing off the nasal airway. Whether or not the superior pharyngeal constrictor muscle produces a soft tissue prominence (Passavant's cushion) in normal infants, thereby aiding in obstructing the nasal airway, is questionable (Fig. 4–5C). Fluoroscopic examination of young infants will frequently show minimal reflux of contrast material into the nasopharynx if the nipple opening is large or if they are taking the liquid contrast material rapidly (Fig. 4–6). As the ingested bolus reaches the valleculae, the larynx has been approximated to the hyoid bone and the epiglottis tipped backwards. Most of the ingested material passes laterally through the food channels on each side of the larynx, and this is facilitated by forward movement of the larynx. In the concluding phase of deglutition, the tongue arches backward into the pharynx and the posterior pharyngeal walls and soft tissue moves forward to meet it. This motion is from above downward and is accompanied by pushing of the food material caudally. Normally the laryngeal lumen is completely closed at this stage, and the epiglottis is pressed over the laryngeal entrance by the pharyngeal peristaltic wave. As the pharynx fills with air, the larynx falls back to the position of rest and the epiglottis moves upward to a more vertical position.

The esophagus is seen to best advantage during fluoroscopic examination with the patient in the right anterior oblique position. In this position the esophagus is clear of the spine and is silhouetted sharply against the aerated lungs. In the upright position the liquid barium is propelled by the act of swallowing into the pharynx, where contraction of the pharyngeal constrictors pushes the contrast material into the upper esophagus. There it drops rapidly by the action of gravity to the stomach, with only slight delay near the level of the esophageal hiatus. Infants are of necessity examined in the recumbent position, in which the effect of gravity is eliminated, and the contrast material fills the esophagus by rapidly repeated acts of swallowing which inhibit progressive esophageal peristalsis. Less frequent swallows initiate a peristaltic wave which propels the bolus down the esophagus into the stomach. The importance of the gastroesophageal vestibule (lower esophageal segment) in the physiologic activity of the esophagus is discussed in the next chapter.

Because of the slower emptying of the esophagus when the patient is lying down, this position is preferable in the examination of both infants and older children. The variation in caliber of the esophageal

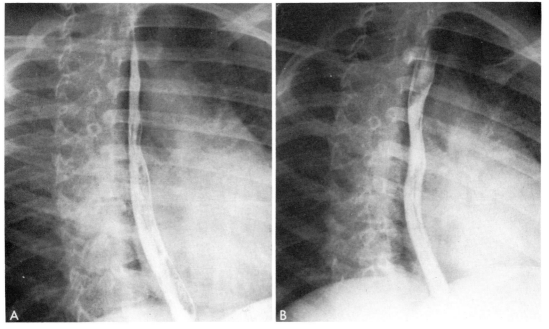

Figure 4–4. Changes in curvature of the esophagus in retrocardiac area on inspiration (A) expiration (B) in a 5-year-old child. The posterior displacement of the esophagus during expiration should not be mistaken for left atrial dilatation.

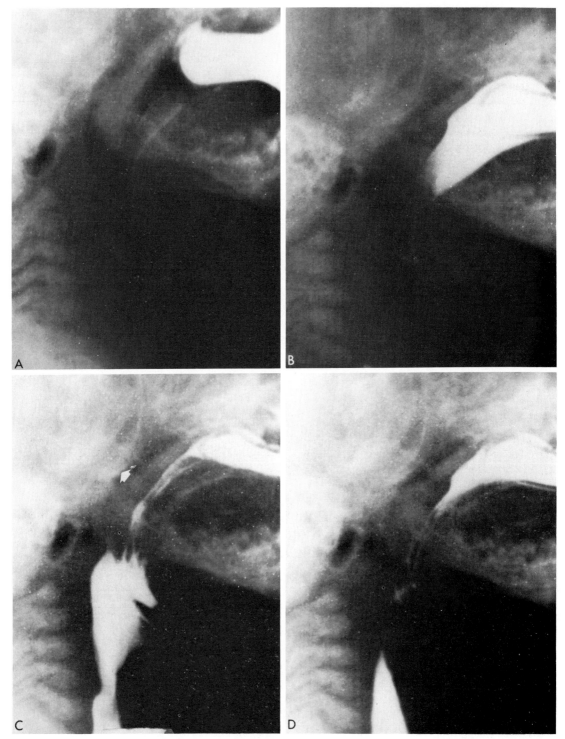

Figure 4–5. Continued on the opposite page.

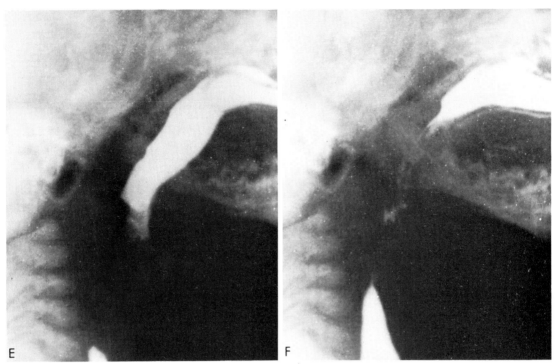

Figure 4–5. Normal process of deglutition in a young infant. *A,* The infant's tongue begins upward pressure on the nipple, compressing it between the tongue and palate. *B,* Further compression results in barium entering the mouth and oral pharynx. *C,* The soft palate is elevated, the posterior pharyngeal muscles are contracted, closing off the nasal airway, the epiglottis is tipped posteriorly, the tongue arched backward into the pharynx, and the bolus of contrast material passed into the upper esophagus. The normal soft tissue pad probably produced by the superior pharyngeal muscle is not prominent (arrow). *D,* The tongue has moved forward and the cycle is repeated, with beginning compression of the tongue on the lower portion of the nipple. *E,* Further compression results in the passage of contrast medium into the oral pharynx as noted above. *F,* The act of deglutition is completed and the cycle begins again.

lumen in infants is remarkable, depending to a large extent upon the quantity propelled from the pharynx into the esophagus during each act of swallowing, as well as upon the degree of relaxation of the lower esophagus. In children past early infancy the peristaltic contractions are more prominent and consist of a primary contraction in the upper esophagus accompanied by relaxation of the esophagus distal to this (Fig. 4–7). In the contracted segment, longitudinal striations are usually visible. Peristaltic activity is more prominent if a semisolid mixture of barium is given, the peristaltic waves and the resulting striations of the esophageal mucosa being more noticeable. Relaxation of the lower esophageal segment is accompanied by superior displacement of this area.

Air bubbles in the esophagus are seen in nearly every examination and should not be confused with filling defects (Fig. 4–8). Occasionally, contractions originating in the midportion of the esophagus with propulsion of barium superiorly as well as down the esophagus are identified. The contractions are similar to the "secondary peristaltic contractions" described originally in the adult patient by Templeton. Similar types of secondary contractions, beginning at the level of the diaphragm with retrograde propulsion of the barium mixture, are often seen in the infant who takes the bottle too fast. Tertiary esophageal contractions have not been reported in normal children but have been seen in infants and children with esophagitis. These contractions appear either

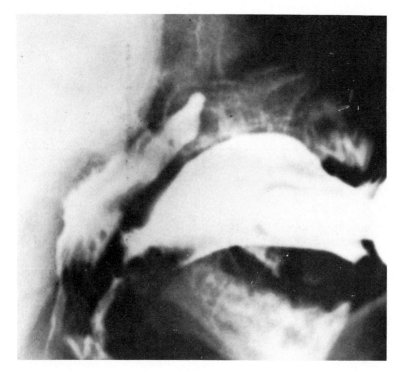

Figure 4-6. Mild pharyngonasal reflux in normal infant who is ingesting the barium rapidly through a large hole in the nipple.

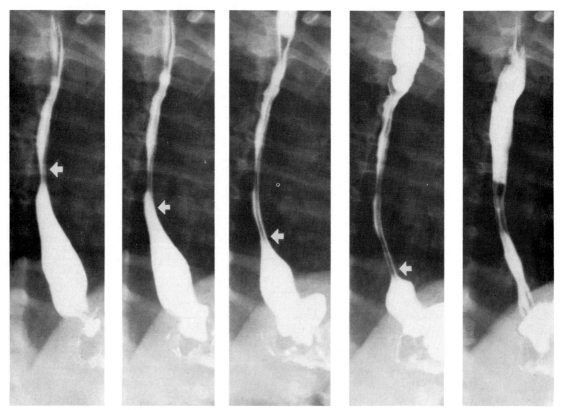

Figure 4-7. Serial films of the esophagus showing caudal progression of the contraction wave accompanied by relaxation of the esophagus distal to it.

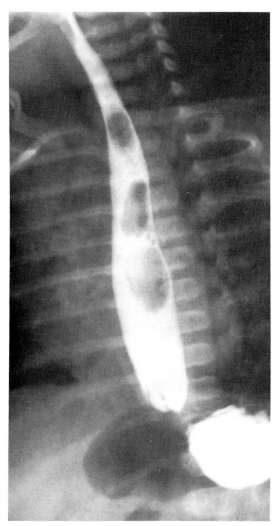

Figure 4–8. Air bubbles in the esophagus, a common finding when barium is administered by nursing bottle.

curately the anatomy of this area with its physiologic activity. An understanding of the normal mechanism is essential to the consideration of those conditions in which the gastroesophageal junction is incompetent in preventing reflux of gastric contents into the esophagus.

Radiologic descriptions of the anatomic and physiologic characteristics of the gastroesophageal junction were published as

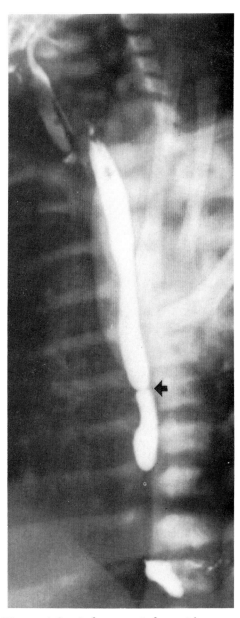

Figure 4–9. Infant, age 1 day, with congenital duodenal stenosis, showing transient narrow constriction in the lower esophagus.

as multiple serrations or as deep indentations. Transitory weblike constrictions in the midesophagus presumably represent a peculiar unexplained localized muscular contraction (Figs. 4–9 and 4–10) and in our experience are asymptomatic.

The normal physiology of the distal portion of the esophagus in the region of the diaphragmatic hiatus and the gastroesophageal junction has been the subject of considerable controversy and differences in opinion, not only in regard to the anatomic structure but especially concerning the physiologic function and its relation to the valvular mechanism. There has been, and is to some extent, a failure to correlate ac-

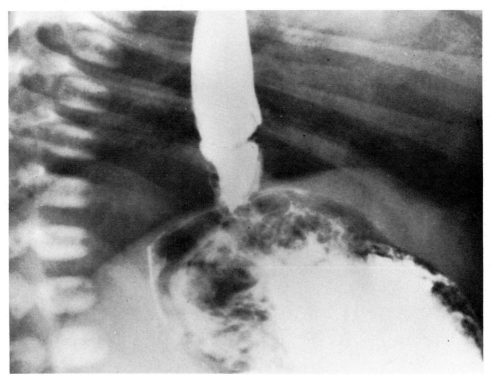

Figure 4–10. Localized constriction of the distal esophagus in a 1-week-old infant. No evidence of reflux. Reexamination one week later showed no abnormality.

early as 1914, when Smith and LeWald described the influence of posture on regurgitation in several infants who apparently had gastroesophageal incompetence. In 1926, Robins and Jankelson reported several cases of "cardioesophageal relaxation" and described in more detail the anatomy of this area. Renewed interest in the subject followed Wyllie's recognition of the clinical significance of gastroesophageal reflux, and especially Neuhauser's description in infants. The attention given mainly by British authors to gastroesophageal incompetence associated with thoracic stomach and a short esophagus has also focused attention sharply on this portion of the alimentary tract. The work of Lerche has helped to clarify the true anatomic and physiologic relationship of the area. The anatomic components which help establish the valvular mechanism in the lower esophagus are the inferior esophageal sphincter, the phrenoesophageal membrane, the constrictor cardiae, the rosette arrangement of mucosa in the area of the gastric cardia, and the acute angle of insertion of the esophagus into the stomach. However, all of these are insignificant compared to the inherent physiologic activity of the gastroesophageal vestibule (lower esophageal segment) (Fig. 4–11). The rhythmic opening and closing of this important and physiologically different segment of the lower esophagus, especially noticeable during fluoroscopic studies of young infants rapidly taking barium from a nursing bottle, emphasize its dominant importance. There have been reliable studies showing that the act of swallowing reflexly produces relaxation and opening of the lower esophageal segment.

The inferior esophageal sphincter is a physiologic constriction in the distal esophagus just above the level of the diaphragmatic hiatus and at the upper border of the gastroesophageal vestibule. It is readily identified during fluoroscopy but is less prominent in infants than in older children. Slight dilatation of the esophagus above the sphincter is seen in infants and children but is much smaller than the typical "phrenic ampulla" so common in adults. The degree of constriction at the inferior esophageal sphincter varies in different in-

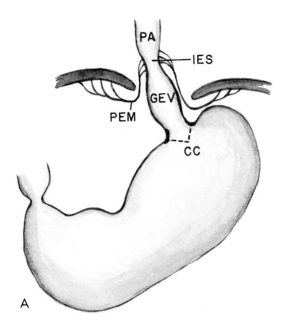

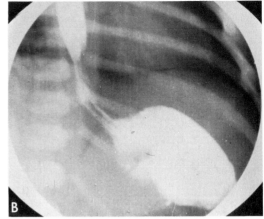

Figure 4–11. Anatomy of the lower esophagus. *A,* Diagrammatic drawing: *PA,* phrenic ampulla; *IES,* inferior esophageal sphincter; *PEM,* phrenoesophageal membrane (ascending limb); *GEV,* gastroesophageal vestibule (lower esophageal segment); *CC,* constrictor cardiae. *B,* Spot film of normal lower esophageal segment.

dividuals and in the same individual during different examinations, and is probably related to the true physiologic gastroesophageal vestibule.

The phrenoesophageal membrane arises from the fascia of the diaphragm and divides into an ascending and descending limb. The descending portion attaches to the musculature of the cardia, and the ascending portion attaches to the esophagus at the level of the inferior esophageal stricture. The constrictive effect of this attachment on the esophagus appears to be especially pronounced during deep inspiration. The attachment of the membrane maintains this portion of the esophagus in a relatively fixed position, and prevents the longitudinal muscle of the esophagus from pulling the lower esophagus and the cardia into the chest. According to Kay, relaxation of the phrenoesophageal ligament allows the stomach to herniate into the chest.

The cardiac sphincter (constrictor cardiae) is the slight constriction at the junction between the vestibule and the stomach and apparently has little sphincteric action, playing an inept role in preventing reflux. Its radiographic location is usually difficult. According to several sources, the competence of the cardia is due to the muscularis mucosae pulling the lax mucosa into a type of fold or valve.

The angle of insertion of the esophagus into the stomach has been and is considered by some authors to be a major component in maintaining competency at the gastoesophageal junction.

The role of the diaphragm in maintaining competency is debatable. Jackson originally described the pinch-cock action of the diaphragm in preventing reflux of stomach contents into the esophagus. Many other investigators support this belief, and consider the sling of the right crus of the diaphragm surrounding the esophageal hiatus to be a major factor in the valvular mechanism. Other authors indicate that the diaphragmatic hiatus has little if any constricting effect on the lower esophagus.

The gastroesophageal vestibule (lower esophageal segment or epiphrenic bell) has been recognized as a unique segment of the distal esophagus, not only in its anatomy but also in its function. The vestibule represents the true gastroesophageal junction and extends from the inferior esophageal sphincter slightly above the diaphragm to the gastric cardia in the abdomen. It cannot strictly be referred to as esophagus because a portion of it is lined with gastric epithelium, the extent largely depending upon the degree of distention of the fundus. By placing metallic clips at the mucous membrane junction of

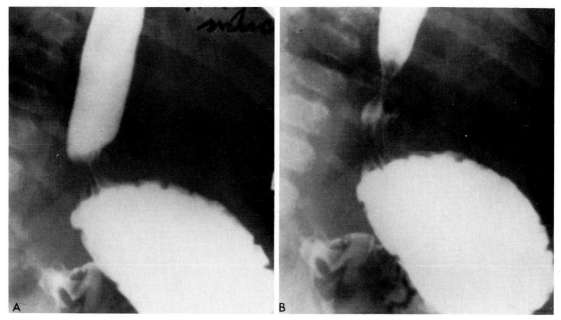

Figure 4–12. Normal 3-month-old infant showing: *A,* Closure of the gastroesophageal vestibule prior to relaxation; *B,* Normal migration of gastric mucosa above the diaphragm.

esophagus and stomach, both Johnstone and Palmer demonstrated considerable variation in the radiographic position of the gastroesophageal junction, apparently as a result of the activity of the muscularis mucosae. If the fundus is distended the junction is in the region of the gastric cardia, whereas if the fundus is contracted the junction is near the diaphragmatic hiatus. More recently Stewart has shown upward movement of the lower esophageal segment as it relaxes, allowing passage of the bolus into the stomach. This explains the frequent normal observation of seeing a small segment of gastric mucosa above the diaphragm during fluoroscopic studies (Fig. 4–12). The physiologic activity of the vestibule is different from that of other portions of the esophagus. Normally it remains in a tonic resting stage, opened by an esophageal peristaltic wave or by sufficient weight of material in the esophagus above it. There is evidence which suggests that it reacts antithetically to the upper esophagus in response to sympathetic and parasympathetic stimuli. Studies of the vestibule in cases of achalasia have shown that the vestibule remains in a contracted state and does not respond to the stimulation of normal peristalsis from the more proximal por-

tions of the esophagus. This suggests that if the vestibule is unable to contract normally, the opposite condition, or gastroesophageal incompetence, would result. Future investigations may well show that it is this form of vestibular dysfunction, possibly due to immaturity of the innervation, which leads to abnormal reflux of stomach contents into the esophagus in the infant age group.

Although each of the components of the gastroesophageal junction described here may act in the prevention of reflux of gastric contents from the stomach into the esophagus, it appears that the most important role is played by the inherent action of the gastroesophageal vestibule.

REFERENCES

Ardran, G. M., and Kemp, F. H. Normal and disturbed swallowing, *Progr. Pediatr. Radiol.,* 2:151, 1969.
Chrispin, A. R. Abnormalities of oesophageal function: some radiologic aspects. *In* Wilkinson, A. W., editor, *Recent Advances in Pediatric Surgery* (2nd ed.; New York: Grune and Stratton, 1969).
Chrispin, A. R., Friedland, G. W., and Wright, D. E. Some functional characteristics of the oesophageal vestibule in infants and children, *Thorax,* 22:188, 1967.

Cimmino, C. V. The distal esophagogastric closing mechanism, *V. M. M.*, 94:131, 1967 (editorial).

Fyke, F. E., Jr., Code, C. F., and Schlegel, J. F. Gastroesophageal sphincter in healthy human beings, *Gastroenterologica*, 86:135, 1956.

Gryboski, J. D., Thayer, W. R., and Spiro, H. M. Esophageal motility in infants and children, *Pediatrics*, 31:382, 1963.

Jackson, C. Diaphragmatic pinchcock in so-called "cardiospasm," *Laryngoscope*, 32:139, 1922.

Johnstone, A. S. Reflections on hiatus hernia and related problems, *Radiology*, 62:750, 1954 (editorial).

Kay, E. B. Inferior esophageal constrictor in relation to lower esophageal disease, *J. Thoracic Surg.*, 25:1, 1953.

Kelley, M. L., Jr., Wilbur, D. L., III, Schlegel, J. F., and Code, C. G. Deglutitive responses in gastroesophageal sphincter of healthy human beings, *J. Appl. Physiol*, 15:483, 1960.

Lerche, W. *The Oesophagus and Pharynx in Action: A Study of Stricture in Relation to Function* (Springfield, Ill.: Charles C Thomas, 1950).

Neuhauser, E. B. D., and Berenberg, W. Cardioesophageal relaxation as cause of vomiting in infants, *Radiology*, 48:480, 1947.

Palmer, E. D. Attempt to localize the normal esophagogastric junction, *Radiology*, 60:825, 1953.

Robins, S. A., and Jankelson, I. R. Cardio-esophageal relaxation, *J.A.M.A.* 87:1961, 1926.

Silverman, F. N. Gastroesophageal incompetence, partial intrathoracic stomach, and vomiting in infancy, *Radiology*, 64:664, 1955.

Smith, C. H., and LeWald, L. T. Influence of posture on digestion in infancy, *Am. J. Dis. Child.*, 9:261, 1915.

Stewart, E. T., and Dodds, W. J. Preliminary observations on the opening mechanism of the lower esophageal sphincter as studied in the feline esophagus. Presented at the Society of Gastrointestinal Radiologists, Chicago, Ill., Nov. 27, 1972.

Strawczynski, H., Beck, I. T., McKenna, R. D., and Nickerson, G. H. The behavior of the lower esophageal sphincter in infants and its relationship to gastroesophageal regurgitation, *J. Pediatr.*, 64:17, 1964.

Templeton, F. E. *X-Ray Examination of the Stomach: A Description of the Roentgenologic Anatomy, Physiology and Pathology of the Esophagus and Duodenum* (Chicago: University of Chicago Press, 1944).

Wolf, B. S. The inferior esophageal sphincter— anatomic, roentgenologic and manometric correlation, contradictions and terminology, *Am. J. Roentgenol. Radium Ther. Nucl. Med.*, 110:260, 1970.

Wyllie, W. G., and Field, E. C. Etiology of intermittent oesophageal regurgitation and haematemesis in infants, *Arch. Dis. Child.*, 21:219, 1946.

Chapter 5

FUNCTIONAL ABNORMALITIES OF THE PHARYNX, ESOPHAGUS, AND THE GASTROESOPHAGEAL JUNCTION

Vomiting and difficulty in feeding are the predominant symptoms in physiologic abnormalities of the pharynx, esophagus, and gastroesophageal junction. Prior to the utilization of cine and videotape studies, these disorders were frequently unrecognized; now, however, they represent a prominent and common group of problems which are easily identified radiologically. These disorders are common in premature and in brain-damaged infants but may occur in normal babies. They may be of mild degree or severe and may be transient or persistent, requiring gastrostomies for feeding purposes.

PHARYNGEAL AND ESOPHAGEAL INCOORDINATION

Physiologic disorders of swallowing are frequently seen in premature infants, and in infants who are debilitated or have brain damage. The disorder may be in the form of pharyngeal or esophageal incoordination or may be a combination of the two. In cases of pharyngeal incoordination the infant has difficulty in swallowing. Under fluoroscopy, contrast material is held in the mouth longer than normal and when deglu-

tition is initiated only a portion enters the esophagus, the remainder being regurgitated into the nose and mouth, and a portion often being aspirated into the trachea. Although a small amount of pharyngonasal reflux is a normal observation at fluoroscopy, especially if the hole in the nipple is large, significant reflux is often seen in a variety of conditions including prematurity, brain damage, generalized muscular diseases, cleft palate, and congenitally short velum (Figs. 5–1 and 5–2). Infants who take their feedings with difficulty and in whom an organic cause cannot be demonstrated should be suspected of having cerebral damage, especially if the physiologic mechanism is altered as described. In addition, any infant with persistent pneumonia or atelectasis of the right upper lobe should be suspected of having a swallowing disorder because of the propensity of involvement of this pulmonary segment in aspiration pneumonitis. Failure of relaxation of the cricopharyngeal muscle with similar choking spells may occur in brain-damaged infants (Fig. 5–3) or may be a transient physiologic disturbance in otherwise normal infants.

In congenital dysautonomia there is apparently a decreased sensitivity to the reflex mechanism of deglutition, with result-

36

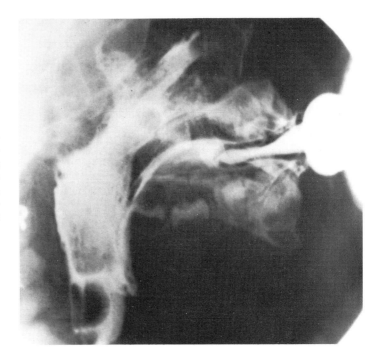

Figure 5–1. Pharyngonasal reflux in a 2-year-old child with cerebral palsy. During deglutition there is extensive reflux of contrast medium into the nasopharynx. Hold-up of barium in the valleculae with periodic aspiration into the trachea was also observed.

ing aspiration into the trachea. Failure of relaxation of the cricopharyngeal muscle in patients with the Riley-Day syndrome has also been incriminated as a cause of aspiration.

Any infant with pneumonia or atelectasis of the right upper lobe should be suspected of having a T-E fistula or a swallowing dysfunction and should be studied fluoroscopically (Fig. 5–4).

Esophageal incoordination is determined fluoroscopically by ineffective to-and-fro

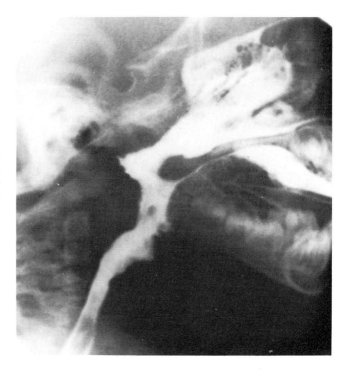

Figure 5–2. Pharyngonasal reflux in an infant with congenital short velum. During deglutition contrast media passed into the nasopharynx because of failure of the short palate to occlude the nasopharyngeal passage.

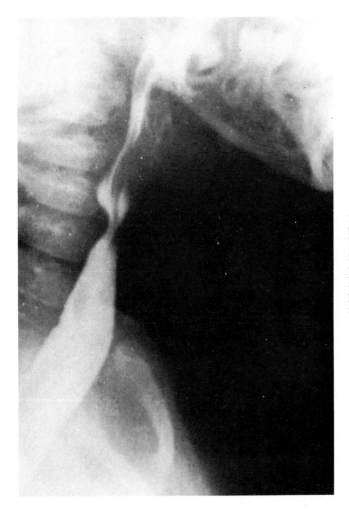

Figure 5–3. Cricopharyngeal spasm in a young infant. Persistent defect on the posterior portion of the esophagus by the cricopharyngeal muscle was identified in this brain-damaged child who had difficulty in swallowing. Similar failure of relaxation of the cricopharyngeal muscle has been reported in congenital dysautonomia.

peristaltic movements, beginning usually in the mid- or lower esophagus and propelling the contrast material back into the pharynx and mouth.

Rumination or merycism is a syndrome consisting of repeated regurgitation and reswallowing (Fig. 5–5). The cause of this rare condition is unknown. It has frequently been attributed to emotional or psychiatric causes and has also been associated with hiatus hernia. However, many infants with hiatus hernia fail to ruminate, and it is difficult to incriminate a psychologic problem in a young infant as being the cause. The possibility of it being a manifestation of some central nervous system abnormality is another consideration.

GASTROESOPHAGEAL JUNCTION (Lower Esophageal Segment)

If one considers the anatomy of the gastroesophageal junction, the explanation for normal periodic regurgitations observed in infants may be as follows. The gastroesophageal vestibule (lower esophageal segment) normally remains in a tonic or contracted state, and manometric studies show that this is an area of higher pressure than the more proximal portion of the esophagus. In the young infant, this condition may be overcome when the intraluminal pressure of the stomach surpasses the energy of the contracted vestibule. This is undoubtedly aided by the normal relaxation of the

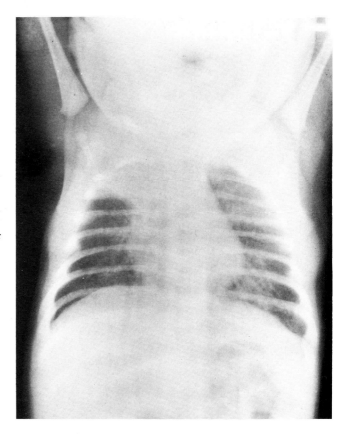

Figure 5–4. Newborn infant with esophageal atresia showing characteristic atelectasis and pneumonia of the right upper lobe. This finding in any young infant should suggest aspiration, and appropriate fluoroscopic studies of swallowing are indicated if the condition is recurrent.

vestibule as it receives the peristaltic wave from the adjoining segment. Consequently, the expulsion of air accompanied by milk from the stomach during the periods of vestibular relaxation seems to be a logical occurrence. Recent experimental evidence suggests that in older patients with lower esophageal segment incompetence there is a diminished release of endogenous gastrin. The application of this pathophysiologic mechanism to the young infant with chalasia is unknown. Regurgitation is especially apt to occur if the infant is placed in the supine position following feeding. In this position the stomach contents collect in the fundus and effectively block the cardia. Thus, during relaxation of the gastroesophageal junction, whether in response to an eructation or to a peristaltic wave from the adjacent esophagus, reflux of liquid into the esophagus and regurgitation are inevitable. Some reports indicate relaxation of the gastroesophageal vestibule reflexly occurs during deglutition. If the infant is put into a prone position, the stomach con-

tents collect in the antrum, the fundus containing only air. Eructation of air occurs easily in this position and is less likely to be accompanied by regurgitation (Fig. 5–6). Fluoroscopic examination of these normal infants shows that the valvular function at the gastroesophageal junction effectively prevents reflux when pressure is applied to the abdomen and when the child is in the Trendelenburg position, thereby differentiating the normal variation of incompetence from the more severe conditions of gastroesophageal relaxation. More severe forms of gastroesophageal incompetence, or chalasia, represent serious conditions which must be considered as distinct and grave illnesses capable of producing esophagitis and irreversible changes in the esophagus. The opposite disorder of the gastroesophageal vestibule is achalasia, a condition which, at least in infants, is due to failure of the normal tonic vestibule to relax with normal esophageal pressures.

Gastroesophageal incompetence (chalasia) is relatively common and may be ei-

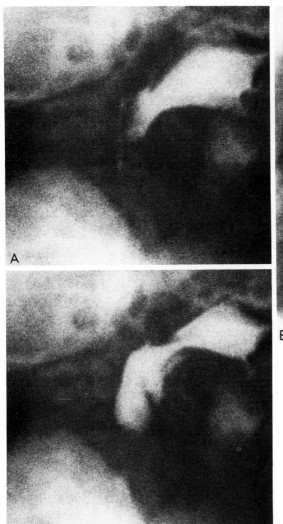

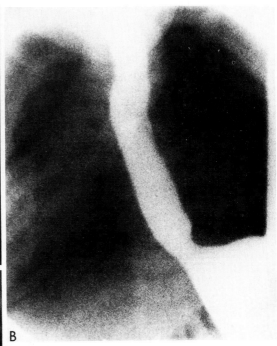

Figure 5-5. Rumination syndrome is an 8-month-old infant. *A*, Contrast media is taken into the mouth and swallowed. *B*, When the material reaches the stomach or lower esophagus, reflux occurs through a patulous lower esophageal segment and passes back into the pharynx and mouth (*C*) where the process is repeated. This phenomenon of rumination is accompanied by a peculiar "clucking-sucking" sound.

ther of mild degree or severe. The predominant symptom of all infants with incompetence of the gastroesophageal junction is vomiting. This is due to reflux of ingested liquids from the stomach into the esophagus. Transient regurgitation of fluid from the stomach into the esophagus is a normal occurrence and is the result of momentary relaxation of the gastroesophageal vestibule. However, persistent chalasia is potentially a serious problem which, unless corrected, leads to chronic aspiration pneumonia and esophagitis. It is most commonly associated with prematurity or central nervous system disorders, and is attributed to neuromuscular dysfunction of the lower esophageal segment. It may also

occur in pyloric stenosis or inflammatory disease of the stomach or duodenum. In the absence of primary causes such as these, the condition is considered idiopathic. In all cases, however, the abnormal patency of the lower esophageal segment is probably the result of neurogenic imbalance or immaturity of the autonomic neurogenous control of the gastroesophageal segment.

Vomiting begins in infants with this condition a few days to a few weeks after birth. The vomiting episodes begin after each feeding and usually are not projectile. The infant fails to gain weight satisfactorily and, moreover, frequently loses weight in spite of a good appetite.

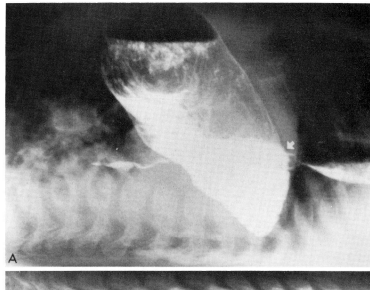

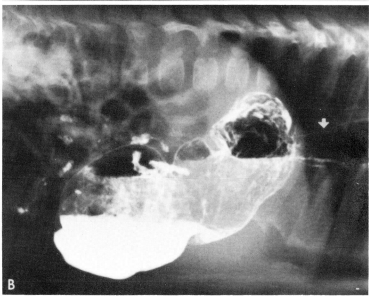

Figure 5–6. Changes in distribution of liquid contents in the stomach with change in position of the infant. *A*, In a supine position, stomach contents collect deep in the fundus of the stomach adjacent to the cardia and gastroesophageal junction (arrow). *B*, In the prone position the air content of the stomach rises to the fundus, the liquid material filling the antrum adjacent to the pyloric canal. This position as well as the upright position facilitates the eructation of air into the esophagus (arrow).

RADIOLOGIC APPEARANCE. Fluoroscopic examination is begun with the infant in the recumbent supine position. A barium mixture having the consistency of the infant's formula is given in a bottle, and the passage of contrast material down the esophagus is carefully observed. In chalasia the esophagus is usually dilated and flaccid, the peristaltic waves are shallow and inadequate, and the contrast material passes without interruption through a wide patent gastroesophageal junction into a normally situated cardia. Pressure applied to the abdomen produces reflux of gastric contents into the esophagus. The same free passage of barium into the

esophagus may be seen during crying or even during inspiration as a result of the increased intra-abdominal pressure during these maneuvers (Fig. 5–7). Also, when the infant is in the Trendelenburg position, barium is observed to pass into the esophagus (Fig. 5–8). In the prone position reflux is not evident, the barium being situated in the antrum rather than at the cardia. The incompetence of the gastroesophageal junction in some cases of chalasia is apparently transitory and repeat radiologic examinations are necessary before reflux can be demonstrated (Fig. 5–9). Additional evidence of periods of normal control of the gastroesophageal junction is seen in the

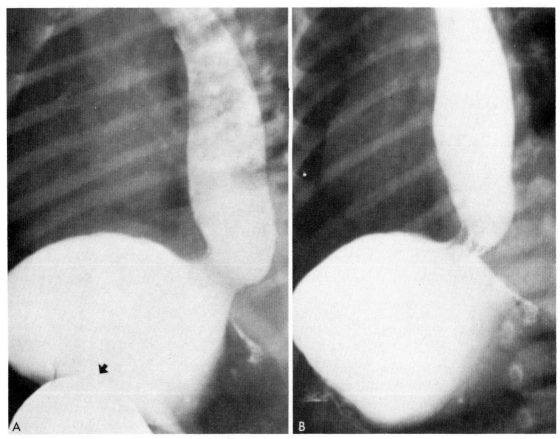

Figure 5-7. Chalasia in a 3-week-old infant with a history of persistent regurgitation. *A,* Pressure applied to the stomach by the gloved hand (arrow) results in an increased amount of reflux with associated widening of the cardia and lower esophageal segment. *B,* Exposure made during fluoroscopy shows reflux of barium into the esophagus.

occasional case in which transitory periods of contraction of the vestibule are followed a few moments later by periods of incompetence. The radiologic examination should always include the stomach and upper small bowel in an effort to determine whether the chalasia is secondary to disease in these areas.

The ingestion of water following barium has been advocated to promote gastroesophageal reflux. This "siphonage test" for gastroesophageal incompetence is unreliable and many normal infants will demonstrate chalasia using this technic. On the other hand, reflux of mild or questionable degree will be enhanced, allowing a more definite diagnosis. Consequently, careful clinical and radiologic correlation is necessary in such cases.

TREATMENT. Improvement is achieved in mild forms by keeping the infant in an upright position after feedings and changing to thicker feedings and semisolid foods. Antispasmodics may be helpful. Severe cases are difficult to manage and usually progress to esophagitis, stricture, etc., requiring replacement of the esophagus by colon bypass.

GASTROESOPHAGEAL INCOMPETENCE WITH HIATUS HERNIA AND PARTIAL SHORT ESOPHAGUS

Previously, the majority of cases of gastroesophageal incompetence with associated hiatus hernia in infants were reported in the medical literature under the title of congenital short esophagus. Howev-

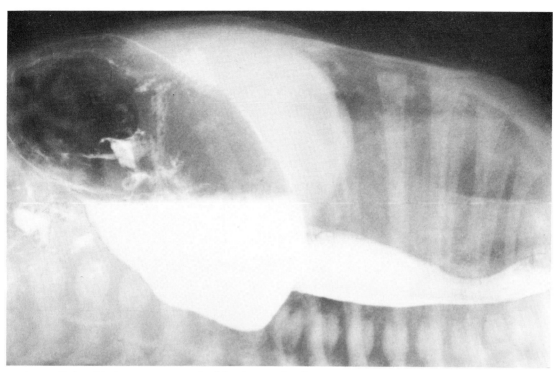

Figure 5–8. Chalasia in a 2-week-old infant with a history of vomiting since birth. Lateral view of the esophagus made of the infant in a partial Trendelenburg position, and after all ingested barium has entered the stomach, shows reflux into the esophagus.

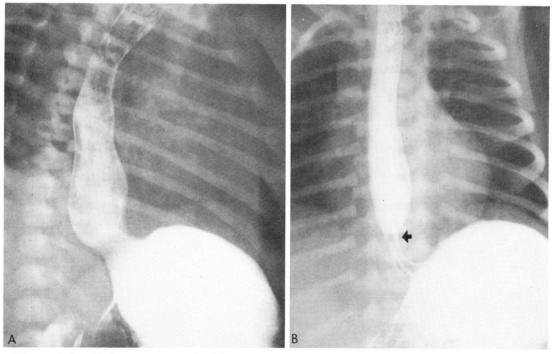

Figure 5–9. Chalasia in a 2-week-old infant with a history of recurrent regurgitation. *A,* Exposure made with pressure on the abdomen shows a patulous cardia and reflux. *B,* Repeat examination the following day fails to demonstrate gastroesophageal incompetence. The lower esophageal segment, the upper part of which is designated by the arrow, is contracted and functions normally.

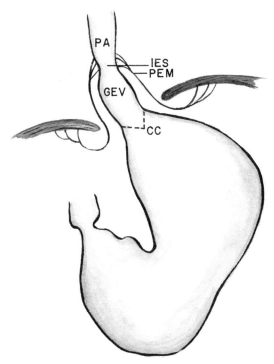

Figure 5-10. Diagram of alteration of the anatomy of the lower esophageal segment following prolonged gastroesophageal reflux and esophagitis. The esophagus is shortened and the gastroesophageal vestibule or lower esophageal segment is retracted into the thorax. See Figure 4–11 for comparison with the normal anatomy.

er, true congenital shortening of the esophagus due to failure of normal longitudinal growth is exceedingly rare. Between the 30th and 39th day of fetal development considerable elongation of the esophagus occurs, concomitant with the caudal migration of the septum transversum. Conceivably, failure of normal development at this stage associated with a defect in the diaphragm may result in an abnormally short esophagus. In theory, if there is an embryonic failure of longitudinal esophageal growth with intrathoracic position of the stomach, the gastric blood supply should be from the thoracic aorta.

It is impossible to determine the number of cases of true congenital short esophagus which have been recorded. Some cases may be the result of cicatricial changes occurring in the esophagus secondary to fetal hypoxia, or stress and resulting ischemia of the esophagus.

The relationship of intractable chalasia and resulting esophagitis, cicatricial changes, and retraction of the cardia into the thorax is well established but ordinarily takes many months to develop (Fig. 5–10). Shortening of the esophagus may occur before the formation of cicatricial changes (Fig. 5–11). Supporting evidence for this is found in experimental studies which have shown that stimulation of the vagus nerve, either directly or through the abdominal viscera, will result in contraction of the lower esophagus, and if the stimulus is marked or continued over a long period, there is displacement of the fundus into the thorax. Therefore, it seems logical to assume that irritation of the esophagus by persistent reflux of acid gastric secretions through an incompetent valvular mechanism at the gastroesophageal junction would lead to reflex shortening of the esophagus before cicatricial changes have time to develop.

Why chalasia with partial thoracic stomach and short esophagus is more commonly reported in the British literature than in this country is not understood. Their method of examination of the lower esophagus is somewhat different and more precise than the usual examination in this country. In addition, the identification of certain signs such as "the beak," "the hole" (the orifice of the cardia seen on end), and delayed reflux are criteria used to denote hiatal hernia in this age group. However, these may well be normal variants. Chalasia is a common finding, but a short esophagus and hiatus hernia in the newborn is rare. Admittedly the radiologic identification of the junction of esophageal and gastric mucosa is difficult and actually may vary in location depending upon the distention of the stomach, the level of the diaphragm, and the phase of peristaltic activity. In fact, the radiologic identification of transient migration of gastric mucosa above the diaphragm is a normal variation and should not be mistaken for hiatus hernia. However, this is quite different from the newborn with symptoms of vomiting, hemetemesis, and radiologic finding of short esophagus, esophageal ulceration, and hiatus hernia. This condition in the newborn must develop in intrauterine life and cannot be attributed to reflux because acid formation does not occur until after birth, reaches a peak during the first few

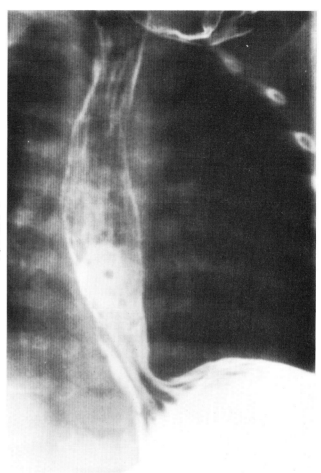

Figure 5–11. A short esophagus with associated chalasia in a 2-month-old male infant. Gastric mucosal folds are identified above the diaphragm and gastroeso-phageal reflux is obvious at the time of fluoroscopic study.

days, and then drops to a normal level. Consequently, one must theorize that in-trauterine vascular insults may affect the esophagus in a manner similar to compar-able changes in the intestinal tract. The resulting scarring, if severe, may produce sufficient retraction of the stomach into the chest and disrupt the competence of the gastroesophageal vestibule.

Symptoms of infants having this condi-tion are similar to those found in chalasia. Vomiting begins shortly after birth, and the vomitus may contain mucus and blood.

RADIOLOGIC APPEARANCE. During fluor-oscopy, the infant usually takes the barium mixture hungrily. The esophagus may be dilated or constricted, and it termi-nates in a small loculus of stomach located above the diaphragm (Figs. 5–12 and 5–13). The loculus is identified by the promi-nence of the gastric rugal folds, usually ar-ranged vertically but sometimes irregu-larly, which converge at the apex and become continuous with the finer longitu-dinal folds of the esophagus. The loculus often fills completely only for a fleeting period, thus making careful fluoroscopy im-perative. There is a free flow of barium from the stomach into the esophagus dur-ing increase in the intra-abdominal pres-sure similar to that described in chalasia. The esophagus is shortened, and loss of the normal angle of insertion of the esophagus may be noted (Fig. 5–14). Additional evi-dence of shortening of the esophagus and hiatus hernia is gained by identifying the inferior esophageal sphincter at a higher than normal level above the diaphragm (Figs. 5–15 and 5–16). Occasionally stric-ture of the lower esophagus with or with-·out evidence of ulceration may be the pre-senting radiologic finding. Chronic esophagitis may result in small mucosal diverticula of the esophagus (Fig. 5–17).

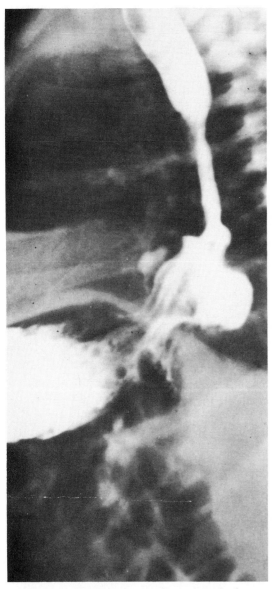

Figure 5-12. Short esophagus with hiatus hernia and gastroesophageal reflux in a 12-day-old infant. These changes in an infant of only 12 days suggests that gastroesophageal reflux and resulting esophagitis is not the cause; some condition, perhaps ischemic changes of the esophagus, occurred in intrauterine life.

time of fluoroscopy should not exclude reflux esophagitis as the pathogenesis (Fig. 5-18).

Treatment of partial thoracic stomach is the same as for chalasia. The infant is maintained in an upright position and semisolid foods are given. Symptomatic improvement usually follows promptly, and as the infant grows older the regulatory mechanism becomes more efficient. After symptomatic improvement, Astley found that the partial thoracic loculus often persisted but reflux did not occur. Patients with intractable reflux who fail to improve on medical management usually develop permanent strictures and an increase in herniation of the stomach. Occasionally the condition is not diagnosed in infancy but is detected later in life, by which time permanent changes have developed. In such cases esophageal replacement by colon is the procedure of choice.

Sandifer's syndrome is a curious clinical and radiographic entity whereby unusual movements of the head and neck are associated with hiatus hernia. It occurs predominately in males and is characterized by peculiar gyrating movements of the upper torso, head, and neck, including hyperextension of these segments of the body followed by side to side motions and marked flexion. These movements usually occur with or soon after meals and disappear during sleep.

This syndrome is very rare and has been mistaken repeatedly for severe neurologic disease. The cause of the unusual movements has not been explained. Radiographically there is little difficulty in demonstrating the hiatus hernia which is frequently associated with free gastroesophageal reflux. Esophagitis, ulceration, and stricture formation may occur as complications of the repeated gastroesophageal reflux. Surgery for the hiatus hernia produces dramatic reversal of symptoms.

These are similar in appearance to congenital bronchial remnants, a rare congential defect resulting from failure of normal mesenchymal differentiation following separation of the tracheal and esophageal anlage. Although gastroesophageal reflux usually can be demonstrated, its absence at the

ECTOPIC GASTRIC MUCOSA

Ectopic gastric mucosa in the supradiaphragmatic portion of an otherwise normal esophagus is a rare cause of esophagitis and vomiting in infants. The irritant secretions formed by the aberrant

Text continued on page 50

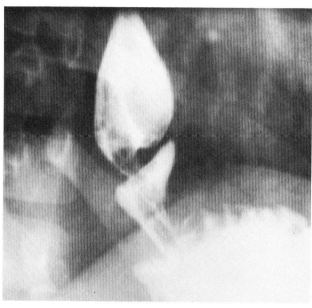

Figure 5–13. Partial intrathoracic stomach and chalasia in a 6-year-old boy with a history of vomiting in infancy and recurrent episodes of dysphagia. A loculus of the stomach is seen above the diaphragm distal to localized stricture.

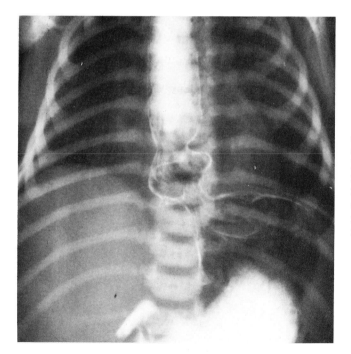

Figure 5–14. Sliding hiatus hernia and gastroesophageal reflux in a 4-day-old infant with persistent regurgitation. Fluoroscopic examination showed free reflux of contrast media from stomach into the esophagus, with alternate changes in the position of the cardia from its normal position into an intrathoracic position.

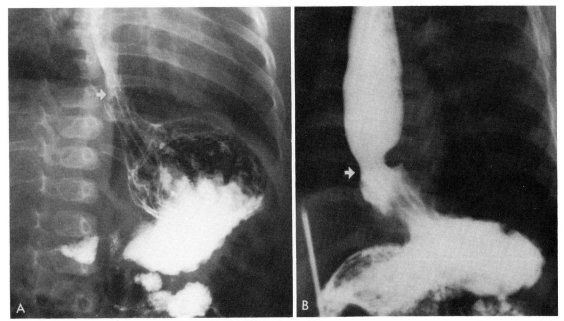

Figure 5–15. Hiatus hernia and short esophagus with associated reflux. *A,* Gastric mucosal folds are identified above the diaphragm, the arrow designating what is thought to be the inferior esophageal sphincter which is at a higher position than normal. *B,* Another infant with hiatus hernia and short esophagus, also showing elevated position of the inferior esophageal sphincter and persistent patency of the lower esophageal segment.

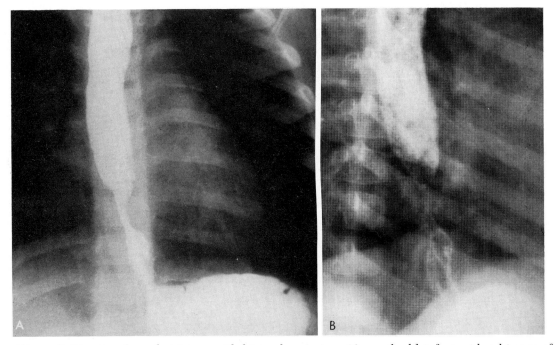

Figure 5–16. Esophageal stricture with hiatus hernia in a 16-month-old infant with a history of repeated vomiting during the first few months of life. *A,* Anteroposterior radiograph shows the esophageal stricture with a small loculus of the stomach above the diaphragm. *B,* With regurgitation of air the gastric mucosal pattern is seen within the herniated loculus beneath the stricture. Both radiographs show loss of the normal angulation of esophagus and cardia.

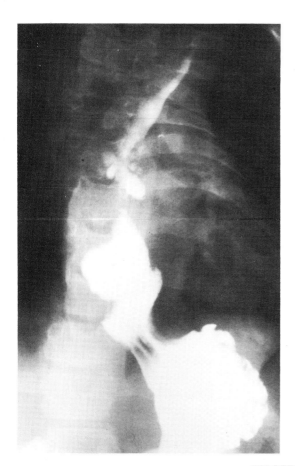

Figure 5–17. Esophageal stricture and hernia with multiple small diverticula in a 16-year-old cerebral palsy patient with chronic gastroesophageal reflux.

Figure 5–18. Esophageal stricture in a 3-year-old boy with a history of vomiting and hematemesis. Lateral view shows the esophageal stricture with ulcer (arrow) in the lower portion of the esophagus. Although the cause is probably that of reflux esophagitis, this could not be demonstrated at the time of fluoroscopy.

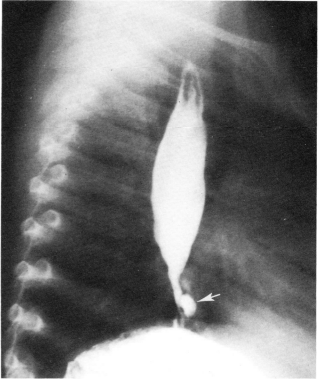

tissue cause esophagitis and contraction of the esophagus, making differentiation from partial thoracic stomach impossible by radiologic means. The only reliable method of differentiation is histologic examination of the lower esophagus and the finding of isolated areas of gastric mucosa in the esophagus, separated from the normal gastroesophageal junction by esophageal epithelium.

Accurate differentiation of these conditions—chalasia, partial thoracic stomach, and gastric mucosal ectopia—is not as important as realizing that all may be responsible for severe vomiting in infancy. If not

treated the esophagus will be irritated by the gastric juice, and such serious sequelae as esophagitis, esophageal ulceration, hematemesis, growth retardation, and esophageal stricture may develop.

ACHALASIA

Although achalasia is less common than chalasia in the pediatric patient, its occasional occurrence warrants consideration. It may represent a physiologic disturbance in the young infant and be associated with prematurity or central nervous system dam-

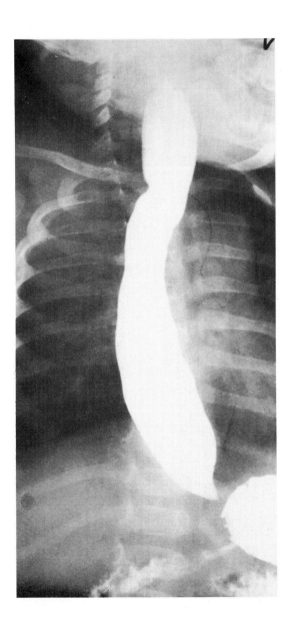

Figure 5–19. Achalasia in a 6-week-old infant with persistent vomiting. The esophagus is dilated and contrast media is held up by the contracted lower esophageal segment. In very young infants this may be a transient phenomenon, but more often dilatation or surgical correction of the defect is required.

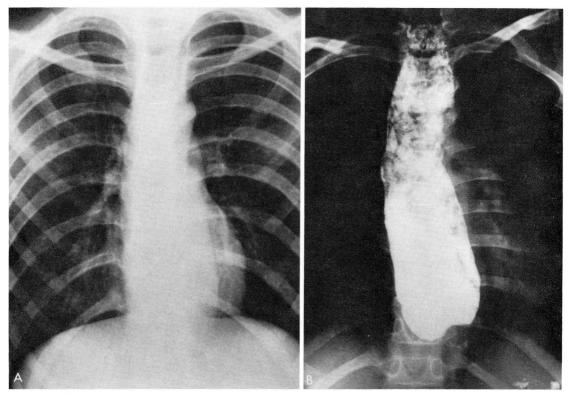

Figure 5-20. Achalasia. *A,* Posteroanterior chest roentgenogram of 10-year-old boy shows dilated esophagus within the cardiac silhouette. *B,* Esophagram shows marked dilatation of the esophagus secondary to achalasia.

age, or may be a transient finding in otherwise normal infants. In the older child its appearance and permanency are similar to that seen in the adult.

The term cardiospasm, commonly used to describe the condition, was introduced by Mikulicz, who thought that the cause was intractable spasm of the lower end of the esophagus. Although older articles suggest that achalasia is a disease of the myenteric plexus of the upper esophagus, it apparently is the result of failure of the normal tonicity of the gastroesophageal vestibule to relax under normal pressures from above, i.e., the opposite of chalasia. For this reason the term achalasia, recommended by Hurst, is preferred. Consequently, the ineffectual peristaltic activity of the esophagus seen fluoroscopically is probably secondary to dilatation and atony rather than to an inherent neuromuscular dysfunction. There is current evidence that in achalasia the lower esophageal segment is supersensitive to endogenous gastrin, with resulting hypertonicity of this structure.

Destruction of the neuromuscular plexuses of the esophagus by *Trypanosoma cruzi* (Chagas' disease) produces radiographic findings indistinguishable from achalasia.

Symptoms in children with achalasia are similar to those found in adults, namely, progressive dysphagia over a long period accompanied by increasing bouts of vomiting, the vomitus often being food ingested several hours previously. Thus, nutrition is poor in these children, and extreme inanition may be present in advanced cases. Emotional and psychogenic problems are common and, although these are probably not causative, add to the severity of the condition.

RADIOLOGIC FINDINGS. In young infants routine frontal and lateral chest films will show air in the esophagus. Ingested barium outlines a mildly dilated esophagus and contrast material drops to the level of

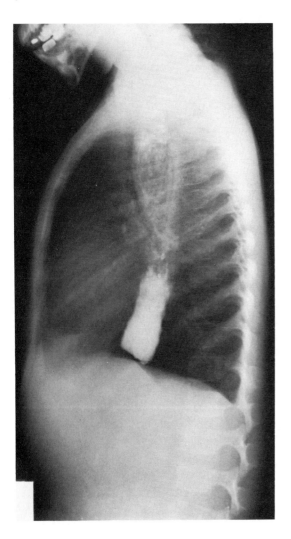

Figure 5-21. Achalasia in a 7-year-old boy. Food particles are identified within the barium, and there is anterior displacement of the trachea by the dilated esophagus.

the gastroesophageal vestibule, where it is held up for a short period of time before trickling into the stomach (Fig. 5–19). Occasionally the gastroesophageal vestibule will suddenly relax, allowing prompt emptying of the esophagus.

In advanced cases the diagnosis is suspected from routine chest films. The dilated esophagus casts a shadow of increased density in the posterior portion of the mediastinum, and the redundancy of the esophagus may be so great as to be identified along the right mediastinal border (Fig. 5–20). Many times an air-fluid level is present in the silhouette of the dilated esophagus. A swallow of contrast material makes the diagnosis obvious and demonstrates accurately the huge size which the esophagus may attain even in children. Food particles are usually seen, appearing as radiolucent filling defects in

the barium column (Fig. 5–21). The distal end is tapered and a thin stream of barium outlines the distal portion of the esophagus and its passage into the stomach. Fluoroscopic examination shows that the primary peristaltic wave which begins in the upper portion of the esophagus with the act of swallowing seldom passes inferior to the level of the aortic arch. If the wave does proceed down the esophagus, it is shallow and ineffectual. Purposeless and segmental contractions may be observed and are probably due to the atonic condition of the esophagus, which has been ineffectual in producing relaxation of the gastroesophageal vestibule. Tertiary esophageal contractions may occasionally be identified (Fig. 5–22). Esophagitis may develop and show irregularity of the lumen and ulceration.

Treatment is directed to the vestibular

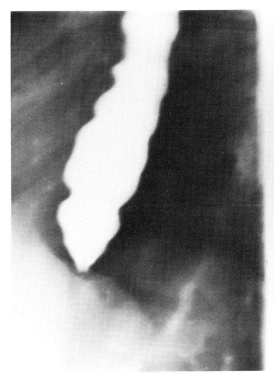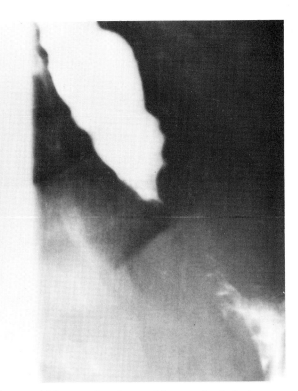

Figure 5–22. Tertiary contractions in a 7-year-old boy with a 3-year history of achalasia.

segment and consists of attempting by dilatation or incision to make this area patulous. Follow-up radiologic studies are useful in estimating the results of treatment, and also in detecting the complicating esophagitis which may occur if the gastroesophageal junction becomes incompetent.

REFERENCES

Pharyngeal and Esophageal Incoordination

Ardran, G. M., Benson, P. F., Butler, N. R., Ellis, H. L., and McKendrick, T. Congenital dysphagia resulting from dysfunction of the pharyngeal musculature, *Dev. Med. Child Neurol.*, 7:157, 1965.

Ardran, G. M., and Kemp, F. H. Normal and disturbed swallowing, *Progr. Pediatr. Radiol.*, 2:151, 1969.

Baghdassarian Gatewood, O. M., and Vanhoutte, J. J. The role of the barium swallow examination in evaluation of pediatric pneumonias, *Am. J. Roentgenol. Radium Ther. Nucl. Med.*, 97:203, 1966.

Herbst, J., Friedland, G. W., and Zboralske, F. F. Hiatal hernia and rumination in infants and children, *J. Pediatr.*, 78:261, 1971.

Lund, W. S. The function of the cricopharyngeal sphincter during swallowing, *Acta Otolaryngol.*, 59:497, 1964.

Margulies, S. I., Brunt, P. W., Donner, M. W., and Silbiger, M. L. Familial dysautonomia. A cineradiographic study of the swallowing mechanism, *Radiology*, 90:107, 1968.

Neuhauser, E. B. D., and Griscom, N. T. Aspiration pneumonitis in children, *Progr. Pediatr. Radiol.*, 1:265, 1967.

Neuhauser, E. B. D., and Harris, G. B. C. Familial dysautonomia of Riley-Day roentgenographic features, Abstract X, International Congr. Radiol. p. 194, 1962.

Seaman, W. B. Cineroentgenographic observations of the cricopharyngeus, *Am. J. Roentgenol. Radium Ther. Nucl. Med.*, 96:922, 1966.

Gastroesophageal Junction

Abrahams, P., and Burkitt, B. F. E. Hiatal hernia and gastroesophageal reflux in children and adolescents with cerebral palsy, *Aust. Paediatr. J.*, 6:41, 1970.

Chrispin, A. R. Abnormalities of oesophageal function: some radiological aspects. In Wilkinson, A. W., editor, *Recent Advances in Pediatric Surgery* (2nd ed.; New York: Grune and Stratton, 1969).

Cohen, S. Hypogastrinemia and sphincter incompetence, *N. Engl. J. Med.*, 289:215, 1973 (editorial).

Edwards, D. A. W. The antireflux mechanism: manometric and radiological studies, *Br. J. Radiol.*, 34:474, 1961.

Gryboski, J. D., Thayer, W. R., and Spiro, H. M. Esophageal motility in infants and children, *Pediatrics*, 31:382, 1963.

Linsman, J. F. Gastroesophageal reflux elicited while drinking water (water siphonage test), *Am. J. Roentgenol. Radium Ther. Nucl. Med.*, 94:325, 1965.

Lipshutz, W. H., Gaslans, R. D., Lukash, W. M., and Sode, J. Pathogenesis of lower-esophageal-sphincter incompetence, *N. Engl. J. Med.*, 289:182, 1973.

Neuhauser, E. B. D., and Berenberg, W. Cardio-esophageal relaxation as cause of vomiting in infants, *Radiology*, 48:480, 1947.

Shopfner, C. E., Kalmon, E. H., and Coin, C. G. The diagnosis of hypertrophic pyloric stenosis, *Am. J. Roentgenol. Radium Ther. Nucl. Med.*, 91:796, 1964.

Silverman, F. N. Gastroesophageal incompetency, partial intrathoracic stomach, and vomiting in infancy, *Radiology*, 64:664, 1955.

Strawcyznski, H., Beck, I. T., McKenna, R. D., and Nickerson, G. H. The behavior of the lower esophageal sphincter in infants and its relationship to gastroesophageal regurgitation. *J. Pediatr.*, 64:17, 1964.

Gastroesophageal Incompetence With Hiatus Hernia and Partial Short Esophagus

Astley, R., and Carre, I. J. Gastroesophageal incompetence in children, with special reference to minor degrees of partial thoracic stomach, *Radiology*, 62:351, 1954.

Berridge, F. R., and Friedland, G. W. Anatomical basis for radiological diagnosis of minimal hiatal herniation, *Ir. J. Med. Sci.*, 6:51, 1967.

Botha, G. S. M. The gastro-oesophageal region in infants: observations on the anatomy, with special reference to the closing mechanism and partial thoracic stomach, *Arch. Dis. Child.*, 33:78, 1958.

Carre, I. J. The natural history of partial thoracic stomach (hiatus hernia) in children, *Arch. Dis. Child.*, 34:344, 1959.

Carre, I. J. Postural treatment of children with partial thoracic stomach (hiatus hernia), *Arch. Dis. Child.*, 35:569, 1960.

Carre, I. J., and Astley, R. The fate of the partial thoracic stomach (hiatus hernia) in children, *Arch. Dis. Child.*, 35:484, 1960.

Chrispin, A. R., and Friedland, G. W. Functional disturbances in hiatal hernia in infants and children, *Thorax*, 22:422, 1967.

Chrispin, A. R., Friedland, G. W., and Wright, D. E. Some functional characteristics of oesophageal vestibule in infants and children, *Thorax*, 22:188, 1967.

Darling, D. B. Hiatal hernia and gastroesophageal reflux in infancy and childhood, *Am. J. Roentgenol. Radium Ther. Nucl. Med.*, 123:724, 1975.

Dey, F. L., Gilbert, N. C., Trump, R., and Roskelley, R. C. Reflex shortening of the esophagus in the experimental animal with the production of esophageal hiatus hernia, *J. Lab. Clin. Med.*, 31:499, 1946.

Friedland, G. W., Dodds, W. J., Sunshine, P., and Zboralski, F. F. The apparent disparity in incidence of hiatal hernias in infants and children in Britain and the United States, *Am. J. Roentgenol., Radium Ther. Nucl. Med.*, 120:305, 1974.

Sutcliffe, J. Torsion spasms and abnormal postures in children with hiatus hernia, Sandifer's syndrome, *Progr. Pediatr. Radiol.*, 2:190, 1969.

Ectopic Gastric Mucosa

Allison, P. R., and Johnstone, A. S. The oesophagus lined with gastric mucous membrane, *Thorax*, 8:87, 1953.

Barrett, N. R. Chronic peptic ulcer of the esophagus and esophagitis, *Br. J. Surg.*, 38:175, 1950.

Burgess, J. N., Payne, W. S., Andersen, H. A., Weiland, L. H., and Carlson, H. C. Barrett esophagus: the columnar-epithelial-lined lower esophagus, *Mayo Clin. Proc.*, 46:728, 1971.

Achalasia

Cloud, D. T., White, R. F., Linker, L. M., and Taylor, L. C. Surgical treatment of esophageal achalasia in children, *J. Pediatr. Surg.*, 1:137, 1966.

Cohen, S., and Lipshutz, W. Lower esophageal sphincter distinction in achalasia, *Gastroenterology*, 61:814, 1971.

Cohen, S., Lipshutz, W. H., and Hughes, W.: The role of gastrin supersensitivity in the pathogenesis of lower esophageal sphincter hypertension in achalasia, *J. Clin. Invest.*, 50:1241, 1971.

Hurst, A. F. Achalasia of the cardia, *Q. J. Med.*, 8:300, 1915.

Magilner, A. D., and Isard, H. J. Achalasia of the esophagus in infancy, *Radiology*, 98:81, 1971.

Sorsdahl, O. A., and Gay, B. R. Achalasia of the esophagus in childhood, *Am. J. Dis. Child.*, 109:141, 1965.

Chapter 6

CONGENITAL MALFORMATIONS OF THE ESOPHAGUS

ESOPHAGEAL ATRESIA AND TRACHEOESOPHAGEAL FISTULA

Radiologic recognition and descriptions of esophageal atresia have been known for many years, but it was not until 1939, when Ladd and Leven independently devised methods of building an antethoracic or "skin tube" esophagus, that interest in the diagnostic aspects were renewed. This interest was further stimulated by Haight's successful method of end-to-end anastomosis of the esophagus and closure of the accompanying tracheoesophageal fistula. The importance of x-ray methods in providing confirmatory evidence of esophageal atresia is attested to by the many reports in the medical literature of the various types of this condition accompanied by preoperative radiographic demonstration. Perfection of the surgical technic has led to a high survival rate in infants with this anomaly, and no other obstructive lesion of the alimentary tract has had such a rapid improvement in mortality figures in recent years. The high incidence of associated anomalies accounts for many of the deaths of infants with esophageal atresia. Because of the high incidence of imperforate anus and esophageal atresia, any newborn infant with imperforate anus should have radiologic studies of the esophagus.

EMBRYOLOGY. In early fetal life the esophagus and trachea are one tube which becomes divided into two structures by the folding in of the lateral walls of the foregut (see Chap. 3). By this process two parallel tubes, the future trachea and esophagus, are formed. Embryologic texts explain that if the folding process is incomplete, and the lateral mesodermal walls fail to meet at any one point, then communication of the trachea and esophagus, i.e., tracheoesophageal fistula, will result. If these lateral folds turn dorsally in their development, thereby cutting through the esophageal lumen, atresia will result. However, intrauterine anoxia or stress with resulting vascular compromise may, as in cases of bowel atresia (see Chap. 12) produce focal necrosis of the esophagus with resulting atresia or tracheoesophageal communication.

CLINICAL PICTURE. During the first few hours of life, these infants frequently have an excessive amount of saliva, which may cause repeated attacks of coughing and strangling as a result of aspiration into the tracheobronchial tree. Attempts to feed the infant produce similar episodes of choking. Abdominal distention secondary to excessive amount of air entering the stomach and intestinal tract in tracheoesophageal fistula without atresia, or in cases of esophageal atresia with fistulous connection of the lower esophageal segment with the trachea, is frequently another clinical observation. If esophageal atresia is present, the passage of a catheter through the infant's nose and down into the esophagus encounters obstruction. If obstruction is not met, tracheoesophageal fistula without atresia is still to be considered. Radiologic procedures will accurately disclose which of the several types of anomalies exist.

Vogt devised the following classification of esophageal atresia (Fig. 6–1):

Type I. — Complete atresia of the esophagus.

Type II. — Atresia of the esophagus with

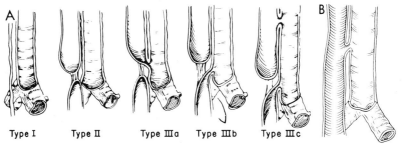

Figure 6–1. Classification of esophageal atresia and tracheoesophageal fistula. *A − I,* Complete atresia of the esophagus. *II,* Localized atresia of the esophagus. *III a,* Esophageal atresia with tracheoesophageal fistula involving the proximal esophageal segment and the trachea. *III b,* Esophageal atresia with tracheoesophageal fistula involving the lower esophageal segment. *III c,* Esophageal atresia with tracheoesophageal fistulae involving both upper and lower esophageal segments. *B,* Tracheoesophageal fistula without esophageal atresia.

an upper and lower esophageal segment, each consisting of a blind pouch.

Type III.—Atresia of the esophagus with associated fistulous communication with the tracheobronchial tree. Three combinations of this condition are recognized: A. fistula between the upper esophageal segment and the trachea; B. fistula between the lower esophageal segment and the trachea or bronchus; C. fistula between both upper and lower esophageal segments and the trachea or bronchus.

To this classification must be added a fourth type (IV) in which tracheoesophageal fistula is present but the esophageal lumen is patent. Type III B is by far the most common of the anomalies, accounting for 85 to 90% of the total.

Tracheoesophageal clefts are high communications which are extremely difficult to diagnose by x-ray examination, usually being mistaken for pharyngeal incoordination and resulting aspiration into the trachea. Infants with these clefts frequently have aphonia, but it should be recognized that brain-damaged babies with pharyngeal incoordination may also be aphonic.

RADIOLOGIC FINDINGS. Before any radiologic studies are begun, one should be certain that oxygen and suction equipment are close at hand. Anteroposterior and lateral roentgenograms of the chest, including the abdomen, should precede the fluoroscopic examination and will give presumptive evidence of the type of abnormality. If gas is present in the stomach or intestinal tract, it may be presupposed that either esophageal atresia is not present or, if

present, there is communication between the lower esophageal segment and the tracheobronchial tree. If air is absent from the intestinal tract, one may conclude that either esophageal atresia alone is present or, if fistula exists, communication is with the upper esophageal segment.

Esophageal Atresia With Fistulous Communication Between Lower Esophageal Segment and Trachea (type III B). Because this is by far the most common type of this group of anomalies, its radiographic characteristics are given first.

The chest roentgenogram will disclose air in the upper esophageal pouch (Fig. 6–2) and the stomach is often distended with gas. However, there are rare exceptions to this rule. If the infant has CNS depression because of brain damage or oversedation of the mother, the amount of gastric air may be normal or diminished. The lateral chest roentgenogram frequently shows the upper esophageal pouch to be distended with air and often displacing the trachea anteriorly (Fig. 6–3). Occasionally on lateral chest films the lower esophageal segment may be identified as a narrow air column (Fig. 6–4). In such cases the site of the fistula can be located directly. Atelectasis and pneumonia of the right upper lobe are present in over 50% of the cases of esophageal atresia because of aspiration of saliva and feedings. The frequency of aspiration into the right upper lobe is due to the lower position of the right upper lobe bronchus, especially when the infant is cradled on the nurse's or mother's left arm during attempted feedings. Pneumonia is also occa-

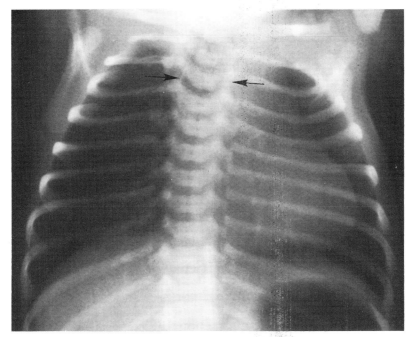

Figure 6-2. Esophageal atresia. Air is identified in the upper esophageal pouch. Air is also present in the stomach, indicating communication between the lower esophageal segment and the tracheobronchial tree.

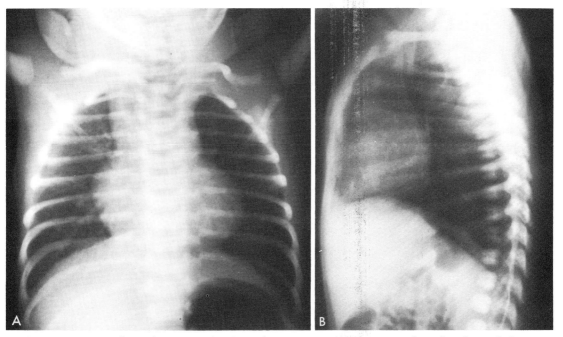

Figure 6-3. Esophageal atresia. *A,* Frontal projection shows air within the distended upper esophageal pouch; the presence of gas in the stomach indicates fistulous communication between the lower esophageal segment and the trachea. *B,* Lateral view shows to better advantage the distended upper esophageal pouch with resulting pressure deformity upon the trachea.

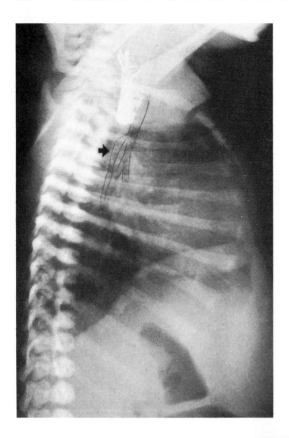

Figure 6–4. Esophageal atresia with lower tracheoesophageal fistula. A small amount of contrast media outlines the upper esophageal pouch. The arrow denotes a small amount of air in the proximal portion of the lower esophageal segment (enhanced for greater clarity).

Figure 6–5. Esophageal atresia with tracheoesophageal fistula (type III B). The presence of pneumonia and atelectasis in the right upper lobe is a common finding and is secondary to aspiration.

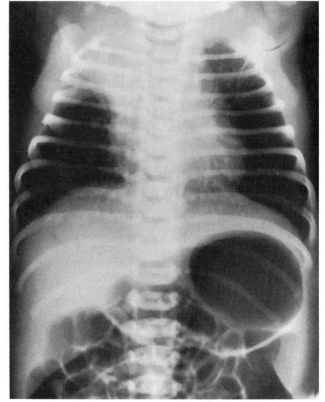

sionally seen in the lower lobes and left perihilar area, and results from either aspiration or reflux of gastric contents from the lower esophageal segment into the respiratory tree (Fig. 6–5).

Following the radiographic examination of the chest and abdomen, the infant is placed uner the fluoroscopic screen and a No. 8 or 10F catheter is passed into the nose and down the esophagus. If this is not done under fluoroscopy, misconception of the location of the obstruction is possible as a result of the catheter coiling on itself (Fig. 6–6). It is also possible to pass the catheter through the larynx, into the trachea, and then through the esophageal fistula into the stomach. Appropriate fluoroscopic evaluation and spot films will avoid this mistake. Once obstruction is encountered, the infant is placed on his right side and slightly prone with the head of the table lowered, and a small amount of Dionosil is injected into the catheter distending the esophagus (Fig. 6–7). Careful fluoroscopic observation, perferably with videotape or cine recordings, is important in determining if contrast material seen in the

trachea is the result of aspiration through the larynx or if there is a fistula between the esophagus and trachea. Appropriate spot films should be made, preferably in rapid sequence. Overhead radiographs after the fluoroscopic study are less reliable. It is neither necessary nor advisable to examine the infant supine because of the facility of aspiration of the contrast material in this position. Also, if fistula is present, it naturally will arise from the anterior esophageal wall and will be demonstrated more easily with the child in the prone position.

Another method of examination is to place the x-ray table upright and to observe the injection of contrast material while the infant is lying prone on the elevated footrest. The use of Dionosil rather than Lipiodol has helped to overcome the complication of lipoid pneumonia. Barium is an acceptable contrast medium but water-soluble iodine solutions are pulmonary irritants. After fluoroscopic examination the contrast material is withdrawn from the esophagus and the catheter removed. The lower level of the upper esophageal pouch

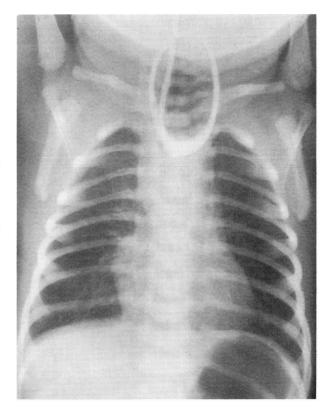

Figure 6–6. Esophageal atresia (type III B). The catheter is coiled within the upper esophageal pouch, giving the erroneous impression that it has passed to a lower level, thereby indicating the importance of passing the catheter into the esophagus under fluoroscopic visualization.

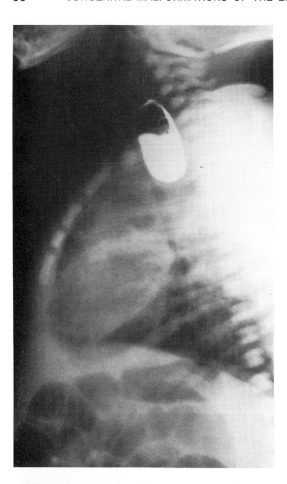

Figure 6–7. Esophageal atresia (type III B) showing a small amount of Dionosil in the upper esophageal pouch.

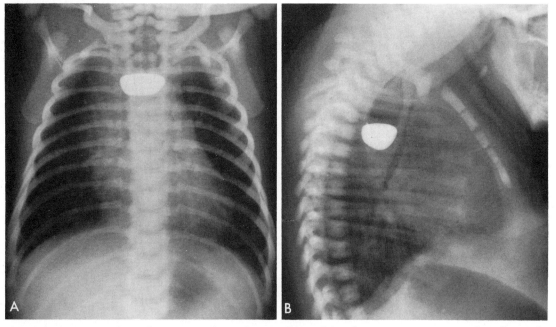

Figure 6–8. Esophageal atresia with tracheoesophageal fistula. *A*, Contrast material outlines the inferior portion of the upper segment. *B*, Note distinction of upper pouch and anterior displacement of the trachea.

usually is located opposite the second or third dorsal vertebral body, but this is not always an accurate index of the actual level found at the time of thoracotomy (Fig. 6–8). This is largely due to the change in position of the pouch with respirations. If contrast material has been aspirated, a bronchogram will result and frequently disclose the location of the lower esophageal segment. However, it is neither desirable nor necessary to demonstrate this.

Esophageal Atresia Without Tracheoesophageal Fistula (type II). In this type there will be complete absence of gas in

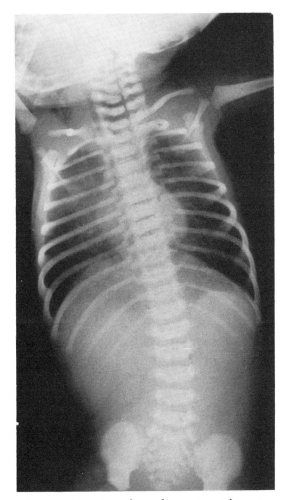

Figure 6–9. Esophageal atresia without tracheoesophageal fistula between the lower esophageal segment and the tracheobronchial tree. There is complete absence of gas in the stomach and intestinal tract. The exclusion of a fistula between the upper esophageal segment and the trachea cannot be made without fluoroscopic studies.

the stomach and intestinal tract. However, other indications of obstruction, such as inability to pass the catheter down the esophagus and demonstration of an upper blind pouch after instillation of a small amount of Dionosil into the catheter will be the same as in the more common type just described (Figs. 6–9 and 6–10).

Esophageal Atresia With Fistulous Communication Between Both Upper and Lower Esophageal Segments (type III C). In these cases there will be gas in the intestinal tract. Instillation of contrast material into the esophagus discloses the upper esophageal pouch and, in addition, evidence of communication of this pouch with the tracheobronchial tree. Occasionally the fistulous tract may be so minute that accurate identification by fluoroscopy as well as by spot films is impossible. In such cases, however, the identification of contrast material in the tracheobronchial tree, with the assurance that at the time of fluoroscopy aspiration of the medium over the glottis did not occur, is presumptive evidence that this type of tracheoesophageal fistula and esophageal atresia is present. Differentiation between a high tracheoesophageal fistula and a laryngeal cleft is frequently impossible, but in cleft anomalies swallowed contrast material enters the trachea more easily than in cervical tracheoesophageal fistulas.

Esophageal Atresia With Communication Between Only the Upper Esophageal Pouch and Trachea (type III A). These rare cases are identical with the type just described except that gas is not present in the gastrointestinal tract (Fig. 6–11). If the fistulous communication between the upper esophageal segment and the trachea is situated very high, it may be virtually impossible to determine whether fistula is present or whether the contrast material reaches the tracheobronchial tree by aspiration or through a laryngeal cleft.

Tracheoesophageal Fistula Without Esophageal Atresia. Diagnosis of this condition may be very difficult. Any child who has a history of choking on liquid feedings and recurrent episodes of pneumonia without apparent cause should be suspected of having the condition and examined accordingly. The stomach and intestinal tract are commonly distended with air and the esophagus is also frequently identified by

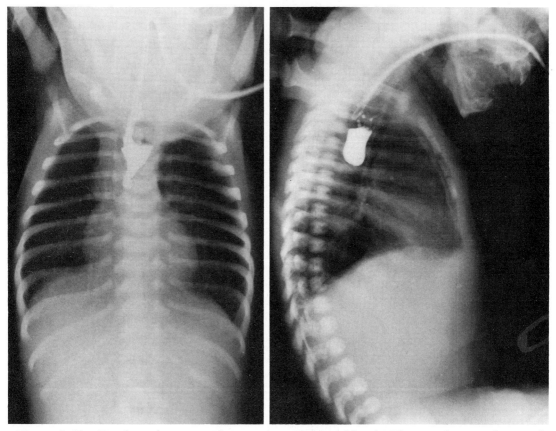

Figure 6–10. Esophageal atresia without tracheoesophageal fistula. There is absence of gas in the stomach, and anteroposterior and lateral projections show no evidence of tracheoesophageal fistula between the upper esophageal segment and the trachea.

its air content. Respiratory efforts and equation of pressures in the trachea and esophagus allow free entrance of air into the esophagus and stomach.

The fistulous tract arises from the anterior wall of the esophagus and extends to the posterior wall of the trachea (Fig. 6–12) or to the left main stem bronchus. However, the communication is usually high and above the thoracic inlet (Fig. 6–13). A catheter passed down the esophagus does not encounter obstruction. The catheter should then be withdrawn to the upper esophageal level above the carina, and with the infant in the lateral position a small amount of Dionosil or thin barium mixture is injected into the catheter. Barium is preferred because of its lower viscosity and the better chance of its passing through a narrow fistula. Again, careful attention should be paid to the passage of the contrast material

down the esophagus, not only to determine if communcation with the trachea is present but also to look for associated abnormalities of the esophagus. Lateral visualization with the infant in a prone position is preferable for demonstrating the fistula (see Fig. 2–6).

The head of the infant should be lowered because of the usual cephalad direction of the fistula, resulting from the proportionately greater growth of the esophagus during embryonic life. If the caliber of the fistula is very small, the viscosity of the contrast medium may prevent its passage. Therefore, if a patient is suspected of having a fistula and during fluoroscopy neither the tract nor trachea becomes opacified, we have used a small amount of water-soluble iodide contrast material successfully, presumably because of its lower viscosity. Admittedly, this medium is more irritating to the lungs

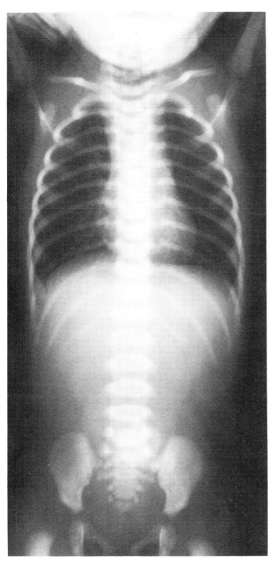

Figure 6-11. Esophageal atresia with communication between the upper esophageal pouch and trachea (type III A). Subsequent fluoroscopic studies showed evidence of tracheoesophageal fistula in the cervical portion of the esophagus.

fluoroscopic study utilizing a nursing bottle containing barium. This not only permits an evaluation of deglutition but also may demonstrate a cervical tracheoesophageal fistula. Presumably this is due to the fistula assuming a more horizontal position with upward movement of the esophagus during the act of swallowing. The fistula may also be demonstrated by utilizing a Foley cath-

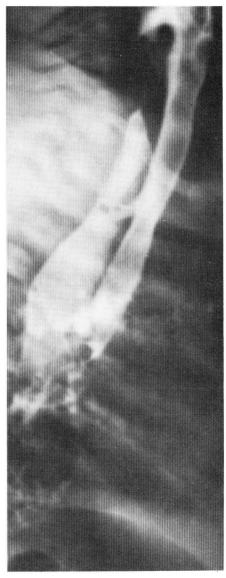

Figure 6-12. Tracheoesophageal fistula without esophageal atresia. The fistula arises from the anterior portion of the esophagus and passes cephalad to the posterior portion of the trachea. These lesions are usually high and can frequently be corrected by a cervical approach.

and must be used in small amounts. The success of the examination depends upon careful observation at the time of fluoroscopy and on adequate spot films and videotape recordings to be certain that if contrast material is seen in the tracheobronchial tree, it reaches there via the fistula and not by aspiration over the glottis (Fig. 6-14).

Any infant suspected of having a tracheoesophageal fistula should also have a

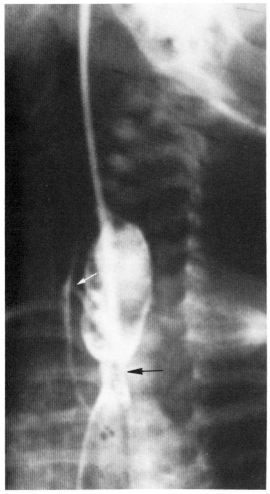

Figure 6–13. Postoperative examination of esophageal atresia and lower tracheoesophageal fistula showing a second congenital tracheoesophageal communication between the esophagus and the cervical portion of the trachea (white arrow). The mild esophageal stenosis represents the point of surgical anastomosis (black arrow).

eter which is inserted into the esophageal inlet and the balloon inflated. This prevents reflux and aspiration of the contrast material. Occasionally the fistula may be so small as to require repeated examination for identification.

It is important to recognize that any infant with atelectasis and/or pneumonia of the right upper lobe is probably aspirating or has a tracheoesophageal fistula, and appropriate radiologic studies of deglutition and of the esophagus should be performed.

If gastrostomy is performed prior to oper-

ative repair, the injection of contrast material will usually reflux into the lower esophageal segment and determine the length of the atretic segment (Fig. 6–15). The use of repeated catheter bougies placed in the upper and lower esophageal segments for the purpose of approximating the ends of the esophagus is helpful preoperatively in possible primary anastomoses.

Postoperative radiologic studies are of value in determining the success of the anastomosis as well as the development of complications. Surgical correction of the defect is usually made through a right transpleural approach, this method affording the surgeon greater access to the defect than the older retropleural approach. The tracheoesophageal fistulas without atresia are usually high and are repaired by a cervical extrathoracic approach. On the third

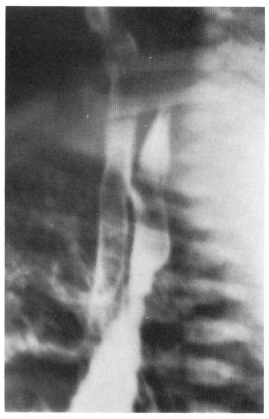

Figure 6–14. Tracheoesophageal fistula without esophageal atresia. The fistula may be extremely short, making a differentiation between this and aspiration of contrast media into the trachea difficult without careful fluoroscopic and videotape recordings.

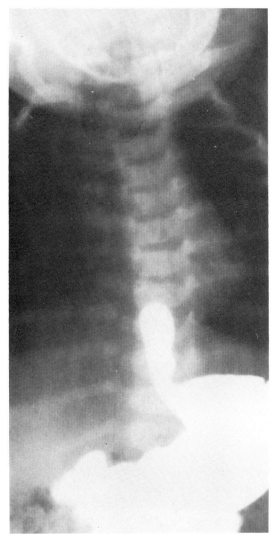

Figure 6–15. Esophageal atresia with barium introduced through a feeding gastrostomy prior to surgical repair of the esophageal defect. There is a reflux into the distal esophageal segment. The upper air-filled pouch marks the lower portion of the upper esophageal pouch. The distance between the two segments is too great for a primary anastomosis.

or fourth postoperative day, the infant is brought to the x-ray department and is fed a small amount of barium under fluoroscopy. Spot films are made as the contrast material reaches the site of anastomosis, and careful attention is paid to the configuration of the anastomosis as well as to the ease with which the barium passes this area of the esophagus. Alteration of the physiology of the reconstructed esophagus

is inevitable. It consists of normal peristalsis above the anastomosis and absence of peristalsis for a variable distance of 2 to 5 cm below it. A back-and-forth or "yo-yo" type of contractile activity may be observed. If there is no evidence of leakage and the ingested contrast material reaches the stomach satisfactorily, oral administration of fluids in small amounts is begun. The examination may be repeated two to three days later and, if the anastomosis appears satisfactory once again, the feedings are increased in amount. Postoperative complications consist of a leak of contrast material localized around the site of anastomosis, and a few will show extension of this leak with the establishment of an esophagopleural or even external esophagocutaneous fistula (Fig. 6–16). The development of either complication, although regrettable, should not be viewed as an operative failure, for most of these fistulas close spontaneously in a few weeks following temporary gastrostomy. However, strictures are more apt to develop in cases showing leakage at the site of anastomosis.

If recurrent bouts of pneumonitis follow successful surgical correction of esophageal atresia and tracheoesophageal fistula, an additional fistula, usually involving the upper portion of the esophagus, should be suspected and searched for carefully. The appearance of the esophagus months and years after successful repair is extremely variable. Most of these individuals have some mild distortion and even narrowing of the esophagus at the site of anastomosis. The degree of distortion varies considerably in different individuals and is not necessarily a reflection of the postoperative course, although infants who have had leakage at the site of anastomosis are more apt to have significant stricture, requiring dilatation. A complication found in many of these patients later in life is obstruction of the esophagus by an ingested foreign body (Fig. 6–17).

STENOSIS

Theoretically, congenital stricture or stenosis of the esophagus may be the result of inadequate canalization of the esophagus early in embryonic life. Rapid proliferation of the epithelial lining of the alimentary

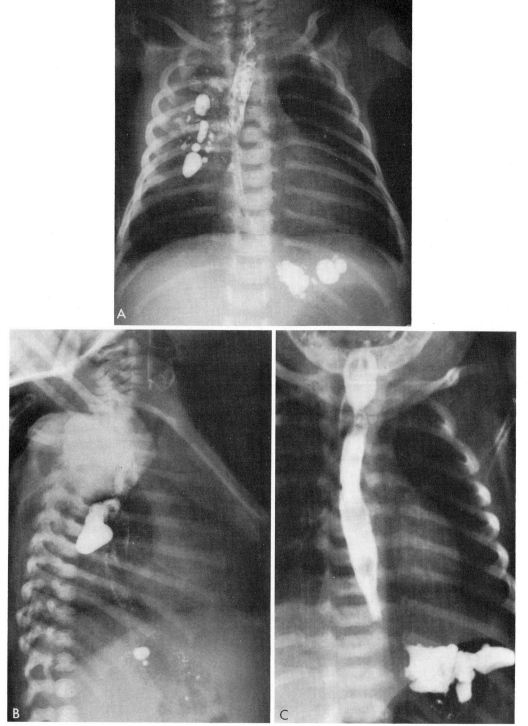

Figure 6–16. Postoperative studies showing complications of surgical repair of esophageal atresia and tracheoesophageal fistula. *A*, Disruption of right lateral wall of esophagus with puddling of contrast material in pleural space. *B*, Another example of breakdown of esophageal anastomosis, showing collection of contrast material in the mediastinum and a sinus tract opening into the esophagus. *C*, Same case as in *B*, repeat esophagram made 10 months later. Narrow defect remains at the site of anastomosis.

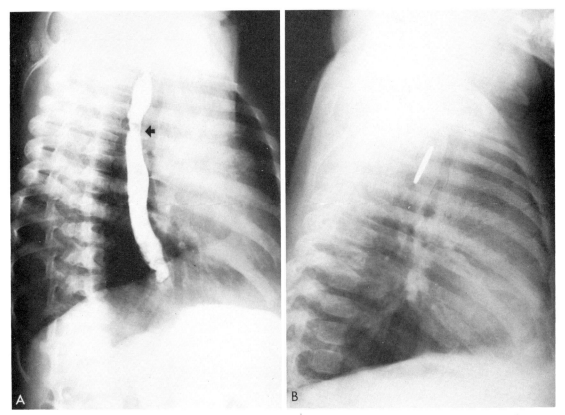

Figure 6-17. Foreign body at the site of stenosis in a 4-year-old child who had esophageal atresia repaired shortly after birth. *A*, Esophagram made at age 3 shows minimal constriction at site of anastomosis. *B*, Coin lodged at point of constriction.

tract occurs about the fifth week of fetal life, converting the lumen into a solid cellular structure. Although a similar proliferation of cells occurs in the esophagus a solid stage apparently does not develop, with a narrow lumen remaining in the cell masses. With growth of the esophagus and with vacuole formation, a normal lumen is established. The failure of normal coalescence of the vacuoles at any one point has been offered as an explanation for congenital stenosis of the esophagus. However, as in the cases of congenital stenosis and atresia of the bowel, a more plausible explanation is the vascular insufficiency occurring in the esophagus in episodes of intrauterine anoxia or stress (see Chap. 12).

Esophageal stenosis is less common than atresia and less often associated with tracheoesophageal fistula. The area of stenosis may form a diaphragm within which is a small perforation, or may consist of a constricted lumen of variable length.

SYMPTOMS. The time of onset and severity of symptoms depends upon the degree of deformity. As a rule, persistent regurgitation begins early, when the infant is put on solid foods. However, the condition may not make itself known until childhood, when a solid object such as a fruit pit or piece of meat becomes lodged in the esophagus. In severe cases the infant fails to gain properly and, in time, if the condition is not recognized and corrected, dilatation of the upper esophageal segment may produce pressure on the adjacent trachea, causing wheezing and respiratory difficulties. Aspiration of the regurgitated material may, as in atresia, lead to aspiration pneumonia.

ROENTGENOLOGIC EXAMINATION. If the infant only has trouble retaining solid foods, milk and liquid feedings causing no difficulty, he is placed under the fluoroscope in a supine position and given a nursing bottle containing a mixture of thin

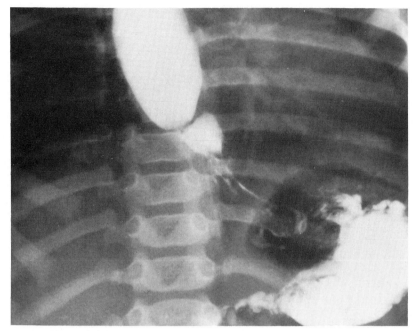

Figure 6–18. Esophageal stenosis in a 10-month-old infant. At operation a thin diaphragm with a small central opening was found.

barium. However, if the infant has a history of vomiting after liquid feedings, or if feedings are accompanied by choking spells suggestive of fistula, a catheter is inserted under fluoroscopic visualization into the upper esophagus and a small amount of barium injected. Careful attention is paid to its passage down the esophagus, and spot films of the stenosis are obtained with the infant in the supine and the right anterior oblique positions. Thick barium may be utilized to distend the esophagus more adequately. Following this, an effort should be made to determine if fistula is present by turning the infant into the prone position and again observing the passage of contrast material down the esophagus. The stomach and duodenum should be included in the examination in order to exclude unsuspected abnormalities of these structures. The majority of the congenital strictures of the esophagus are at the junction of the mid and lower thirds of the esophagus and are only 1 or 2 cm long.

The diagnosis of stenosis is based on the persistence of the defect, with failure of the narrowed segment to expand to the degree of the esophageal segments above and below it (Figs. 6–18 and 6–19). The esophagus above the constriction is dilated, and

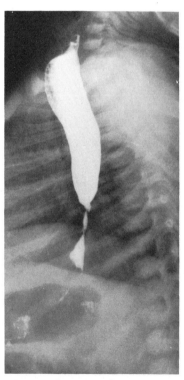

Figure 6–19. Congenital stenosis of esophagus in an 8-month-old infant. Esophagus was found to be normal below constricted area.

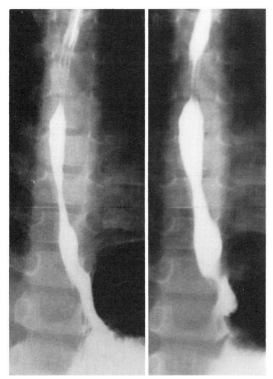

Figure 6–20.   Serial roentgenograms of mild esophageal stenosis involving the proximal and middle thirds of the esophagus.

the amount of contrast material delayed in passing the point of constriction depends upon the size of the narrowed lumen. Occasionally the area of stenosis is so slight as to be scarcely noticeable. In such cases, it is an incidental finding during fluoroscopy for other reasons (Fig. 6–20). If the stricture is in the lower part of the esophagus near the esophageal hiatus of the diaphragm, it may be impossible to differentiate it from achalasia or from acquired strictures resulting from gastroesophageal incompetence or ectopic gastric mucosa.

Follow-up fluoroscopy and radiographic studies are invaluable in following the results of treatment, whether it be by dilatations or by resection of the stenosis and anastomosis.

ESOPHAGEAL BRONCHUS

An esophageal bronchus is a rare foregut malformation whereby a bronchus extends from the esophagus or stomach into a sequestered segment of the lung. Whether this develops as a bronchial bud from the esophagus or in some way is due to incom-

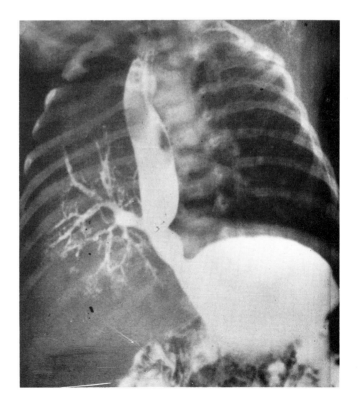

Figure 6–21. Bronchopulmonary foregut malformation. An anomalous bronchus arises from the distal esophagus and supplies a portion of the right lower lobe. (From Singleton, E. B., et al: Radiographic evaluation of lung abnormalities, *Radiol. Clin. North Am., 10*:333, 1972. Courtesy of B. R. Girdany, Pittsburgh, Pa.)

plete cleavage of the trachea and esophagus is not known. However, the close association of the foregut and the respiratory tree explains the embryonic defects which frequently accompany both systems. The affected pulmonary segment does not have a normal bronchial communication and its arterial blood supply is from the aorta, similar to other forms of sequestrations. Clinically there is an area of pulmonary parenchymal density which may or may not be partially aerated depending upon air flow from the adjacent pores of Kohn. Chronic infection invariably is present and, fluoroscopically, the aberrant bronchus fills with ingested contrast material flooding the area of lung which it enters (Fig. 6–21).

DUPLICATIONS (Neurenteric Cysts)

The esophagus is the second commonest site of duplications in the alimentary tract, the most common being the ileum. The duplication rarely communicates with the adjacent esophagus and is most often located in the right hemithorax.

EMBRYOLOGY. The origin of duplications of the esophagus as well as of duplications elsewhere in the alimentary tract has been proposed by Bremer to result from incomplete recanalization of the alimentary tract lumen. In the fifth or sixth week of intrauterine life, rapid proliferation of epithelial cells of the alimentary tract takes place, convering the lumen of the tract into a solid core. The solid stage probably never affects the entire intestinal tract at one time but apparently involves most of it during a 5- to 6-week period of embryonic development. In the esophagus the solid stage is never reached, with a minute lumen being retained, surrounded by a thick wall of massed epithelial cells. At the tenth week of intrauterine life, vacuoles begin to appear. If one or more connections of these vacuoles fail to occur, duplication results. Consequently, a duplication may arise in any portion of the alimentary tract from the base of the tongue to the anus.

The high incidence of anomalies of the cervical and upper thoracic spine and esophageal duplication is not readily explained by this process of development. Consequently, Veeneklaas proposed the theory that in such cases there is adherence of the foregut to the notocord, with the result that as the stomach descends, with growth of the alimentary tract, the traction at the point of adherence leads to anomalous development of the future vertebral bodies (notocord), and the corresponding adherent portion of the foregut becomes pinched off, forming the duplication. Additional evidence of the intimate development of the gut and the notocord is given by Neuhauser, et al. These authors support Bremer's hypothesis that those duplications which arise from the foregut and connect with the meninges and spinal cord through a defect in the vertebral bodies are derived from persistence of an accessory neurenteric canal. Normally, in the early development of the human embryo, there is a communication from the gut to the dorsal surface of the embryo, the neurenteric canal of Kovalevsky. The final location of the remnant of this structure is at the coccyx. Accessory neurenteric canals may exist and, if one of these fails to become obliterated, it persists as a cyst lined by intestinal epithelium and connecting with the meninges through a defect in the vertebral bodies. There are on record several examples of duplications of the foregut with anomalous vertebra, but without operative or necropsy evidence of communication between the duplication and the spinal cord. However, because the remnant of the accessory neurenteric canal may be in the form of a fibrous cord, which could be easily overlooked at operation or necropsy, one should consider the possibility that all duplications of the foregut in which there are also vertebral anomalies represent neurenteric cysts.

PATHOLOGY. The duplicated segment has a thick wall of smooth muscle and is lined with mucosa similar to some other portions of the alimentary tract. Because of the variations in the type of mucosa lining the duplicated segment, numerous terms, including reduplication, enterogenous cysts, gastroenterogenous cysts, gastroenteric cysts, and thoracic cysts of enteric origin, have appeared in the medical literature, all being synonymous with duplications. Many of these cysts are lined with gastric mucosa, in which case peptic ulceration of the duplication is a common finding.

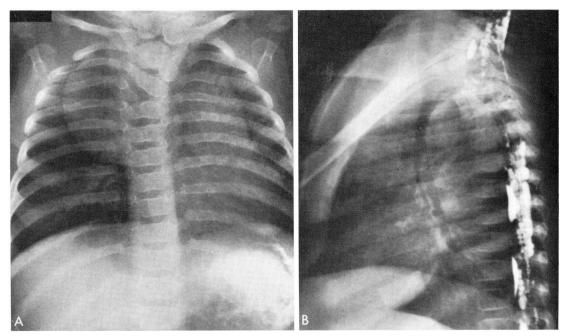

Figure 6-22. Duplication of esophagus in a 2-month-old infant with recurrent episodes of vomiting. A, Posteroanterior chest roentgenogram showing large right superior mediastinal mass with associated vertebral anomalies. B, Lateral chest roentgenogram, localizing mass from posterior mediastinum displacing trachea anteriorly, A myelogram was performed to exclude an anterior meningocele. (Courtesy of Dr. J. F. Holt, Univ. of Michigan.)

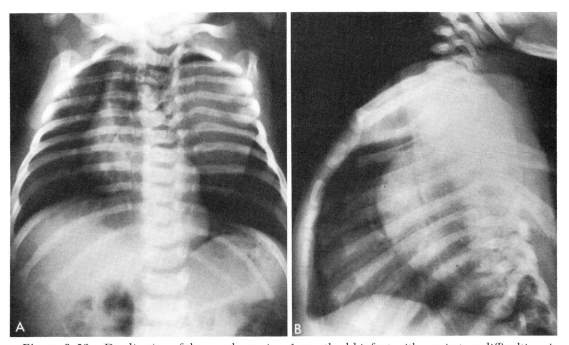

Figure 6-23. Duplication of the esophagus in a 1-month-old infant with respiratory difficulties. A, Posteroanterior chest roentgenogram, showing large mass in left hemithorax displacing mediastinum to the right. Note associated vertebral anomalies. B, Lateral chest roentgenogram, indicating posterior location of the mass. Pathology report: duplication of esophagus lined with gastric mucosa.

SYMPTOMS. In the newborn and infant, symptoms are due to pressure on the adjacent lung or tracheobronchial tree, leading to respiratory difficulties, or to pressure on the esophagus, resulting in dysphagia and vomiting. Chest pain may also occur, owing to increased pressure in the cyst or to ulceration. If the duplicated segment communicates with the esophagus, there may be hematemesis secondary to ulceration.

ROENTGENOLOGIC EXAMINATION. Posteroanterior and lateral chest roentgenograms disclose a mass in the posterior mediastinum with encroachment on the adjacent lung (Figs. 6–22 and 6–23). The most common location is the right side, and the mass may occupy most or all of the hemithorax with displacement of mediastinal structures to the opposite side.

Barium studies show the esophagus to be displaced to the side opposite the mass and usually anteriorly. In the occasional case with communication with the esophagus some of the contrast material may enter the duplicated segment. However, even in the rare communicating type, the orifice may be so minute as not to afford entrance of the contrast material. The lateral border of the mass is usually sharply defined against aerated lung and may extend the entire length of the mediastinum. The majority of patients have associated anomalies of the thoracic spine.

DIFFERENTIAL DIAGNOSIS. Any posterior mediastinal mass, including neoplasms arising from the sympathetic chain, anterior meningoceles, hemangiomas, pulmonary sequestrations, pericardial cysts, and even aneurysms of the descending aorta, should

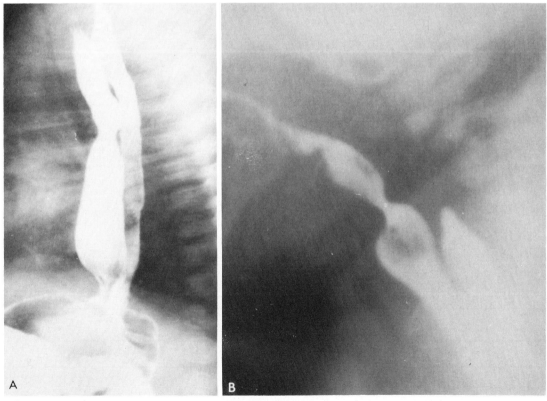

Figure 6–24. Infant with complete esophageal duplication presenting with recurrent vomiting and pulmonary infection. *A*, Lateral view of the chest showing complete duplication of the esophagus. Barium readily fills the normal esophagus and stomach. There is subsequent regurgitation into the posteriorly placed duplication which apparently fills from the gastric cardia. *B*, Film of the nasopharyngeal area demonstrates passage into the normal anteriorly placed esophagus and subsequent filling of the duplication which ends blindly in the neck. (Courtesy of Dr. L. Swischuk.)

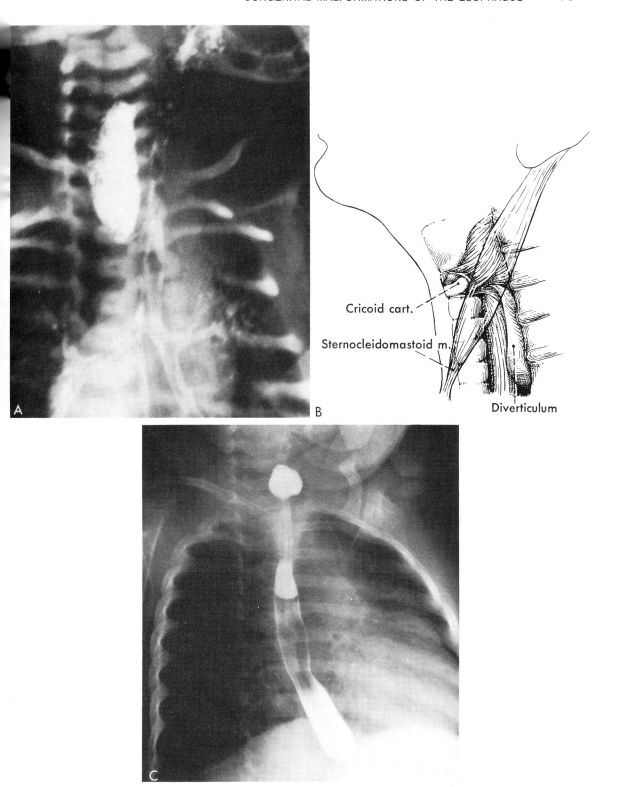

Cricoid cart.

Sternocleidomastoid m.

Diverticulum

Figure 6-25. Congenital diverticulum of the hypopharynx in a newborn. *A*, Contrast material in diverticulum simulating esophageal atresia. *B*, Drawing of diverticulum as found at surgery. (Courtesy of Dr. E. S. Brintnall, Iowa State University.) *C*, 2-year-old with small diverticulum of cervical esophagus.

be included in the list of differential possibilities. Investigative procedures, including angiography, myelography, and bronchography, may be helpful in excluding these conditions, but in most instances a definite diagnosis of esophageal duplication is made only after thoracotomy and surgical excision.

Complete duplication of the esophagus is an extremely rare malformation and is often associated with gastric duplication. Visualization of the duplicated segment depends upon communication with the normal esophagus or stomach, and complete esophageal duplication may not be appreciated until after surgical treatment for the gastric component.

The complete, tubular form of esophageal duplication is often not recognized on plain radiography nor does there appear to be a high incidence of associated vertebral body abnormalities (Fig. 6–24). This feature might further suggest more than one etiology of esophageal duplication.

PHARYNGEAL DIVERTICULUM

Congenital diverticulum of the hypopharynx is extremely rare, but because of its intimate association with the esophagus, it is considered here. This type of diverticulum is similar in appearance to Zenker's pulsion diverticulum seen in adults (Fig. 6–25). A cephalic diverticulum is an extremely rare lesion with extension of the esophagus superior and posterior to the hypopharynx (Fig. 6–26).

The majority of esophageal diverticula in the newborn are secondary to trauma and are discussed in the next chapter. Differentiation as to etiology may be difficult. The

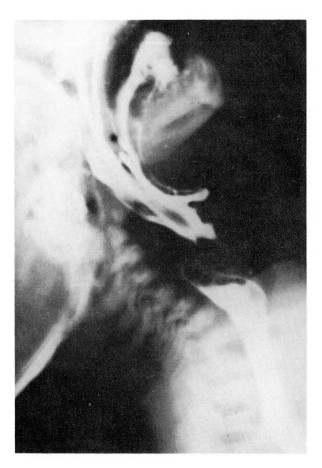

Figure 6–26. Cephalic diverticulum of the esophagus. There is communication of the hypopharynx with the cervical portion of the esophagus but there is abnormal extension of the proximal portion of the esophagus into the retropharyngeal space. Pharyngonasal reflux is also pronounced. (From Singleton, E. B.: The gastrointestinal tract in children. *In* Margulis, A. R., and Burhenne, H. J. (eds.): Alimentary Tract Roentgenology. 2nd ed. St. Louis: C. V. Mosby Co., 1973; courtesy of Dr. John Fawcitt.)

true congenital type contains a muscular wall and a lining of stratified epithelium.

The embryological fault leading to development of a congenital diverticulum is perhaps similar to that of duplications. However, the absence of adherence of the body of the diverticulum to the adjacent alimentary tube does not entirely support this assumption. According to Bremer, diverticula develop as buds from the epithelial lining of the gut and extend through the bundles of the inner circular muscle beyond the boundaries of the gut wall. Extension of the cyst within the submucosa will lead to encroachment on the patent lumen and will ultimately cause obstruction.

SYMPTOMS. The severity of symptoms depends upon the size of the pouch. There are regurgitation of saliva and food from the diverticulum, and dysphagia due to pressure on the adjacent esophagus. These lesions are usually mistaken for esophageal atresias.

ROENTGENOLOGIC EXAMINATION. Lateral views of the infant's neck may show a soft tissue mass in the retropharyngeal area displacing the trachea and larynx anteriorly. With the child in a supine position on the fluoroscopy table, a swallow of contrast material will fill the diverticulum, which in turn will be clearly identified when the patient is turned to a lateral position.

COMPRESSION BY VASCULAR MALFORMATIONS

Compression and displacement of the esophagus as a result of anomalous development of the aorta and its branches are not uncommon in the pediatric patient. A detailed discussion of the complex variety of these anomalies has been given by many authors. Only the more common anomalies and their relation to the esophagus are included here.

The most serious of these defects is the *double aortic arch*, which consists of an anterior and a posterior arch encircling the trachea and esophagus in a tight ring, the double arches joining to form a common descending aorta (Fig. 6–27). Infants with this anomaly have, as a rule, severe respiratory symptoms and some swallowing difficulty. Dysphagia produced by vascular anomalies is occasionally referred to as dysphagia lusoria. Pulmonary infection is common, and chest roentgenograms usually show some degree of obstructive emphysema. Fluoroscopy with barium in the esophagus discloses a horizontal defect on the posterior wall of the esophagus at the level of the third or fourth thoracic vertebra. This defect is formed by the posterior arch, usually the larger of the two, as it passes behind the esophagus. Aortic pulsa-

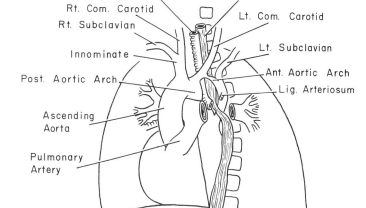

Figure 6–27. Diagram of double aortic arch.

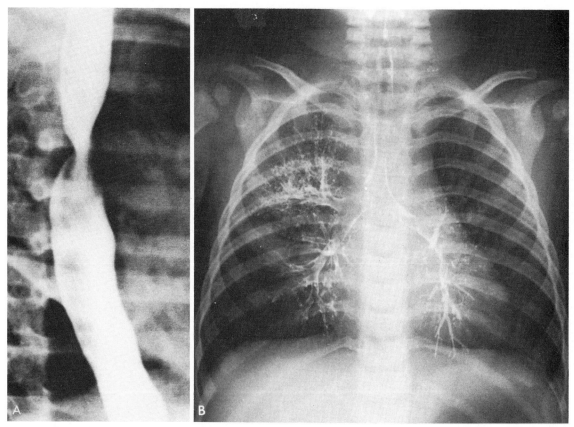

Figure 6-28. Double aortic arch. *A,* Oblique view of the esophagus showing compression defects on anterior and posterior walls. *B,* Tracheogram, showing similar constrictive defects on trachea.

tions are visibly transmitted to the esophagus at the site of compression. Tracheal compression is usually evident on lateral chest films, but at times tracheograms aid in confirming the diagnosis by demonstrating the indentation on the anterior and right lateral portion of the trachea (Fig. 6-28).

A *right aortic arch with a left descending aorta* and ligamentum arteriosum in another type of vascular ring, producing symptoms similar to those of a double aortic arch. The right aortic arch may be identified, or at least suspected, on posteroanterior roentgenograms of the chest by the soft tissue prominence in the right superior mediastinum and by displacement of the trachea to the left. After ingestion of contrast material, the right aortic arch is identified by the indentation it makes on the right lateral wall of the esophagus. The ligamentum arteriosum is attached between the pulmonary artery and the base of

the left subclavian artery and is identified by its impression on the anterolateral wall of the esophagus (Fig. 6-29). Once again, tracheograms are of help in establishing the presence of the true ring.

An *aortic diverticulum with right aortic arch* may produce deformity of the esophagus similar to a right aortic arch which descends on the left. The diverticulum usually gives rise to the left subclavian artery and therefore is believed to result from traction by the ligamentum arteriosum on the base of the subclavian artery at its origin from the aortic arch. Another theory is that there is failure of complete obliteration of the embryologic anterior arch, to unobliterated segment persisting as a dilatation or diverticulum. Angiocardiograms or retrograde aortograms are necessary to identify this type of abnormality (Fig. 6-30).

A *right aortic arch without a ring* produces a characteristic indentation on the esophagus (Fig. 6-31). The abnormal

Text continued on page 81

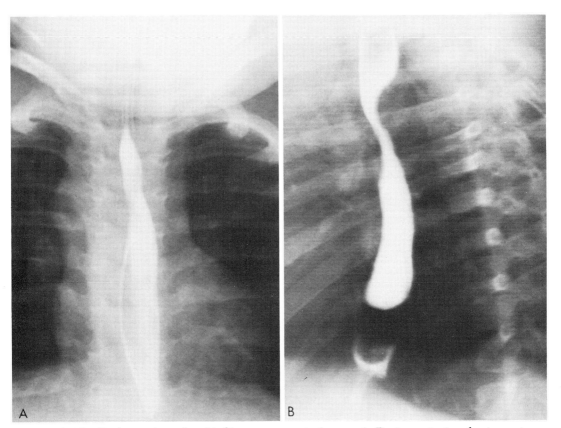

Figure 6-29. Right aortic arch with ligamentum arteriosum. *A,* Posteroanterior chest roentgeno-gram, showing fullness in right superior mediastinum with compression on right lateral wall of esophagus by right arch. *B,* Lateral view showing defect in posterior wall of esophagus by posterior arch. Operation disclosed a right arch with left descending aorta and ligamentum arteriosum.

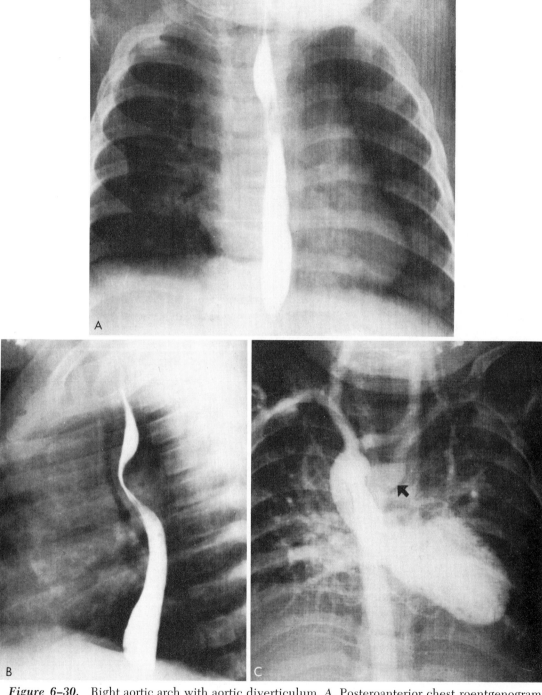

Figure 6–30. Right aortic arch with aortic diverticulum. *A,* Posteroanterior chest roentgenogram, showing compression of right wall of esophagus by right aortic arch. *B,* Lateral view, showing anterior displacement of esophagus simulating defect found with a right aortic arch which passes posterior to the esophagus to descend on the left. *C,* Angiocardiogram, showing descending aorta on right and esophageal defect to be due to an aortic diverticulum (arrow). (Courtesy of Dr. M. Figley.)

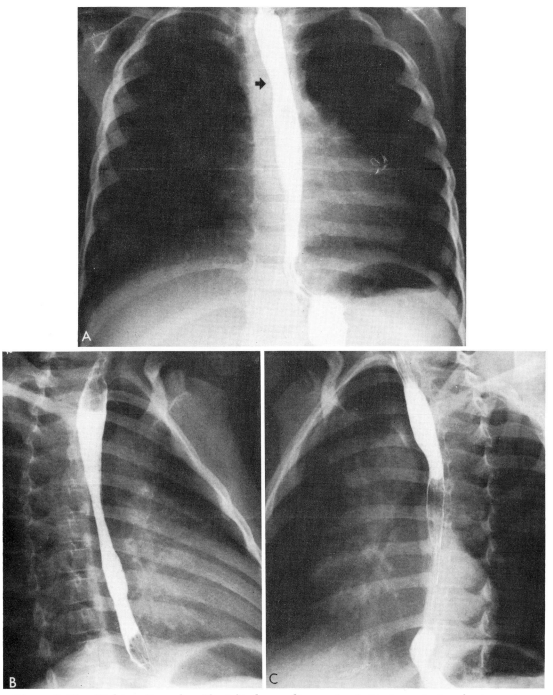

Figure 6-31. Right aortic arch with right descending aorta. *A,* Posteroanterior chest roentgenogram, showing fullness in right superior mediastinum and compression on right lateral wall of esophagus (arrow). *B,* Right anterior oblique view, showing no evidence of compression on anterior esophageal wall, usually seen with left arch. *C,* Left anterior oblique view, showing indentation on anterior esophageal wall by right aortic arch.

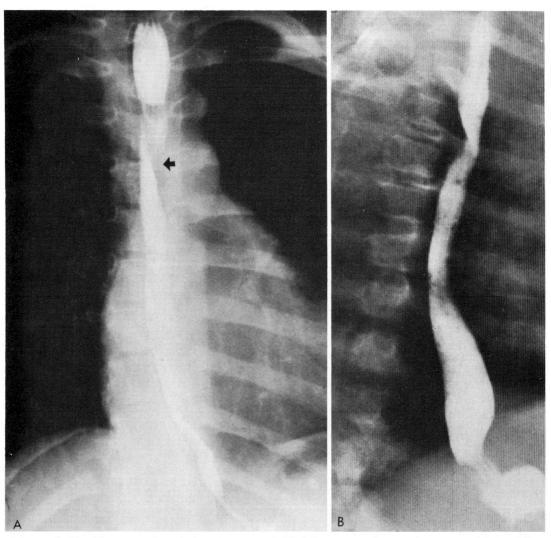

Figure 6–32. Ectopic right subclavian artery. *A*, With barium in the esophagus, an oblique filling defect is identified passing cephalad from left to right (arrow). *B*, Lateral view, showing defect to the posterior to the esophagus.

location of the arch may be suspected on posteroanterior chest films from absence of the normal prominence of the aortic knob and fullness in the right paratracheal region due to displacement of the superior vena cava and adjacent structures. With barium in the esophagus, instead of the indentation on the left anterior wall of the esophagus produced by a normal left arch, there is an indentation on the opposite side. If the aorta crosses behind the esophagus at this level to descend on the left, anterior displacement of the esophagus will be evident, but more often the aorta crosses to the left at a lower level.

The most common of the aortic arch anomalies is an *aberrant subclavian artery,* which arises from the left side of the aortic arch and then passes behind the esophagus to its normal position, producing a characteristic and actually pathognomonic indentation on the esophagus. As is the case with other arch anomalies, the abnormality is seen to best advantage during fluoroscopy after a swallow of contrast material. The aberrant artery makes an oblique filling defect passing posterior to the esophagus and extending from left to right (Fig. 6–32). Occasionally the vessel passes anterior to the esophagus, in which case the filling defect involves the anterior rather than the posterior esophageal wall. This condition rarely causes symptoms, except for occasional mild dysphagia.

Coarctation of the aorta when the coarctation is just distal to the left subclavian artery produces a characteristic indentation on the esophagus as a result of the poststenotic dilatation (Fig. 6–33). The dilatation displaces the esophagus to the right and anteriorly below the level of the aortic arch. This sign is the earliest and most reliable radiologic evidence of this type of abnormality.

Left pulmonary artery sling anomaly is another vascular defect which may be responsible for respiratory disturbances or recurrent pneumonia, and may also produce

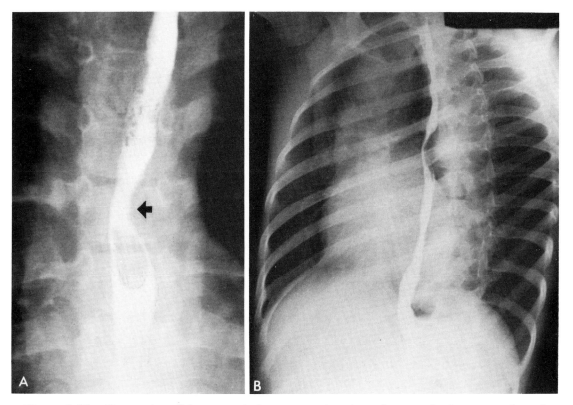

Figure 6–33. Coarctation of the aorta. *A,* Anteroposterior view, showing displacement of esophagus to right below level of aortic arch (arrow). *B,* Lateral view, showing characteristic anterior displacement of esophagus by poststenotic dilatation of the aorta.

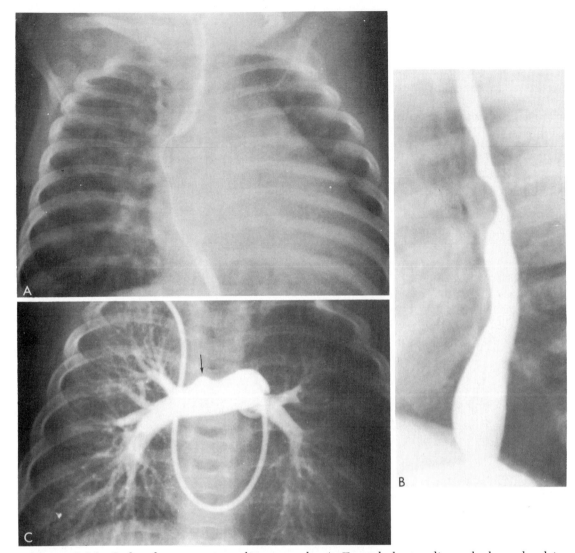

Figure 6–34. Left pulmonary artery sling anomaly. *A,* Frontal chest radiograph shows local indentation upon the left side of the barium column. *B,* Lateral radiograph shows anterior indentation of the esophagus by the aberrant left pulmonary artery. *C,* Angiocardiogram shows ectopic origin of the left pulmonary artery (arrow). (Reprinted from *Radiologic Atlas of Pulmonary Abnormalities in Children* [Philadelphia: W. B. Saunders Co., 1971].)

a pressure defect upon the esophagus. In this condition the left pulmonary artery passes over the right bronchus, behind the trachea and in front of the esophagus, thereby depressing and compressing the right main stem bronchus and the adjacent anterior wall of the esophagus. Routine films may show an increased distance between the esophagus and tracheal air column, and the right lung is frequently overinflated as a result of partial obstruction by the ectopic left pulmonary artery

(Fig. 6–34). Angiocardiography will accurately demonstrate the lesion.

REFERENCES

Esophageal Atresia and Tracheoesophageal Fistula

Felman, A. H., and Talbert, J. L. Laryngotracheo-
   esophageal cleft, *Radiology, 103*:641, 1972.
Griscom, N. T. Persistent esophagotrachea; the most
   severe degree of laryngotracheo-esophageal cleft,

Am. J. Roentgenol., Radium Ther. Nucl. Med., 97:211, 1966.

Gwinn, J. L. Tracheo-esophageal fistula with and without esophageal atresia—special aspects, *Progr. Pediatr. Radiol.*, 2:170, 1969.

Haight, C., and Towsley, H. A. Congenital atresia of the esophagus with tracheoesophageal fistula, extrapleural ligation of fistula and end-to-end anastomosis of esophageal segment, *Surg. Gynecol. Obstet.*, 76:672, 1943.

Holt, J. F., et al. Congenital atresia of esophagus and tracheo-esophageal fistula, *Radiology*, 47:457, 1946.

Kirkpatrick, J. A., Cresson, S. L., and Pilling, G. P. The motor activity of the esophagus in association with esophageal atresia and tracheoesophageal fistula, *Am. J. Roentgenol., Radium Ther. Nucl. Med.*, 86:884, 1961.

Kirkpatrick, J. A., Wagner, M. L., and Pilling, G. P. A complex of anomalies associated with tracheo-esophageal fistula and esophageal atresia, *Am. J. Roentgenol., Radium Ther. Nucl. Med.*, 95:208, 1965.

Ladd, W. E. Surgical treatment of esophageal atresia and tracheoesophageal fistula, *N. Engl. J. Med.*, 230:625, 1944.

Leven, N. L. Congenital atresia of the esophagus with tracheoesophageal fistula: report of surgical extrapleural ligation of fistulous communication and cervical esophagostomy, *J. Thorac. Cardiovasc. Surg.*, 10:648, 1941.

Neuhauser, E. B. D., and Griscom, N. T. Aspiration pneumonitis in children, *Progr. Pediatr. Radiol.*, 1:265, 1967.

Singleton, A. O., and Knight, M. D. Congenital atresia of esophagus, with tracheo-esophageal fistulae: Transpleural operative approach, *Ann. Surg.*, 119:556, 1944.

Swischuk, L. E. Demonstration of the distal esophageal pouch in esophageal atresia without fistula, *Am. J. Roentgenol., Radium Ther. Nucl. Med.*, 103:277, 1968.

Vogt, E. C. Congenital esophageal atresia, *Am. J. Roentgenol. Radium Ther. Nucl. Med.*, 22:463, 1929.

Stenosis

Greenough, W. G. Congenital esophageal strictures, *Am. J. Roentgenol., Radium Ther. Nucl. Med.*, 92:994, 1964.

Lister, J. Blood supply of the oesophagus in relation to the oesophageal atresia, *Arch. Dis. Child.*, 39:131, 1964.

Esophageal Bronchus

Gerle, R. D., Jaretzki, A., Ashley, C. A., and Berne, A. S. Congenital bronchopulmonary-foregut malformation: pulmonary sequestration communicating with the gastrointestinal tract. *N. Engl. J. Med.*, 278:1413, 1968.

Lane, S. D., Burko, H., and Scott, H. W. Congenital bronchopulmonary-foregut malformation, *Radiology*, 101:291, 1971.

Duplications (Neurenteric Cysts)

Abrami, G., and Dennison, W. N. Duplication of the stomach, *Surgery*, 49:794, 1961.

Bremer, J. L. Diverticula and duplications of the intestinal tract, *Arch. Pathol.*, 38:132, 1944.

Gross, R. E., Holcomb, G. W., Jr., and Farber, F. Duplications of the alimentary tract, *Pediatrics*, 9:449, 1952.

Moir, J. D. Combined duplication of the esophagus and stomach, *J. Can. Assoc. Radiol.*, 21:257, 1970.

Neuhauser, E. B. D., Harris, G. B. C., and Derrett, A. Roentgenographic features of neurenteric cysts, *Am. J. Roentgenol., Radium Ther. Nucl. Med.*, 79:235, 1958.

Veeneklaas, G. M. Pathogenesis of intrathoracic cysts, *Am. J. Dis. Child.*, 83:500, 1950.

Pharyngeal Diverticulum

Bremer, J. L. *Congenital Anomalies of the Viscera: The Embryological Basis* (Cambridge, Mass.: Harvard University Press, 1957).

Brintnall, E. S., and Kridelbaugh, W. W. Congenital diverticulum of posterior hypopharynx simulating atresia of esophagus, *Ann. Surg.*, 131:564, 1950.

MacKellar, A., and Kennedy, J. C. Congenital diverticulum of the pharynx simulating esophageal atresia, *J. Pediatr. Surg.*, 7:408, 1972.

Compression By Vascular Malformations

Berdon, W. E., and Baker, D. H. Vascular anomalies in the infant lung: rings, slings, and other things, *Semin. Roentgenol.*, 7:39, 1972.

Capitanio, M. A., Ramos, R., and Kirkpatrick, J. A. Pulmonary sling; roentgen observations, *Am. J. Roentgenol., Radium Ther. Nucl. Med.*, 112:28, 1971.

Gross, R. E., and Neuhauser, E. B. D. Compression of trachea on esophagus by vascular anomalies: surgical therapy in 40 cases, *Pediatrics*, 7:69, 1951.

Klinkahmer, A. C. *Esophagography in Anomalies of the Aortic Arch System* (Amsterdam: Excerpta Medica Foundation, Williams and Wilkins, 1969).

Neuhauser, E. B. D. Roentgen diagnosis of double aortic arch and other anomalies of great vessels, *Am. J. Roentgenol., Radium Ther. Nucl. Med.*, 56:1, 1946.

Stewart, J. R., Kincaid, O. W., and Edwards, J. E. *An Atlas of Vascular Rings And Related Malformations of the Aortic Arch System* (Springfield, Ill.: Charles C Thomas, 1964).

Chapter 7

ACQUIRED LESIONS OF THE ESOPHAGUS

ESOPHAGITIS AND STRICTURE

Esophageal stricture may be either congenital or acquired. The congenital type and those secondary to reflux esophagitis have been described in Chapter 5. Strictures in older infants and children result from the ingestion of caustics, surgery on the esophagus, or opportunistic infections in chronically ill children.

One of the more unusual causes of esophageal stricture is epidermolysis bullosa dystrophica (Pasini's syndrome). This is an inherited condition whereby minor trauma to skin and subcutaneous tissues causes detachment of the dermis from the epidermis, with eventual production of bullae, ulceration, and scar formation. Involvement of the extremities often produces severe flexion contracture deformities, while esophageal defects result in varied degrees of stricture.

Ingestion of Caustics

The ingestion of a caustic substance, usually strong, alkaline cleaning materials, is the most common cause of esophageal stricture in the pediatric patient. The concentrated alkali produces extensive damage to the mucosa of the mouth, pharynx, and esophagus, the damage to the mouth being as a rule superficial in that contact of the irritant in this region is less prolonged than in the esophagus. The mucosal and submucosal layers of the esophagus are edematous, congested, and show localized areas of ulceration. This is followed by sloughing and denudation of the involved segments and necrosis of portions of the muscularis. The resulting cicatricial changes lead to severe strictures. The stomach is seldom significantly involved, due to the neutralizing effect of the gastric acid. However, in poisoning with concentrated acids, involvement of the stomach is often severe and surpasses the degree of damage to the esophagus. Antral or pyloric stenosis may result in such cases.

ROENTGENOLOGIC FINDINGS. After the mouth lesions have subsided so that the child is able to swallow without too much discomfort, he is placed in the supine position on the fluoroscopy table and given a swallow of flavored barium. The material is then observed as it passes down the esophagus, and spot films are obtained. With the patient turned partially onto his left side the esophagus is freed from the image of the vertebral column and is seen to better advantage. In the early stages of the condition, small areas of ulceration may be observed, and there may be marked narrowing of the esophageal lumen as a result of spasm and edema. The areas of constriction may involve any level of the esophagus or the entire structure.

The ends of the involved segments are usually tapered, the transition from involved to normal esophagus being gradual. After the acute stage has passed the areas of previous stenosis often show an increase in the width of the lumen, indicating relaxation of the spasm. In other areas which originally appeared less seriously involved, severe cicatricial changes may develop. Prediction of the extent and degree of stricture is impossible in the acute stage. Only by frequent follow-up examinations can the permanent changes be estimated accurately (Figs. 7–1 and 7–2).

Treatment of severe strictures by dilatation is frequently disappointing and the clinical and radiologic improvement only temporary. Consequently, the current treatment of choice is replacement of the damaged esophagus by a segment of the colon, usually the transverse portion, which is

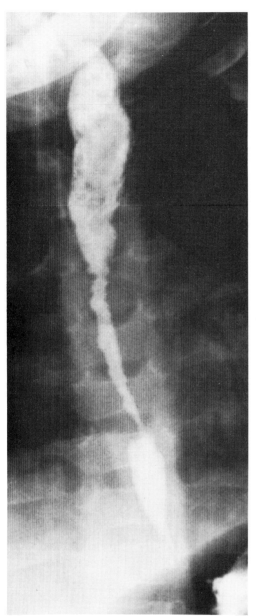

Figure 7-1. Lye stricture. Esophagram made 7 days after ingestion of lye, showing constriction of midportion of the esophagus, and irregularity of esophageal wall secondary to edema and multiple ulcerations.

anastomosed to the proximal esophagus and the stomach. Postoperative chest radiographs of these patients are frequently interesting in demonstrating widening of the mediastinum and air in the intrathoracic colon conduit. Barium studies are also of interest and helpful in postoperative evaluation (Fig. 7-3).

Fluoroscopically, after the barium is swallowed, the esophageal-colic anastomosis is easily identified by a slight constriction, as well as by the anatomic differences of the two structures. Contrast material passes into the stomach by gravity, colonic peristalsis being inactive and consisting mainly of infrequent, segmental contractions rather than peristaltic waves. Foreign materials and ingested food, especially pieces of meat, may become lodged at the anastomotic site and are easily identified by esophagrams. A unique complication is the growth of a juvenile polyp in the colon transplant.

Reflux Esophagitis

Reflux esophagitis is secondary to incompetence of the gastroesophageal junction (chalasia) and may be associated with hiatal hernia. In severe cases chronic esophagitis with subsequent cicatricial changes results in retraction of the cardia into the chest (Fig. 7-4). Reflux esophagitis may also be a postoperative complication of surgical repair of esophageal atresia, particularly if the anastomosis requires upward traction of the lower esophageal segment (Fig. 7-5). Aberrant gastric mucosa in the lower esophagus may produce similar changes. These conditions have been described in Chapter 5.

Ulceration Without Apparent Cause

Acute esophageal ulceration without obvious cause is occasionally found as an unsuspected lesion on postmortem examination of newborn infants. Any young infant who has hematemesis should be suspected of having esophagitis with ulceration. This type of ulceration is seldom deep enough to be identified roentgenologically, but other signs of esophagitis, such as spasm and constriction, are often present. Rarely, however, the ulcer may be large enough to be identified (Fig. 7-6). The pathogenesis in such cases is probably vascular insufficiency produced by the "dive reflex," and may occur in any stress situation accompanying such conditions as brain damage, subdural hematoma, meningitis, and encephalitis.

Spontaneous esophageal rupture in the newborn (Boerhaave's syndrome) is a rare

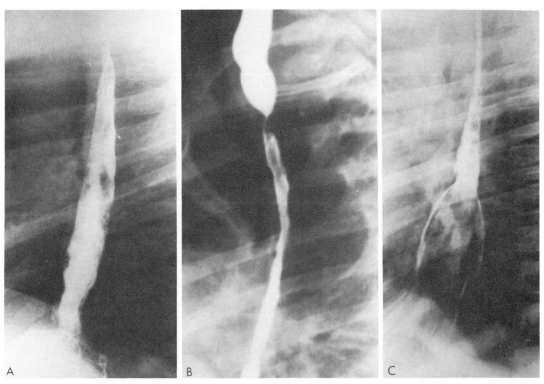

Figure 7–2. Ingestion of Drano in 2-year-old child. *A,* Initial esophagram made several hours after ingestion of the caustic shows ill-defined mucosa probably due to edema and mucus. *B,* Repeat esophagram 3 weeks later shows constriction of the thoracic portion of the esophagus with more severe stricture in the proximal portion and dilatation of the cervical esophagus. *C,* Repeat esophagram 3 months later shows esophageal stricture with retraction of the gastric cardia into the chest.

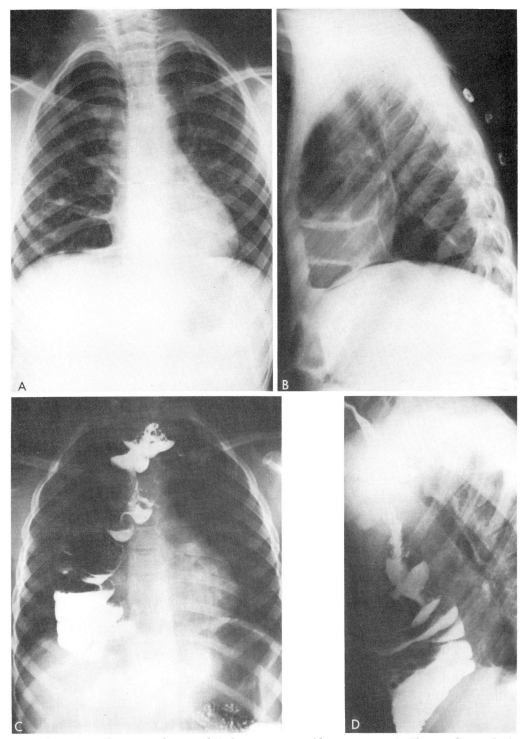

Figure 7–3. Intrathoracic colon conduit for treatment of lye stricture. *A,* Chest radiograph shows air in the interposed colon. *B,* Lateral view showing the usual anterior position of the conduit. *C* and *D,* Barium swallow shows the position of the colon extending between the cervical esophagus and the stomach.

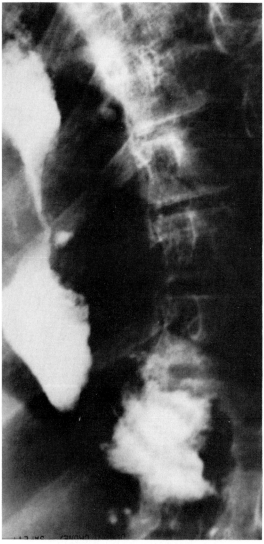

Figure 7–4. Sixteen year old boy with cerebral palsy. Barium esophagram demonstrated a large hiatal hernia with reflux esophagitis and stenosis of the distal esophagus. A large lower esophageal ulcer can be seen.

lesion that is clinically manifested mainly as respiratory distress. The radiographic features include tension pneumothorax or hydropneumothorax, usually on the right, and occasionally pneumomediastinum. Examination of the esophagus often demonstrates an irregular tortuous tract arising from the perforated lower esophagus and extending to the pleural space. The cause is uncertain, but this condition may well be secondary to anoxia similar to necrotizing enterocolitis.

Alimentary tract bleeding may occur in infants with consumptive coagulopathy, a condition in which there is inappropriate intravascular clotting due to a variety of causes. The radiologic identification of the bleeding points is not possible.

Infectious Esophagitis

Esophagitis due to thrush (monilia esophagitis) is usually seen in infants with immunologic deficiencies who have been on prolonged antibiotic therapy or in children with leukemia (Figs. 7–7 and 7–8). The entire esophagus is often affected. Ordinary thrush affecting the mouth, pharynx and esophagus of otherwise normal infants rarely produces radiologic changes. Older children on prolonged antibiotic therapy may develop similar esophagitis (Fig. 7–9).

FOREIGN BODIES

There are three sites in the normal esophagus where foreign bodies usually lodge. The most common is the cervical segment, the narrowest portion of the esophagus, just above the thoracic inlet. Other sites of lodgment are the level of the left main stem bronchus where it impinges on the esophagus, and the inferior portion of the esophagus above the diaphragmatic hiatus. Metallic coins are the objects most often swallowed. They pass down the esophagus with the broad plane parallel to the anterior and posterior surfaces of the body (Fig. 7–10), in contradistinction to foreign bodies in the trachea, which are seen on edge in the frontal plane. Occasionally an ingested coin may lodge in a position suggesting it is in the trachea (Fig. 7–11). Lateral views of the chest frequently show that more than one coin has been swallowed, and consequently this view should always be obtained (Fig. 7–12). Radiolucent objects are naturally more difficult to see, but by careful fluoroscopic studies may appear as radiolucent defects surrounded by swallowed barium (Fig. 7–13).

Although a general anesthesia and removal of the coin by esophagoscopy is the accepted treatment, we have successfully accomplished this fluoroscopically by passing a small Foley catheter beyond the object,

Text continued on page 92

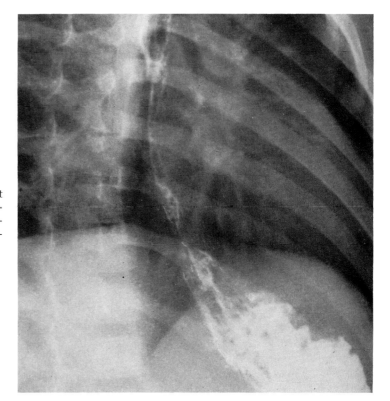

Figure 7–5. 1-year-old infant with gastroesophageal incompetence and hiatus hernia secondary to previous repair of esophageal atresia.

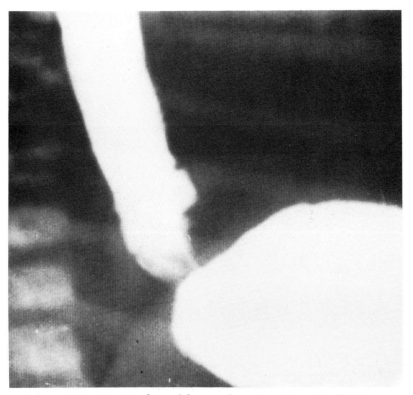

Figure 7–6. Anoxic ulcer of the esophagus in a 1-week-old infant.

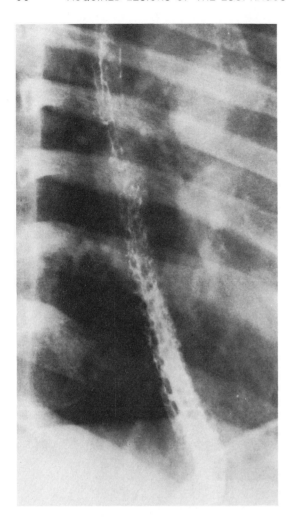

Figure 7–7. Monilia esophagitis in boy aged 11 with advanced lymphosarcoma. Esophagram shows multiple serrated ulcerations and granulomatous areas involving the entire esophagus.

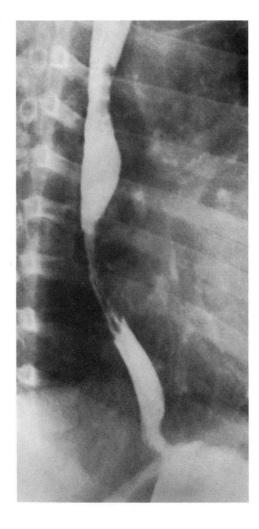

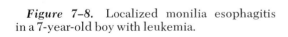

Figure 7–8. Localized monilia esophagitis in a 7-year-old boy with leukemia.

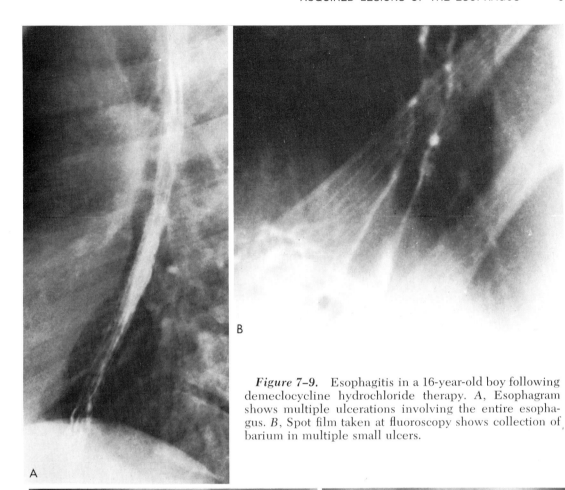

Figure 7–9. Esophagitis in a 16-year-old boy following demeclocycline hydrochloride therapy. *A*, Esophagram shows multiple ulcerations involving the entire esophagus. *B*, Spot film taken at fluoroscopy shows collection of barium in multiple small ulcers.

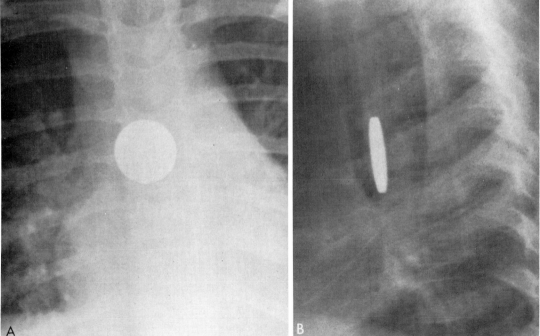

Figure 7–10. Penny lies at level of main stem bronchus. *A*, Anteroposterior and *B*, lateral views.

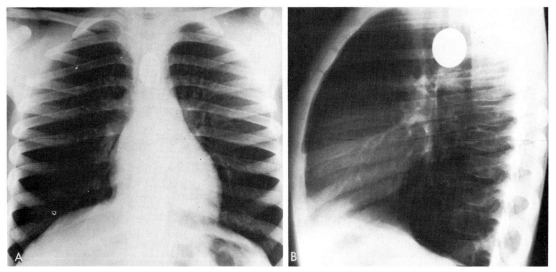

Figure 7–11. Metallic coin lies in the esophagus at the level of the aortic arch. *A*, Frontal projection shows the coin on edge. *B*, Lateral view shows its flat surface, a position opposite that usually seen of coins in the esophagus.

inflating the bag with opaque material and, with the patient prone, withdrawing the catheter and the coin into the pharynx where it is either removed or coughed out (Fig. 7–14). In such cases it is advisable to have an experienced laryngoscopist on hand in case the coin is aspirated into the trachea.

Any other type of object capable of being swallowed may be lodged in the esophagus

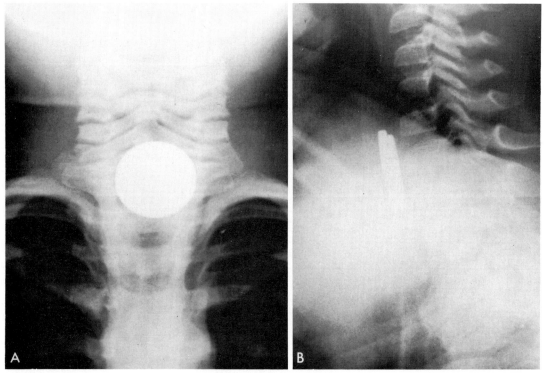

Figure 7–12. Two coins lodged in the esophagus at thoracic inlet. *A*, In anteroposterior position only one coin is visible. *B*, In lateral view two coins are identified.

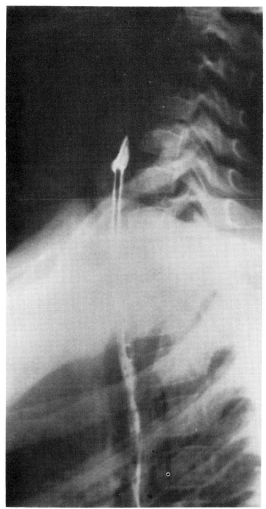

Figure 7–13. Lateral view of the esophagus following barium shows a plastic disc in the esophagus at the thoracic inlet.

at the aforementioned sites (Figs. 7–15 and 7–16). Sharp-pointed objects such as pins and tacks, may perforate the esophageal wall, leading to esophagitis and even mediastinitis. Foreign bodies may go unrecognized and eventually erode the esophageal wall. Posterior erosion results in a retropharyngeal or retroesophageal abscess, and erosion anteriorly may produce tracheoesophageal fistula (Figs. 7–17 and 7–18). As a rule most objects pass into the stomach satisfactorily following ingestion of food. However, it is frequently necessary to remove open safety pins by esophagoscopy. If the safety pin lies in the esophagus with the open end directed caudally, it probably had passed into the stomach and been regurgitated into the esophagus.

The utilization of a small magnet within a catheter to remove a foreign body is now rarely possible because of the nonmagnetic properties of present-day metallic objects.

Nonopaque foreign bodies cannot be directly identified by radiologic means but they may be identified in the esophagus by inducing the child to swallow a pledget of cotton impregnated with barium. The small cotton bolus will frequently become lodged at the site of the foreign body. After surgical repair of esophageal atresia or cicatricial changes that follow ingestion of caustic substances, foreign bodies frequently become lodged at the point of stricture, and in such cases esophagoscopy is usually required for removal (Fig. 7–19). Occasionally congenital esophageal stenosis is not detected until a foreign body is ingested, at which time attention is directed to the stenotic segment.

Stenosis is a common sequel of surgical procedures on the esophagus. It consists of a narrow segment of constriction of varying degree and configuration. The alignment is frequently altered, especially if fistula develops during the postoperative course. The history of the previous surgery serves to differentiate this type of stricture from other forms. Mediastinitis complicating surgical procedures on the esophagus or trachea may produce tracheoesophageal fistula.

TRAUMA

In the newborn traumatic perforation of the pharynx or esophagus produced by a nasogastric tube, suction equipment, or the obstetrician's finger in the infant's mouth at the time of delivery (Smellie-Veit maneuver) may produce radiographic findings simulating a diverticulum. The symptoms are usually those of esophageal atresia and the passage of a nasogastric tube may enter the perforation and extend blindly into the retroesophageal space, giving the erroneous impression of esophageal atresia (Fig. 7–20). Spasm of the cricopharyngeal muscle may theoretically be associated with the original perforation as well as with the passage of the catheter through the site of injury. Retropharyngeal abscess and mediastinitis frequently follow traumatic perforations of the posterior pharynx or upper esophagus (Figs. 7–21 and 7–22).

Text continued on page 97.

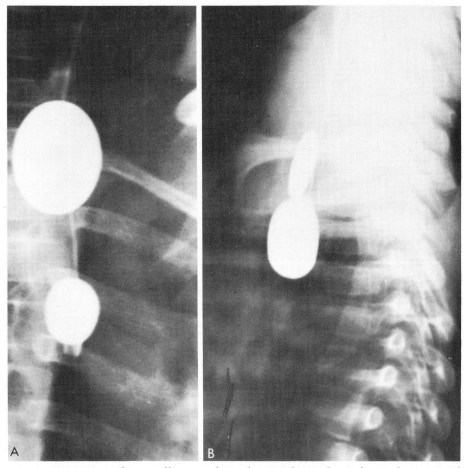

Figure 7–14. Extraction of a metallic coin from the esophagus by Foley catheter. *A,* The Foley catheter has been passed distal to the metallic coin and partially inflated with opaque contrast medium. *B,* The catheter has been withdrawn and has made contact with the inferior surface of the coin prior to complete extraction.

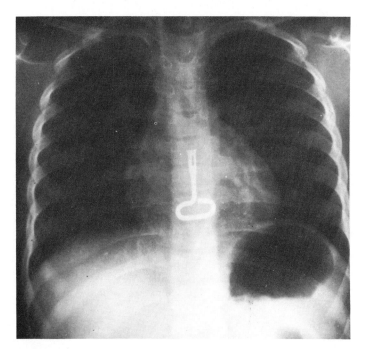

Figure 7–15. 3-year-old child who swallowed a can opener key which lodged in the lower esophagus.

Figure 7–16. A lateral chest roentgenogram of an infant who swallowed the clip part of a link chain. The slit in this type of object commonly catches in the esophageal mucosa and, in spite of its small size, is frequently difficult to dislodge.

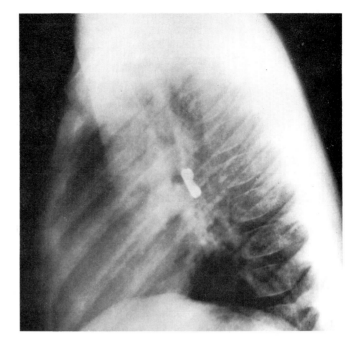

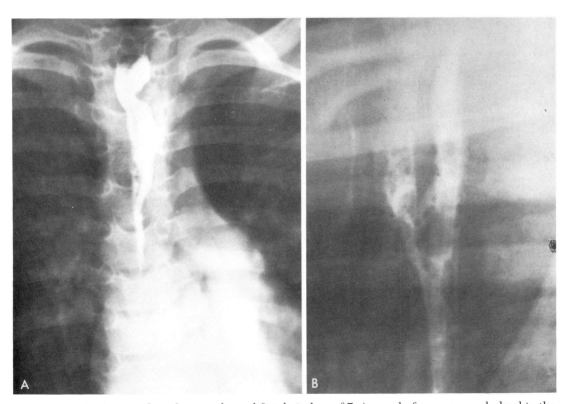

Figure 7–17. Acquired tracheoesophageal fistula in boy of 7. A year before, a penny lodged in the trachea for an unknown period and had been removed by tracheostomy. *A,* Chest roentgenogram with contrast material in esophagus, showing cicatricial change in esophagus, presumably due to mediastinitis. *B,* Spot film with patient in Trendelenburg position, showing tracheoesophageal fistula.

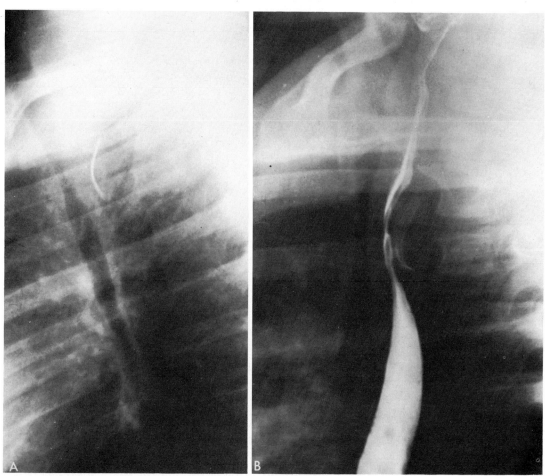

Figure 7–18. 2-year-old infant with history of dysphagia and coughing for several weeks. *A,* Chest radiograph shows curved metallic object posterior to the trachea below the thoracic inlet. There is constriction of the tracheal air column at this level. *B,* Esophagram shows inflammatory stricture of the esophagus with the lower portion of the thin metallic foreign body projecting posterior to the esophageal lumen. The object was found at thoracotomy to be a beer can pull tab opener.

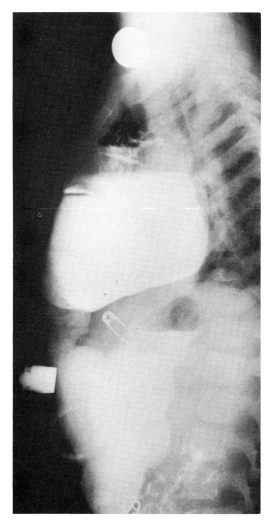

Figure 7–19. Penny lodged at the site of esophagocolic anastomosis following replacement of esophagus by colon conduit for treatment of lye stricture.

ACQUIRED DIVERTICULA

Acquired diverticula of the esophagus are uncommon in pediatric patients, although two types are occasionally seen, the pulsion diverticulum which occurs in the superior portion of the esophagus near the region of the cricopharyngeal muscle, and the traction type which is usually located near the carina of the trachea. A third, the congenital type, is described in Chapter 4. Radiologically it is similar in appearance to the pulsion type.

Pulsion or Zenker's diverticulum is much more common in adults but may occur in older children. The lesion is apparently the result of herniation of the mucosa and submucosa through the fibers of the cricopharyngeal muscle. Symptoms are regurgitation of ingested food and, if the diverticulum becomes large, dysphasia and resulting malnutrition.

Lateral roentgenograms of the child's neck may show a gas-distended pouch in the posterolateral portion of the upper esophagus and upright films will, if the diverticulum is large enough, disclose an air-fluid level in this area. The trachea may be displaced forward by the diverticulum, depending upon its size. The diagnosis is apparent after a swallow of contrast material, the medium collecting in the diverticulum and spilling over into the esophagus when filled. In our experience the pulsion diverticulum is usually a complication of chronic obstruction lower in the esophagus or possibly is due to spasm of the cricopharyngeal muscle (Fig. 7–23). However, we have seen it as an isolated lesion (Fig. 6–25).

Traction diverticulum is due to traction on the esophagus by an adjacent inflammatory process, usually granulomatous lymph nodes below the carina. As a result of the traction, all layers of the esophageal wall are included. The diverticulum is generally small and located on the anterior surface of the esophagus. The condition is usually asymptomatic. Esophageal diverticula in the subcarinal area may occur in severe esophagitis. Whether this is due to destruction of the muscularis with herniation of the mucosa through the muscularis or the result of traction by affected adjacent lymph nodes is unknown (Fig. 7–24).

The diverticulum is usually an incidental finding during examination of the upper gastrointestinal tract. As the contrast material passes down the esophagus, the small diverticulum is observed on the anterior wall near the bifurcation of the trachea and may be missed unless the patient is turned to an oblique or lateral position. Occasionally it may be identified only during distention of this portion of the esophagus by the passing bolus, the esophagus appearing perfectly normal in the relaxed contracted state. Rarely, the traction diverticulum is perforated as a result of the adjacent inflammatory process or impaction of a foreign body in the diverticulum.

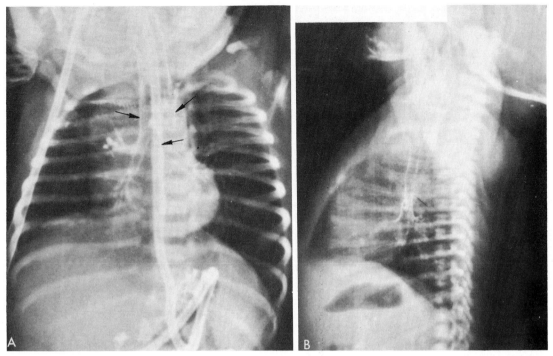

Figure 7–20. Traumatic rupture of the oral pharynx in a newborn. *A*, 1-day-old infant with traumatic pseudodiverticulum of pharynx. Frontal view of chest shows nasogastric tube in esophagus and opaque material outlining the tracheobronchial tree and pseudodiverticulum. *B*, Lateral radiograph of chest of a 1-day-old infant with traumatic pseudodiverticulum of pharynx. Barium is seen to fill the tracheobronchial tree and the posteriorly located pseudodiverticulum. (Courtesy of Dr. Bertram Girdany, Pittsburgh, Pa. Reprinted from the *N. Engl. J. Med.*, **28**:237, 1969.)

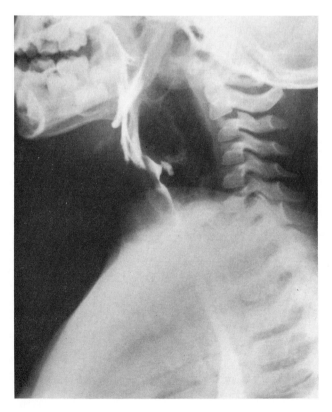

Figure 7–21. Retropharyngeal abscess in child aged 3 years. Pharynx is displaced anteriorly by the abscess, which contains gas. Ingestion of contrast material discloses outline of small perforation above cricopharyngeal muscle.

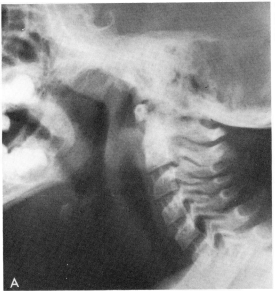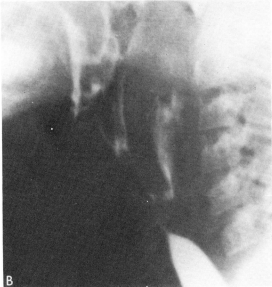

Figure 7–22. Traumatic perforation of the upper esophagus by lollypop stick. *A*, Lateral neck radiograph shows gas within the retropharyngeal and upper retroesophageal space. *B*, Following ingestion of contrast medium the perforation and abscess are opacified.

Transitory Diverticulum

Another form, the transitory type, is similar to the traction diverticulum and may be seen in various portions of the esophagus. Its exact etiology is unknown, but it too is probably a result of traction of adjacent structures on the esophagus and is noted only during distention of the esophagus at the time of passage of contrast material.

ESOPHAGEAL VARICES

Varicosities of the esophagus are nearly always secondary to portal hypertension. In the pediatric patient this is usually due to cirrhosis complicating neonatal hepatitis or omphalitis with resulting portal vein thrombosis. Cirrhosis may also be a complication of pancreatic fibrocystic disease or be associated with renal tubular ectasia. Consequently any child with esophageal varices should have a sweat test and an intravenous pyelogram. Congenital malformations of the portal vein may also produce portal hypertension and esophageal varices. The principal symptoms are recurrent hematemesis, tarry stools, and systemic signs of hemorrhage.

ROENTGENOLOGIC EXAMINATION. The fluoroscopic examination should be carried out with the patient in the recumbent posi-

tion. After the mouthful of barium paste is swallowed, the child is turned slightly to the left in order for the esophagus to clear the spine. In this position the varices are identified as multiple filling defects in the lower end of the esophagus (Fig. 7–25). They are most noticeable after the major portion of the bolus has passed and the esophagus is less distended. The filling defects, which are usually numerous and often vermiform in shape, rarely extend to the cardia of the stomach. However, in advanced cases the cardia may be involved, and extension cephalad may include most of the esophagus. If the child is old enough to cooperate, Valsalva's maneuver may show the varices to best advantage. The Valsalva maneuver may be accomplished involuntarily if the infant is made to cry. Fluoroscopic examination with the child in the prone position with the left side elevated is equally advantageous in examination of the esophagus. Spot films and videotape recordings are invaluable in documenting the fluoroscopic impression. The distortion and enlargement of mucosal folds in the lower esophageal region in cases of gastroesophageal incompetence may simulate the radiographic appearance of varicosities, and one should therefore be very cautious in making a diagnosis of esophageal varices in the infant patient. Percutaneous splenic injection of suitable water-signs of hemorrhage. Celiac and superior mesenteric angiography is now considered a safer and equally adequate diagnostic approach.

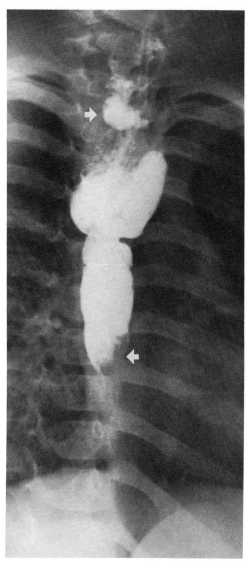

Figure 7–23. Esophagram of infant with old lye stricture at mid- and lower portions of esophagus. An olive pit is lodged at the lower level of the barium column (lower arrow). There is a small pulsion diverticulum in the superior portion of the esophagus (upper arrow).

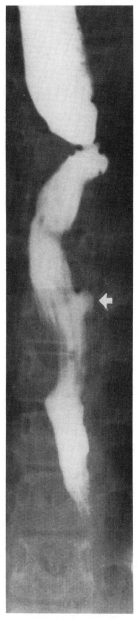

Figure 7–24. Traction diverticulum (arrow). Five months earlier, the tuberculin reaction became positive and a primary Ghon complex was observed to develop. Contriction at the superior portion of the esophagus is secondary to surgical repair of esophageal atresia. (Courtesy of Dr. J. F. Holt, Univ. of Michigan.)

soluble iodide contrast media is an ideal way of directly visualizing the varices, but because of the danger of severe splenic hemorrhage following such a procedure, this examination is recommended only prior to laparotomy for splenectomy. If splenectomy is not performed immediately, the child should be carefully observed for

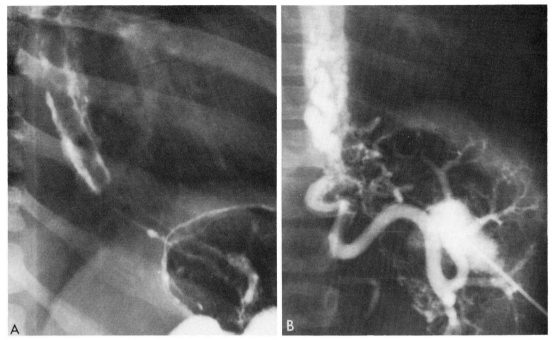

Figure 7-25. Esophageal varices. *A*, Large filling defects in esophagus. *B*, Percutaneous splenic injection of contrast material, demonstrating large dilated veins in esophagus.

REFERENCES

Esophagitis and Stricture

Alpert, M. Roentgen manifestations of epidermolysis bullosa, *Am. J. Roentgenol. Radium Ther. Nucl. Med.*, 78:66, 1957.

Azar, H., Chrispin, A. R., and Waterston, D. J. Esophageal replacement with transverse colon in infants and children, *J. Pediatr. Surg.*, 6:3, 1971.

Becker, M. H., and Swinyard, C. A.: Epidermolysis bullosa dystrophica in children, *Radiology*, 90: 124, 1968.

Dupree, E., Hodges, S., Jr., and Simon, J. L. Epidermolysis bullosa of the esophagus, *Am. J. Dis. Child.*, 117:349, 1969.

Franken, E. A., Jr. Caustic damage of the gastrointestinal tract: roentgen features, *Am. J. Roentgenol. Radium Ther. Nucl. Med.*, 118:77, 1973.

Goldberg, H. I., and Dodds, W. J. Cobblestone esophagus due to monilial infection, *Am. J. Roentgenol. Radium Ther. Nucl. Med.*, 104:608, 1968.

Irving, L., Scholander, P. F., and Grinnell, S. W. The regulation of arterial blood pressure in the seal during diving, *Am. J. Physiol.*, 135:557, 1942.

Kaufmann, H. J. Candida oesophagitis in children with malignant disorders, *Ann. Radiol.*, 13:157, 1970.

Martel, W. Radiologic features of esophagogastritis secondary to extremely caustic agents, *Radiology*, 103:31, 1972.

Sherman, C. D., Jr., and Waterston, D. Oesophageal reconstruction in children using intrathoracic colon, *Arch. Dis. Child.*, 32:11, 1957.

Sullivan, B. H., Jr., Geppert, L. J., and Renson, R. F. Esophageal ulcer in very young infants, *Am. J. Dis. Child.*, 87:49, 1954.

Foreign Bodies

Alexander, W. J., Kadish, J. A., and Dunbar, J. S. Ingested foreign bodies in children, *Progr. Pediatr. Radiol.*, 2:256, 1969.

Shackelford, G. D., McAlister, W. H., and Robertson, C. L. The use of a Foley catheter for removal of blunt esophageal foreign bodies in children, *Radiology*, 105:455, 1972.

Trauma

Ecklof, O., Lohr, G., and Okmian, L. Submucosal perforation of the esophagus in the neonate, *Acta Radiol.*, 8:187, 1969.

Girdany, B. R., Sieber, W. K., and Osman, M. Z. Traumatic pseudodiverticulum of the pharynx in newborn infants. *N. Engl. J. Med.*, 280:237, 1969.

Harell, G. S., Friedland, G. W., Daily, W. J., and Cohn, R. B. Neonatal Boerhaave's syndrome, *Radiology*, 95:665, 1970.

Acquired Diverticula

Dohlman, G., and Mattsson, O. The endoscopic operation for hypopharyngeal diverticula, *Arch. Otolaryngol.*, 71:744, 1960.

Meadows, J. A., Jr. Esophageal diverticula in infants and children, *South. Med. J.*, 63:691, 1970.

Nelson, A. R. Congenital true esophageal diverticulum: report of a case unassociated with other esophago-tracheal abnormality, *Ann. Surg.*, 145:258, 1957.

Esophageal Varices

Auvert, J., Michel, J. R., and Farge, C. The radiological approach to the diagnosis of portal hypertension, *Progr. Pediatr. Radiol.*, 2:99, 1969.

Buonocore, E., Collmann, I. R., Kerley, H. E., and Lester, T. L. Massive upper gastrointestinal hemorrhage in children, *Am. J. Roentgenol. Radium Ther. Nucl. Med.*, 115:289, 1972.

Rosch, J., and Dotter, C. T. Extrahepatic portal obstruction in childhood and its angiographic diagnosis, *Am. J. Roentgenol. Radium Ther. Nucl. Med.*, 112:143, 1971.

Chapter 8

THE NORMAL
STOMACH

ROENTGENOLOGIC ANATOMY. Reports concerning the normal anatomy of the infant's stomach and evaluation of its emptying time are recorded in the early annals of pediatrics and radiology. Early observers compared the shape of the infant's stomach with the previously described types of adult stomach, such as the J-shape or fishhook type, the ovoid or Scotch bagpipe shape, the tobacco-pouch shape and the pear-shaped type. There is a difference of opinion in the earlier literature concerning the factors regulating the shape of the stomach, various investigators attributing the shape to the consistency of the food, the quality or quantity of the feedings, the position of the infant during feedings, the size of the air bubble, and the tone of gastric musculature. Obviously there is a wide variation in the size and shape of the infant's stomach depending solely upon anatomic variability irrespective of other factors.

Most of the inconsistencies of opinion in the earlier literature resulted from differences in examination technics, some of the studies being carried out with the infant upright and some with the infant recumbent. Regardless of this, the shape and position of the stomach are now subject to many individual or anatomic variations. Generally speaking, however, the stomach of the newborn and young infant occupies a transverse or horizontal position in the abdomen (Fig. 8–1). The normal horizontal position in infants is aided to some extent by the upward displacement of the stomach resulting from the accumulation of air in the small intestine. Occasionally, however, the stomach of a young infant occupies a more vertical or J-shaped position (Fig. 8–2) and, unquestionably, if more examinations are made with the infant upright, a greater percentage of the vertical configurations will be

seen. Just what effect the individual habitus has on the position of the infant's stomach is not definitely known. The infant who matures into a sthenic or hypersthenic type of individual probably maintains a more transverse type of stomach than the asthenic or hyposthenic individual, whose stomach assumes a more vertical position (Fig. 8–3). Regardless of the position, for purposes of description the stomach may be divided into three areas. The fundus is that portion superior to the cardiac orifice, and the body or pars media extends between the fundus and the third portion, which is the prepyloric segment or antrum. The junction between the body and the antrum is marked on the lesser curvature by the angularis incisura and on the greater curvature by a line parallel to the left vertebral border (Fig. 8–1D). These demarcations are less definite in the infant than in the older child. Although the fundus lies intimately under the left hemidiaphragm in the older child and adult, there is a normal gap between the fundus and the diaphragm in the infant. This variation should be recognized and not mistaken for a subphrenic lesion or subpulmonic effusion.

As the infant grows older and more active, the pars media expands caudally and the stomach assumes a more vertical or J-shaped position such as one usually sees in the older child and adult. This probably results from the effect of gravity on the greater curvature, the duodenum remaining relatively fixed, and from the increase in size of the abdominal cavity and the decrease in small bowel gas which occur when the infant spends fewer hours in the recumbent position. Although with growth and activity the J-shaped stomach becomes more characteristic, the wide variations in shape and position persist and increase as puberty is approached.

When radiographs of the barium-filled

103

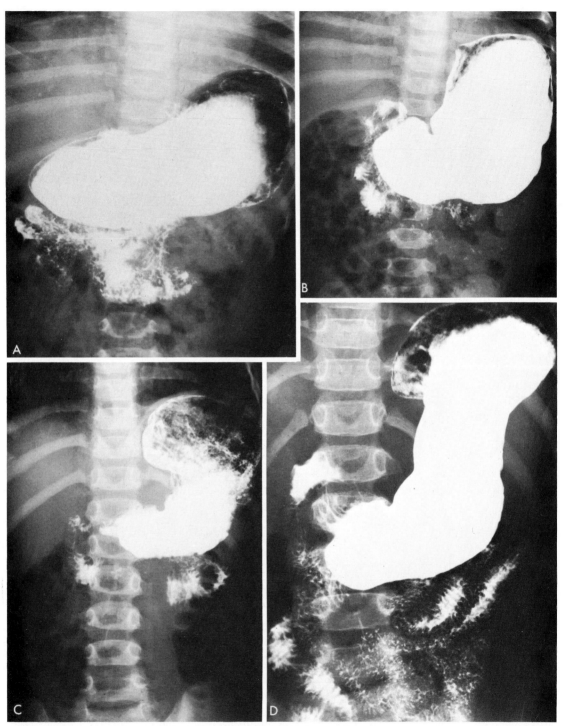

Figure 8-1. Variations in configuration of the stomach at different ages. *A,* Transverse position of stomach of 1-week-old infant. *B,* At 1 year of age the stomach has a somewhat more vertical position. *C,* At 2 years of age the stomach is more vertically situated, approximating the usual adult position. *D,* Normal vertical stomach of 6-year-old child.

stomach are made with the patient lying on his abdomen, a compression defect produced by the adjacent vertebrae (Fig. 8–4) is frequently evident in the antral region. This is most often seen in tall thin children.

The gastric mucosal pattern is poorly defined in the infant, and in the newborn few rugae can be identified. By the age of 1 year, however, the rugal pattern, especially in the fundus and on the greater curvature, becomes more prominent and the increase continues during childhood. Occasionally the mucosal pattern in the stomach of a young infant, especially if the stomach is not distended by barium or air, is unusually conspicuous (Fig. 8–5). The site of opening of the esophagus into the stomach may sometimes be identified as a ring of barium through the gas-distended fundus (Fig. 8–6A). This opening probably marks the site of the constrictor cardiae. A stellate configuration of gastric mucosal folds is commonly identified as the point of esophageal entrance (Fig. 8–6B).

During the initial opacification of the an-

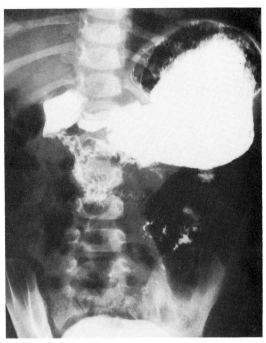

Figure 8–3. Transverse type stomach of hypersthenic child, aged 6 years. Compare with Figure 8–1D.

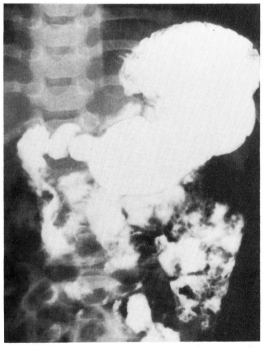

Figure 8–2. Stomach of this infant, aged 6 weeks, occupies more of a vertical than horizontal position in the abdomen. This is less common than the transverse position but is frequently seen.

trum the gastric rugae may appear unusually prominent but smooth out as peristalsis becomes more active (Fig. 8–7).

A rare finding in children undergoing upper gastrointestinal studies is a "bubbly" pattern in the antrum. This has been called the area gastricae (Fig. 8–8). Normally the gastric mucosa is composed of small polygonal elevations 16 mm in diameter, but because mucus usually fills the crevices between these fine elevations, the area gastricae is infrequently demonstrated. This is probably a normal finding but in older individuals may represent atrophic gastritis.

In the newborn and young infant, the amount of ingested air affects the size of the stomach to a remarkable degree. If the stomach is distended by an excess amount of air swallowed during crying or during feeding, without allowing intervals for "burping," the stomach may be distended to several times the size of its relaxed state, the pylorus extending nearly to the right lateral wall of the abdomen (Fig. 8–9). Voluntary and involuntary air swallowing may produce marked dilatation of the stomach and associated clinical findings of abdominal distention, nausea, and vomiting (Fig. 8–10). Once solids are started, the

Text continued on page 109.

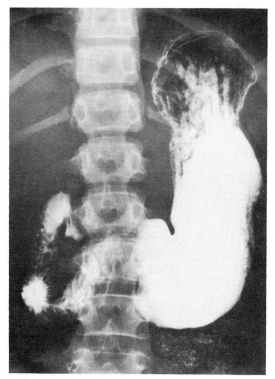

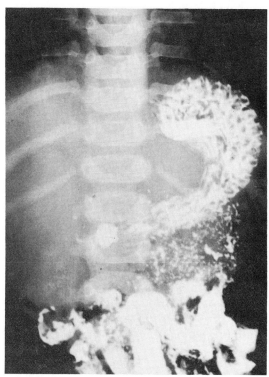

Figure 8–4. Compression defect of antrum in child, aged 11, produced by pressure of vertebral bodies.

Figure 8–5. Unusually prominent rugae in stomach of normal infant, aged 9 months.

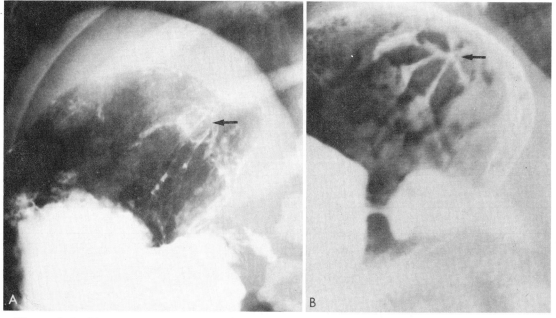

Figure 8–6. Variation in appearance of opening of esophagus into stomach. *A*, Ring-shaped area of density represents barium coating open orifice of esophagus (arrow). *B*, Stellate pattern represents barium in mucosal folds of constricted esophageal orifice (arrow).

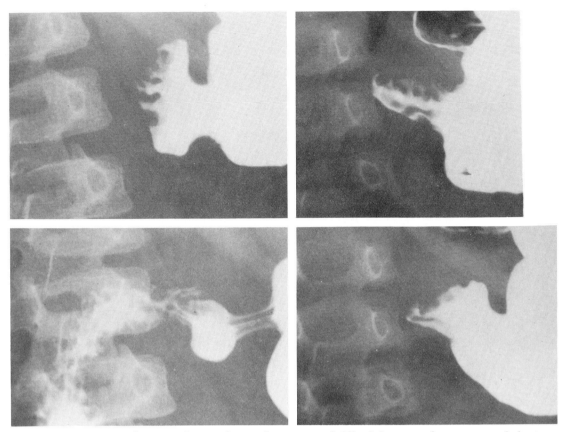

Figure 8–7. Normal mucosal irregularity during initial fill of the prepyloric area with barium. Subsequent sequential films show effacement of these folds during gastric peristalsis.

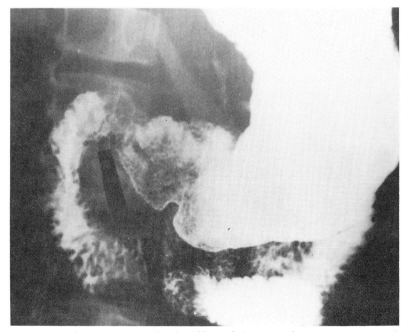

Figure 8–8. 12-year-old boy with multiple filling defects in the gastric antrum (area gastricae). Probably a normal variation.

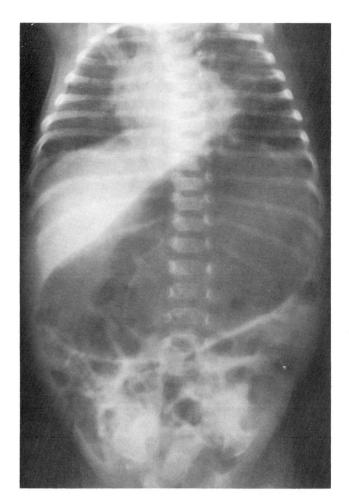

Figure 8–9. Excessive air swallowing in normal infant. Stomach is markedly distended, the antrum extending to right abdominal wall.

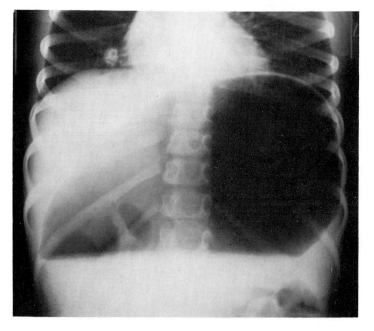

Figure 8–10. Acute gastric distention in a 10-year-old boy who was competing in air swallowing and "belching" contest.

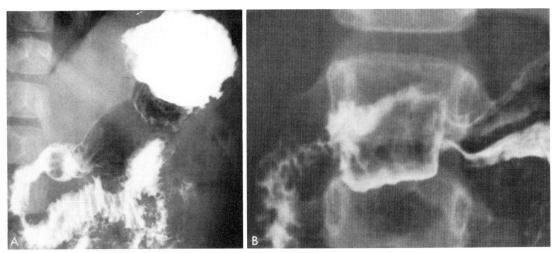

Figure 8–11. Double contrast effect of air and barium obtained by films made with the patient supine and the right side elevated. *A,* Stomach shown to good advantage. *B,* Duodenal bulb in detail.

enormous amounts of air seen with liquid feedings are not so frequently encountered. With ingestion of liquids, more air is swallowed; this is readily appreciated during fluoroscopy if the comparison is made when the infant is offered a bottle followed by a teaspoon of thicker barium. The simple

act of sucking is apparently not accompanied by swallowing of air, as demonstrated by infants nursing a pacifier who do not swallow the quantity of air seen during the ingestion of formula from a bottle. The air content of the stomach may be used advantageously by obtaining films with the pa-

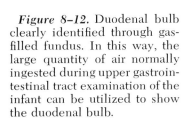

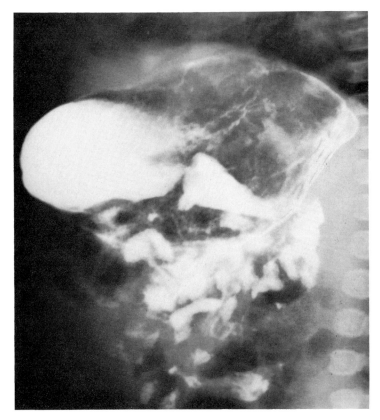

Figure 8–12. Duodenal bulb clearly identified through gas-filled fundus. In this way, the large quantity of air normally ingested during upper gastrointestinal tract examination of the infant can be utilized to show the duodenal bulb.

tient supine and with the right side elevated. This affords a double contrast effect of barium and air in the antrum and duodenal bulb (Fig. 8–11).

The pylorus and duodenal bulb are often difficult to examine fluoroscopically and radiographically in the infant because of their posterior position and the transverse position of the stomach. Thus, when the infant is rotated so as to show the pyloric canal and bulb in profile, the fundus often obscures the detail of this region. However, because of the usual distention of the fundus by swallowed air, the pyloric canal and duodenum can be identified satisfactorily through the gas-distended segment, if not posterior to it, with the infant rotated into a nearly lateral position (Fig. 8–12). As infancy is passed and the stomach assumes a more vertical position, this difficulty is overcome, the duodenum being easily examined by turning the patient into slight degrees of obliquity.

ROENTGENOLOGIC PHYSIOLOGY. A review of the literature relating to the normal physiology of the neonatal and infant stomach discloses nearly as great a nonconformity of opinion as there are authors. This is attributable in part to different methods of examination, with some investigators using a milk-bismuth or barium meal, others adding fats or casein, some comparing human milk and cow's milk, and some keeping the infant in a prone and others in a supine position between roentgenograms. Consequently, reports on the normal emptying time of the stomach vary from approximately 2 to over 24 hours. The emptying time of stomachs is prolonged when various foods are added to the barium-water meal, or when the stomach contains previously ingested food. Consequently, an accurate evaluation of the normal emptying time can be determined only by using water as the vehicle for the barium meal. Nevertheless we have not found that a small amount of chocolate or other flavoring added to the barium significantly interferes with the emptying time of the child's stomach.

The amount of air in the stomach and the position in which the infant is kept after

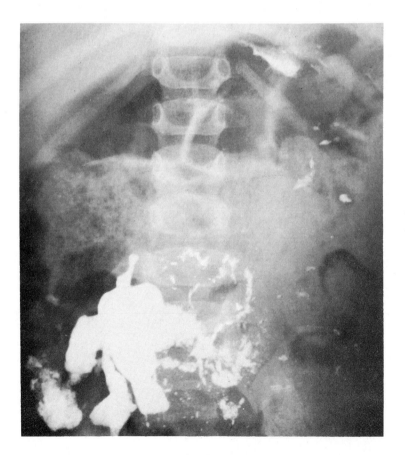

Figure 8–13. Normal emptying of stomach in child. After two hours only a small residuum is present in the stomach.

feeding also greatly affect the length of time the stomach requires to evacuate its contents. This is readily explained by considering the position of the air and ingested material in relation to each other and how this is affected by change of position of the infant. With the infant supine, the air rises to the anterior portion of the stomach, i.e., the body and antrum, whereas the fluid content assumes the dependent position in the fundus. In this position the air acts as an obstacle to the passage of fluids into the small bowel, and the relatively weak peristalsis in the fundus is ineffectual in forcing the fluid into the body and antrum. Similarly, in this position the air cannot be eructated, the fluid blocking the cardia. With the infant in the prone or upright position the situation is reversed, with the air rising to the fundus where it is easily eructated and the fluid contents passing into the antrum where peristaltic movements propel it into the duodenum. Therefore, if the infant is kept in the prone posi-

tion before the examination in order to eliminate most of the air from the stomach, and is returned to this position between the taking of serial roentgenograms, the normal emptying time is usually between 2 and 4 hours. We have found that after the ingestion of barium and with the infant kept either lying on his right side or prone, only a small residuum of barium is seen at 2½ hours (Fig. 8–13). Considerable retention of barium (40 to 50%) has been found after 10 hours in infants who had not been placed in the prone position either before or during the examination. Reexamination of the same infants, when kept in the prone position, showed nearly complete evacuation at the end of 2½ hours. Unless the proper position of the infant is maintained during the roentgenographic studies after the feedings, gastric residues at 8, 12, and even 24 hours cannot be interpreted as evidence of organic pyloric obstruction.

In the ambulatory child, the gastric emptying time is similar to that of the adult. At

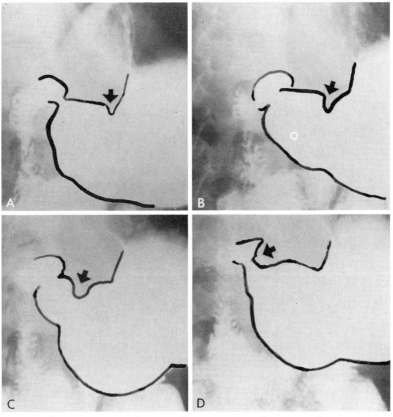

Figure 8–14. Normal progression of peristalsis. *A*, Peristaltic wave begins at angularis incisura (arrow) and progresses toward the pyloric canal as shown in *B*, *C*, and *D*.

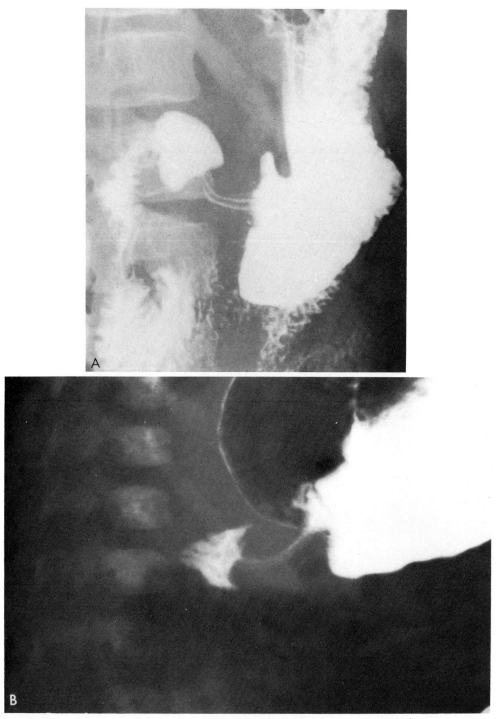

Figure 8-15. A, Normal peristaltic contraction in the prepyloric area. This is a transitory state following passage of a peristaltic wave and conceivably might be misdiagnosed as hypertrophic pyloric stenosis. Fluoroscopic evaluation is important in recognizing the longitudinal mucosal folds as being a part of antral systole rather than elongation of the pyloric canal. *B*, Another example of normal antral systole in a young infant.

the end of 2½ hours, 80 to 90% of the ingested barium has left the stomach.

Motor activity of the stomach differs in the infant and the older child. In the first few days of life peristaltic waves are shallow, widely spaced, and intermittent. Rarely is more than one wave seen at a time. The contractions begin in the pars media and become slightly deeper as they pass toward the pylorus (Fig. 8–14). The greater the gaseous distention of the stomach or small bowel, the less active the gastric peristalsis. Apparently, gaseous distention of the small intestine reflexly inhibits gastric peristaltic activity. Spontaneous contractions are occasionally seen in the antrum and less often in the body. Contraction of the prepyloric area occasionally suggests an elongated pyloric canal (Fig. 8–15) and may be mistaken for pyloric stenosis. The pyloric canal begins at the end of

the stomach, but only by fluoroscopically observing the termination of a gastric peristaltic wave can one determine the origin of the pyloric canal (Fig. 8–16).

Frequently, active peristalsis develops after the ingestion of barium mixture, only to dissipate and be followed by a few minutes of inactivity before normal peristalsis is resumed. In the older infant peristaltic waves are often prominent and pass from the body of the stomach to the pylorus in rapid succession.

In the child past the infant stage gastric motility is similar to that of the adult. Active waves appear a few minutes after barium enters the stomach. The initial swallow may pass by action of gravity through an open pylorus into the duodenum, or temporarily collect in the antrum until the onset of peristalsis opens the pylorus. Occasionally, several minutes of

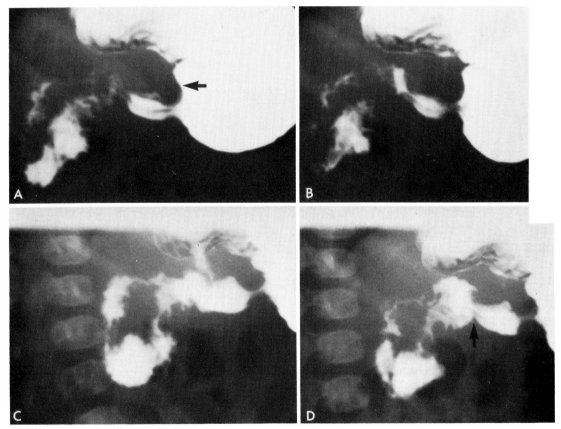

Figure 8–16. Fluoroscopic spot films show variations in the size of the prepyloric area during gastric peristalsis. Initial observations (*A* and *B*) show contraction of the prepyloric area with questionable indentation (arrow) on the antrum by hypertrophied pyloric muscle. Later observations (*C* and *D*) show distention of the prepyloric area with a normal pyloric canal (arrow).

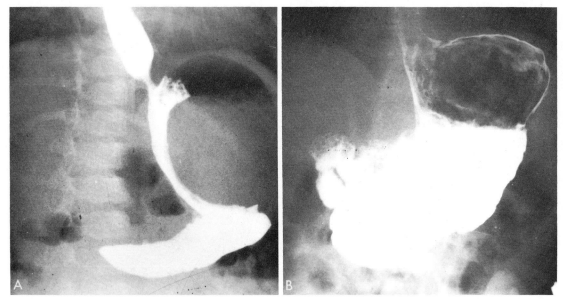

Figure 8–17. *A,* Upper gastrointestinal study in an infant whose stomach is filled with food. The first ingested barium has flowed along the lesser curvature, suggesting an intraluminal mass. *B,* Later films show normal distention of the stomach with incidental gastroesophageal reflux of air.

vigorous peristaltic activity ensue before barium enters the duodenum. This increased tone of the pylorus is probably related to the emotional tension of the patient. If the stomach is filled with food, the initial barium swallow may flow along the lesser curvature and produce the appearance of an intraluminal mass (Fig. 8–17).

REFERENCES

Bouslog, J. S., Cunningham, T. D., Hanner, J. P., Walton, J. B., and Waltz, H. D. The roentgenologic studies of the infant's gastrointestinal tract, *J. Pediatr.,* 6:234, 1935.

Henderson, S. G. The gastrointestinal tract in the healthy newborn infant, *Am. J. Roentgenol. Radium Ther. Nucl. Med., 18:*302, 1942.

Hood, J. H. Effect of posture on amount and distribution of gas in the intestinal tract of infants and young children, *Lancet,* 2:107, 1964.

Margulis, A. R., and Burhenne, H. J., editors, *Alimentary Tract Roentgenology* Vol. 1, p. 456 (1st ed., St. Louis: C. V. Mosby Co., 1967).

Silverio, J. Gastric emptying time in the newborn and the nursling, *Am. J. Med. Sci.,* 47:732, 1964.

Chapter 9

CONGENITAL ABNORMALITIES OF THE STOMACH

The stomach is relatively immune to the formation of congenital anomalies, it being a less common site of anomalous development than any other part of the alimentary tract.

SITUS INVERSUS

In complete situs inversus the thoracic and abdominal organs occupy a mirror image position of the normal. Less usual is partial situs inversus, in which the thoracic viscera are in a normal position but the gastrointestinal tract is reversed, with the stomach beneath the right hemidiaphragm and the cecum in the left lower quadrant (Fig. 9–1). Transposition of the intestinal tract is presumably the result of reversal of the initial rotation of the gut. This should not be confused with reversed rotation as described in Chapter 12. Eventration of the right hemidiaphragm is frequently present and, rarely, the stomach may lie posterior to the liver.

Abnormal visceral situs (complete or partial) associated with bilateral three-lobed lungs (right pulmonary isomerism), congenital heart disease, and asplenia is known as Ivemark's syndrome (Fig. 9–2). Abnormal visceral situs may also be associated with bilateral two-lobed lungs (left pulmonary isomerism), congenital heart disease, and polysplenia. Similar left pulmonary isomerism is seen in females with anisosplenia, congenital heart disease and, occasionally, abnormal visceral situs. Reversed visceral situs with congenital heart disease, a left eparterial bronchus, and right hyparterial bronchus is still another complex syndrome. Consequently, any patient with abnormal visceral situs should be investigated for associated cardiac abnormality.

DIVERTICULA

Gastric diverticula, although not uncommon in the adult, are rare in the pediatric patient. Diverticula which contain all elements of the bowel wall in normal proportions are probably incomplete duplications formed early in fetal life in a manner similar to that of duplications elsewhere in the intestinal tract. Because of their configuration, however, they are usually classified as diverticula. They may involve any portion of the stomach from the fundus to the pylorus and cause such symptoms as abdominal pain, vomiting, or hematemesis only when they are the site of ulceration, perforation, or intussusception.

False diverticula consist mainly of a wall of mucosa or submucosa, the muscular layers being deficient. They are believed to occur in congenitally weak areas of the muscular coat secondary to prolonged increased intraluminal pressure. In adults they are commonly found in the posterior portion of the cardia and are usually asymptomatic. They are very rare in children but have been reported on the greater curvature and near the pylorus, and in such cases may be related to an intrauterine vascular occlusion to the stomach.

Differentiation between true and false diverticula can be made only by microscopic examination to determine the components of the wall of the diverticulum.

ROENTGENOLOGIC FINDINGS. Radiologically, the two types are similar and are identified only after contrast material has passed into the stomach. The collection of

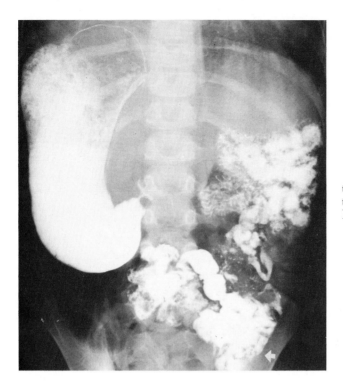

Figure 9–1. Situs inversus of gastrointestinal tract. Stomach is on the patient's right and cecum is in the left lower quadrant (arrow).

Figure 9–2. 1-day-old infant with dextrocardia and intermediate position of the stomach (arrow). Note area of density in the left mid-lung field, suggesting a left middle lobe. Postmortem examination revealed bilateral trilobed lungs, splenic agenesis, abdominal situs inversus, and complex congenital heart disease consisting of dextrocardia, transposition of the great vessels, single ventricle, and pulmonary valvular atresia (Ivemark's syndrome). (Reprinted with permission from *Radiol. Clin. North Am.,* **10**:344, 1972.)

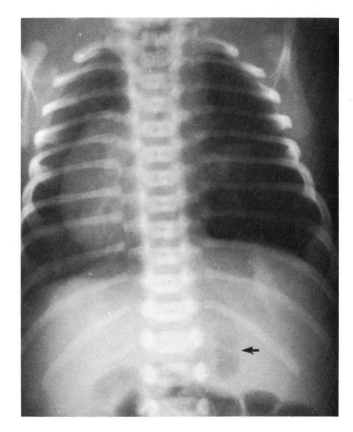

barium in the diverticulum may closely simulate an ulcer and differentiation may be difficult. Diverticula in the region of the fundus and cardia may be missed if the patient is not placed in the recumbent position, and then turned to the left to inspect the posterior portion of the cardia.

DUPLICATIONS

Duplications of the stomach are rare. They usually lie along the greater curvature and are lined with gastric mucosa. They may possibly develop as a result of failure of complete coalescence of the vacuoles during the recanalization of the intestinal lumen in early intrauterine life (see Duplication of Small Intestine). At birth the duplication is usually small but may enlarge rapidly as a result of the accumulation of secretions, in a short time becoming even larger than the stomach. The presenting symptom usually is abdominal pain caused by distention or ulceration of the duplication. Perforation into the peritoneal cavity or adjacent bowel may be a complication of the ulceration. Vomiting and hematemesis may occur and, if the mass becomes sufficiently distended, it may be palpated through the abdominal wall. Theoretically, pressure of the mass on the adjacent stomach may produce gastric obstruction. Unusual types have been reported in which the gastric duplication communicated with the ileum via a Meckel's diverticulum. Combined duplication of the stomach and esophagus has been reported (see Chap. 6).

ROENTGENOLOGIC FINDINGS. Communicating duplications are similar in appearance to gastric diverticula (Fig. 9–3).

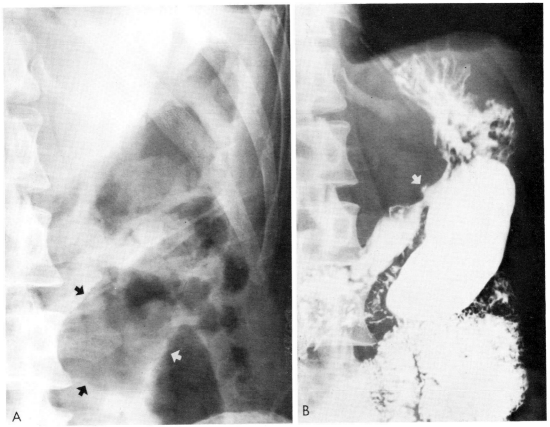

Figure 9–3. Duplication of stomach. *A,* Plain film of abdomen, showing collection of gas (arrows) beneath silhouette of the stomach. *B,* After ingestion of barium, the duplication and its communication with the greater curvature is identified. There is a gastric ulcer on the lesser curvature of the stomach (arrow) opposite the mouth of the duplication. The patient is an adult, but the lesion was undoubtedly present during childhood.

Other duplications are usually visualized only indirectly as a result of displacement and encroachment on the adjacent segments of the alimentary tract. If the duplication communicates with the adjacent stomach, ingested barium may reveal it; otherwise it can only be suspected radiologically from the deformity of the stomach.

DEVELOPMENTAL OBSTRUCTIVE DEFECTS

Developmental defects of the stomach which obstruct the gastric lumen are very rare, with only a few isolated cases reported in the literature. In such cases the obstruction is usually due to a transverse septum of mucosa in the prepyloric region which separates the stomach into two compartments. Extrinsic pressure by congenital peritoneal bands or by annular pancreatic tissue in the gastric wall may cause obstruction of the antrum.

In cases of obstruction involving the stomach, the predominant symptom is vomiting, the vomitus being free of bile.

ROENTGENOLOGIC FINDINGS. A scout film of the abdomen may show distention of the stomach proximal to the obstruction and absence or decrease of gas in the small bowel, depending upon the degree of obstruction. The appearance may be confused with duodenal obstruction, particularly if there is persistent spasm of the circular musculature of the antral inlet. The introduction of contrast material into the stomach will aid in determining the exact location of the obstruction. Several forms of gastric obstruction are recognized. Pyloric atresia is obviously a severe form, causing distention of the stomach and absence of gas in the small bowel (Fig. 9–4). Prepyloric septum or diaphragm without complete obstruction may not be detected until after the newborn period and the initial scout film may be normal. Barium studies should identify the membranous defect (Fig. 9–5).

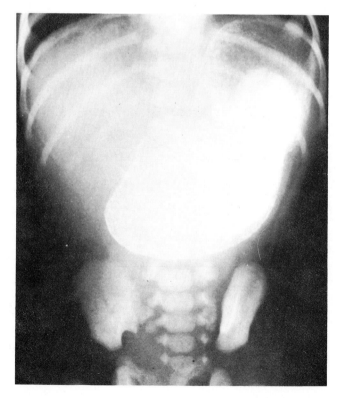

Figure 9–4. Pyloric atresia in a newborn infant. There is complete obstruction at the pyloric canal.

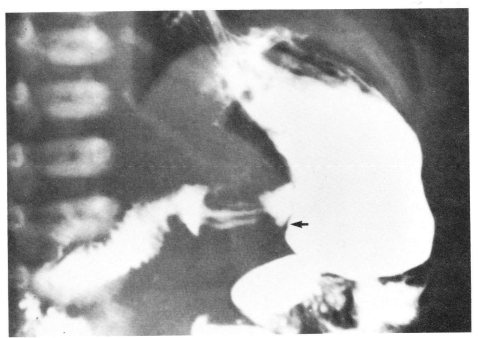

Figure 9–5. Membranous septum partly obstructing the gastric antrum in a 2-day-old infant. (Reprinted with permission from *Semin. Roentgenol.*, 8:341, 1973.)

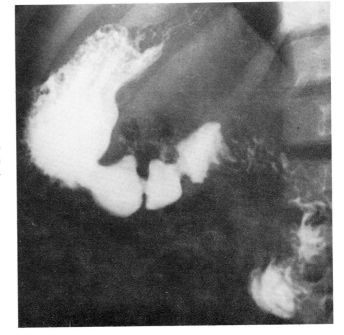

Figure 9–6. Antral stenosis in an 8-year-old boy. The circular defect in the antrum was present on repeat examination and confirmed at surgery.

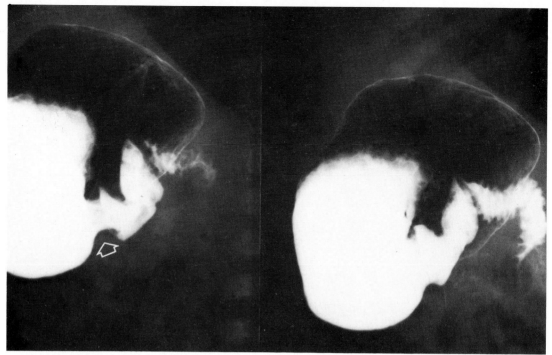

Figure 9–7. Transient circular constriction in the antrum of a 6-month-old infant (arrow). Repeat examination failed to confirm these findings.

Antral stenosis is another form of obstruction, producing a localized circular defect in the gastric antrum. The appearance suggests local constriction of the circular muscle (Fig. 9–6). The condition is rare but when persistent can be relieved by surgical correction. However, we have seen similar defects which have been transient (Fig. 9–7). Aberrant pancreatic tissue in the stomach wall may produce a filling defect, the identity of which can be determined only after laparotomy.

MUSCULAR DEFECTS

Congenital muscular defects of the stomach with perforation have been reported in the newborn infant. They are discovered only during laparotomy or at autopsy. The condition should be considered in any infant in whom spontaneous pneumoperitoneum develops. In all probability these defects develop in intrauterine life, similar to other focal vascular insults arising from intrauterine stress situations.

MICROGASTRIA

Congenital microgastria is an unusual anomaly of the stomach occurring as an isolated anomaly or, more frequently, with asplenia syndromes. The stomach is markedly underdeveloped, without differentiation into fundus, body, and antrum. The greater and lesser curvatures have failed to develop, and the small tube-shaped stomach functions as a straight communication between the esophagus above and the duodenum below (Fig. 9–8). Gastroesophageal reflux is an expected finding in this condition. The gastroesophageal junction is competent and the esophagus appears to take over the storage function of the inadequate stomach. When asplenia accompanies microgastria, associated congenital heart disease, abnormal visceral situs, and pulmonary isomerism are to be expected.

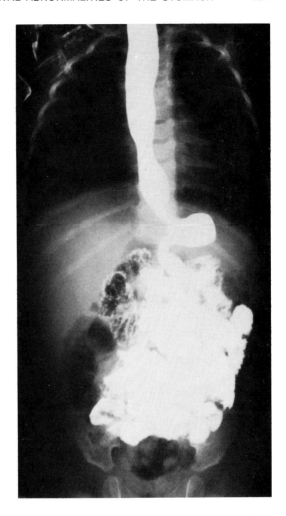

Figure 9–8. Congenital microgastria. The stomach is a rudimentary structure. There is marked incompetence of the gastroesophageal junction with dilatation of the esophagus. (Courtesy of Dr. Fred Lee, Children's Hospital, Los Angeles, California. Reprinted with permission from: *Semin. Roentgenol.,* **6**:221, 1971.)

GASTRIC TORSION

Gastric volvulus or torsion in the pediatric patient is usually associated with eventration or paralysis of the diaphragm, or occasionally is seen after repair of a diaphragmatic hernia. We have not seen this condition without an elevated left hemidiaphragm. The torsion may be along the transverse or longitudinal axis. Symptoms in the pediatric age group usually consist of recurrent episodes of vomiting.

Radiographically the stomach is distended with gas, and the antrum is beneath the elevated diaphragm. The pylorus is directed to the right and often inferiorly (Fig. 9–9). If obstruction is present it is more often at the pylorus although obstruction at the cardia may occur, but less commonly than in the adult patient. If congenital malrotation is also present the ligament of Treitz will not be in a normal identifiable position (Fig. 9–10).

ECTOPIC PANCREAS

Ectopic pancreatic tissue may be found at various sites in the gastrointestinal tract. When located in the stomach it may appear radiographically as a nodular defect or as a larger intraluminal mass (Fig. 9–11).

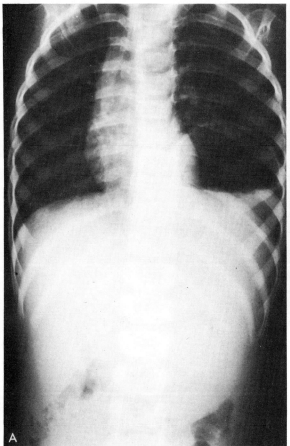

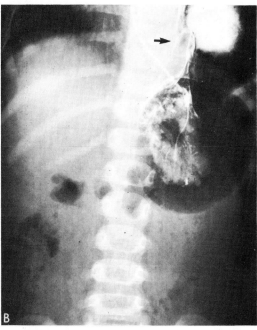

Figure 9–9. Gastric volvulus in a 3-year-old girl with eventration of the left hemidiaphragm. *A*, Initial radiograph shows eventration of the diaphragm with air-fluid level in the adjacent stomach. *B*, Upper gastrointestinal tract studies show the antrum to be beneath the diaphragm with obstruction at the pyloric canal (arrow).

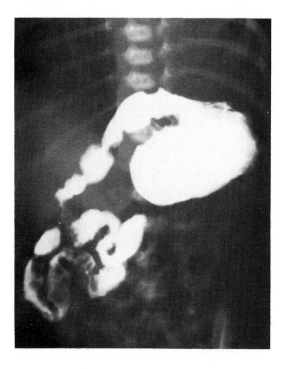

Figure 9–10. Gastric volvulus in a newborn infant following repair of foramen of Bochdalek hernia. The fundus is inferior to the antrum and the jejunum is in an abnormal position.

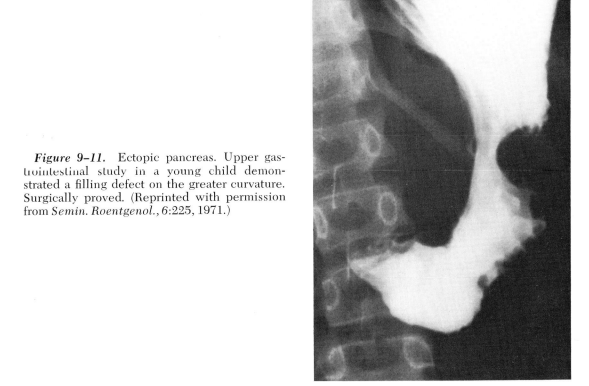

Figure 9–11. Ectopic pancreas. Upper gastrointestinal study in a young child demonstrated a filling defect on the greater curvature. Surgically proved. (Reprinted with permission from *Semin. Roentgenol.*, 6:225, 1971.)

REFERENCES

Situs Inversus

Landing, B. H. Syndromes of congenital heart disease with tracheobronchial anomalies, *Am. J. Roentgenol. Radium Ther. Nucl. Med.*, 123:679, 1975.

Landing, B. H., Lawrence, T-Y.K., Payne, V. C., and Wells, T. R. Bronchial anatomy in syndromes with abnormal visceral situs, abnormal spleen and congenital heart disease, *Am. J. Cardiol.*, 28:456, 1971.

Singleton, E. B., Dutton, R. V., and Wagner, M. L. Radiographic evaluation of lung abnormalities, *Radiol. Clin. North Am.*, 10:333, 1972.

Diverticula

Dodd, G. D., and Sheft, D. Diverticulum of the greater curvature of the stomach: a roentgenologic curiosity, *Am. J. Roentgenol. Radium Ther. Nucl. Med.*, 107:102, 1969.

Ogur, G. L., and Kolarsick, A. J. Gastric diverticula in infancy, *J. Pediatr.*, 39:723, 1951.

Palmer, E. D. Collective review: gastric diverticula, *International Abstracts of Surgery*, 92:417, 1951.

Duplications

Abrami, G., and Dennison, W. M. Duplication of the stomach, *Surgery*, 49:794, 1961.

Gray, D. H. Total reduplication of the stomach: a rare anomaly, *Aust. N. Z. J. Surg.*, 41:130, 1971.

Grosfeld, J., Boles, E. T., Jr., and Reiner, C. Duplication of pylorus in the newborn: a rare cause of gastric outlet obstruction, *J. Pediatr. Surg.*, 5:365, 1970.

Gross, R. E., Holcomb, G. W., and Faber, S. Duplications of the alimentary tract, *Pediatrics*, 9:449, 1952.

Kremer, R. M., Lepoff, R. B., and Izant, R. J. Duplication of the stomach, *J. Pediatr. Surg.*, 5:360, 1970.

Moir, J. D. Combined duplication of the esophagus and stomach, *J. Can. Assoc. Radiol.*, 21:257, 1970.

Developmental Obstructive Defects

Brandon, F. M., and Weidner, W. A. Antral mucosal membrane; a congenital obstructing lesion of the stomach, *Am. J. Roentgenol. Radium Ther. Nucl. Med.*, 114:386, 1972.

Bronsther, B., Nadeu, M., and Abrams, M. Congenital pyloric atresia: a report of three cases and review of the literature, *Surgery*, 69:130, 1971.

Farman, J., Cywes, S., and Werbeloff, L. Pyloric mucosal diaphragms, *Clin. Radiol., 19*:95, 1968.

Felson, B., Berkmen, Y. M., and Hoyumpa, A. M. Gastric mucosal diaphragm, *Radiology, 92*:513, 1969.

Muscular Defects

Inouye, W. Y., and Evans, G. Neonatal gastric perforation: a report of six cases and a review of 143 cases, *Arch. Surg., 88*:471, 1964.

Lloyd, J. R. The etiology of gastrointestinal perforation in the newborn, *J. Pediatr. Surg., 4*:77, 1969.

Nice, C. M., Jr., and Mouton, R. A. Congenital defect of gastric muscle, *Am. J. Roentgenol. Radium Ther. Nucl. Med., 89*:1038, 1963.

Shaw, N. A., Blanc, W. A., Santulli, T. V., and Kaiser, G. Spontaneous rupture of the stomach in the newborn: a clinical and experimental study, *Surgery, 58*:561, 1965.

Microgastria

Blank, E., and Chisolm, A. J. Congenital microgastria, a case report with a 26 year follow-up, *Pediatrics, 51*:1037, 1973.

Schulz, R. D. Congenital microgastria, *Ann. Radiol., 14*:285, 1971.

Schulz, R. D., and Niemann, F. Kongenitale mikrogastrie in Verbindung mit Skelettmissbildungen — ein neues Syndrom, *Helv. Paediatr. Acta, 26*:185, 1971.

Shackelford, G. D., McAlister, W. H., Brodeur, A. E., and Ragsdale, E. F. Congenital microgastria, *Am. J. Roentgenol. Radium Ther. Nucl. Med., 118*: 72, 1973.

Gastric Torsion

Campbell, J. B., Rappaport, L. N., and Skerker, L. B. Acute mesentero-axial volvulus of the stomach, *Radiology, 103*:153, 1972.

Cole, B. C., and Dickinson, S. J. Acute volvulus of the stomach in infants and children, *Surgery, 70*:707, 1971.

Kilcoyne, R. F., Babbitt, D. P., and Sakaguchi, S. Volvulus of the stomach. A case report, *Radiology, 103*:157, 1972.

Ectopic Pancreas

Eklof, O., Lassrich, A., Stanley, P., and Chrispin, A. R. Ectopic pancreas, *Pediatr. Radiol., 1*:24, 1973.

Rooney, D. R. Aberrant pancreatic tissue in the stomach, *Radiology, 73*:241, 1959.

Singleton, E. B., and King, B. A. Localized lesions of the stomach in children, *Semin. Roentgenol., 6*: 220, 1971.

Chapter 10

ACQUIRED LESIONS OF THE STOMACH

HYPERTROPHIC PYLORIC STENOSIS

The first report of the roentgenologic examination of infants with pyloric stenosis was made by LeWald, who emphasized the delay in gastric emptying. The first radiologic description of the elongation of the pyloric canal was published in 1932 by Meuwissen and Sloof.

Characteristically, the disease has its onset between 3 and 6 weeks of age, although it is not unusual to find the condition at slightly younger and older ages. For some unknown reason the condition is more common in males than in females (ratio is 4 to 1). Wallgren found the incidence in 25,500 children in Sweden to be 4 per 1000. More recent studies from the Pittsburgh area in this country indicate an incidence of 1.26 per 1000 in whites and 0.48 per 1000 in blacks.

Usually the onset is sudden after three to four weeks of normal development and is characterized by vomiting which at first is little more than regurgitation, but soon becomes projectile and is especially severe after each feeding. Over a period of a few days the vomiting becomes more frequent and severe. Jaundice due to pressure of the hypertrophied pyloric muscle on the common bile duct or hepatic artery has been implicated in the past; however, recent studies suggest that this is due to temporary decrease in hepatic glucuronyl transferase activity. As a rule, active peristaltic waves are visible on the anterior abdominal wall, and frequently a small olive-shaped tumefaction may be palpated over the right portion of the epigastrium. Because of these rather characteristic physical findings many patients are subjected to laparotomy without roentgenologic examination. However, because of the frequent inconsistency of these findings, radiologic examination is of the utmost importance. Those of us who have practiced in an active pediatric institution cannot fail to be impressed by the number of suspected cases of pyloric stenosis having the physical signs of visible peristalsis and a tumor that is thought to be palpable in which the radiologic examination excludes this condition. There is an equal number of cases which are not typical clinically, but which by x-ray examination are shown to have pyloric stenosis. Other conditions such as chalasia, pylorospasm, and vomiting due to central nervous system damage may be mistaken clinically for pyloric stenosis, but if the time is taken for radiologic evaluation accurate differentiation can be established immediately.

PATHOLOGIC ANATOMY. This consists of hypertrophy and elongation of the circular muscle of the pyloric canal, which enlarges to involve not only the pyloric canal but the prepyloric segment of the stomach (Fig. 10–1). The caliber of the lumen of the gastric outlet is consequently reduced, and partial or complete obstruction results. The cause of the muscular hypertrophy is unknown. Previously it was considered to be congenital because it seemed illogical that an acquired lesion could develop in so short a time. Advocates of the congenital theory believed that the congenitally enlarged muscle did not cause vomiting until the underlying mucosa became edematous as a result of mechanical irritation produced by the passage of milk curds. However, Wallgren's work concluded that it could not be congenital after examining the upper gastrointestinal tract of 1000 consecutive newborn boys. No abnormality was found in five of the infants, in whom characteristic clinical and radiographic evi-

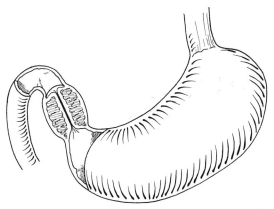

Figure 10-1. Hypertrophic pyloric stenosis. Drawing shows enlargement of pyloric muscle and resulting constriction of pyloric canal and compression defects on antrum and duodenal bulb.

dence of pyloric stenosis developed after the first few weeks of life. Further evidence that the enlargement of the pyloric muscle is not congenital is found in the work of Belding and Kernohan, who described degenerative changes in the ganglion cells of the myenteric plexus of the muscle, suggestive of exhaustion of these cells. This in turn was taken as evidence that the muscular hypertrophy developed secondary to an obstructive lesion in the pylorus, perhaps redundancy of the pyloric mucosa. Another hypothesis is that the hypertrophied muscle is the end result of long-standing pylorospasm secondary to reflex vagal stimulation from disturbances elsewhere.

There have been several reports citing adrenal cortical insufficiency as being responsible for hypertrophic pyloric stenosis and pylorospasm, but in general there has been little substantiating evidence for this. Many cases of congenital adrenal hyperplasia in young infants are accompanied by a salt-losing syndrome and protracted vomiting, with radiologic evidence of obstruction at the gastric outlet simulating hypertrophic pyloric stenosis. Its occurrence in infants with true congenital adrenal hyperplasia, as well as in infants without convincing evidence of such a condition, suggests that it may be a manifestation of severe dehydration due to any cause.

A postmortem study which showed persistence of the hypertrophied pyloric muscle six months after gastrojejunostomy, reported by Morse et al., suggests that chronic obstruction is not responsible for enlargement of the muscle. Injury to the central nervous system has also been considered as a factor. However, there is no confirmatory evidence for this, and the absence of other signs of brain damage discredits the idea. Although neurologic imbalance similar to that in Hirschsprung's disease may be the cause, the number of ganglion cells in the muscle is not decreased and there is no other evidence to support this belief. The essence of these theories suggests that the enlargement of the pyloric muscle is secondary to constant contraction, but whether this is the result of an attempt to overcome some unknown form of obstruction in the pyloric canal or secondary to reflex vagal stimulation initiated elsewhere in the body is not known. The few cases of hypertrophic pyloric stenosis which we have seen in older children and adults have been associated with peptic ulcer. Perhaps superficial ulceration and mucosal edema in the region of the pyloric canal, with partial obstruction of the gastric outlet or reflex vagal stimulation, is responsible for the majority of cases of hypertrophic pyloric stenosis even in young infants.

RADIOLOGIC FINDINGS. A preliminary scout film of the abdomen usually shows the stomach to be markedly dilated, although this is not necessarily so if the infant has recently vomited. Dilatation of the stomach may occur in any infant who cries violently before or during the examination, and consequently gaseous distention of the stomach should not in itself be considered evidence of pyloric obstruction. The amount of gas in the small bowel is usually diminished and, together with gastric dilatation, is suggestive evidence of obstruction at the pylorus. The degree of deficiency of small bowel gas is believed by Feinberg and his associates to be a manifestation of dehydration of the infant rather than of the degree of obstruction at the pylorus. Correction of the dehydration in their cases led to an increase in the amount of small bowel gas. Occasionally, the end of the gas-distended stomach has a conical configuration, the pyloric beak, produced by the indentation of the pyloric muscle on the distal end of the stomach (Fig. 10-2).

Fluoroscopy should begin with the infant in the supine position. The infant is offered

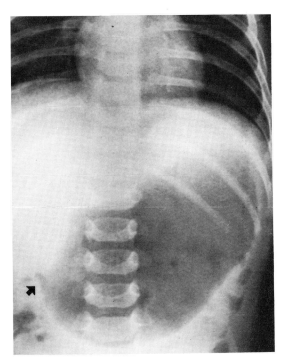

Figure 10-2. Abdominal scout film of infant with hypertrophic pyloric stenosis, showing distention of stomach, decrease in amount of small bowel gas, and antral beak (arrow).

pyloric canal. In our experience the low viscosity of oral Renografin and similar iodide contrast materials, in addition to the hypertonic properties of those materials, makes them less suitable than barium for demonstrating the elongated pyloric canal.

In normal infants, active peristaltic waves begin soon after introduction of the barium into the stomach, and fill of the duodenum occurs within a few minutes after the infant is placed in a right lateral decubitus position. In infants with pyloric stenosis the contractions are very active and are observed immediately. Exceptions to this are noted in infants who have been obstructed for several days; in such cases the stomach may be dilated and atonic, with weak ineffectual contractions. In other cases, the contractions may be very active for a time, only to stop for a brief period before recommencing. There is usually abnormal delay in fill of the duodenum, and frequently the fluoroscopic examination must be delayed before the stomach evacuation begins. However, in such cases, the radiographic identification of the canal is unnecessary, the pyloric beak, active gastric peristalsis, and delay in pyloric obstruction providing sufficient diagnostic information. As barium enters the proximal portion of the constricted pylorus, a beak-like projection may be identified (Fig. 10-3). After a variable length of time, peristalsis succeeds in thrusting barium into the pyloric canal, which is identified as a thin, elongated, stringlike segment of density several times its normal length and frequently angulated cephalad (Fig. 10-4). Often more than one line or "string" of contrast material can be identified and, occasionally, instead of the string sign the canal appears as a narrowed band of contrast material (Fig. 10-5). The elongated canal usually measures 1.5 to 3 cm. in length, and this corresponds fairly accurately to the length of the hypertrophied pyloric muscle. Indentation of this muscle at the base of the duodenal bulb is commonly seen (Fig. 10-6).

The compression of barium between a peristaltic wave and the hypertrophied pyloric muscle produces a transient collection of barium on the lesser curvature in the prepyloric area. This has been referred to as the "teat sign." Also, the "shoulder sign" consists of the prepyloric angle of air

a bottle containing a warm barium mixture, but because of the discomfort of the distended stomach, the infant may refuse the bottle and the barium may have to be introduced into the stomach through a small rubber catheter. In such cases, the air and fluid content of the stomach should be aspirated before injecting the contrast material. Many advocate the routine use of this method of introducing barium into the stomach. It has the advantage of expediency and enables the stomach to be deflated before introducing the contrast material. This is turn affords the examiner a better view of the pyloric canal. However, by allowing the infant to take the bottle, the esophagus can be examined, and although the distended stomach may tend to obscure early fill of the pyloric canal, this can be overcome by proper positioning of the patient. After barium has collected in the fundus, the infant is turned to his right into a right anterior oblique position in relation to the fluoroscopic table while careful attention is given to the distal end of the stomach for evidence of fill of the

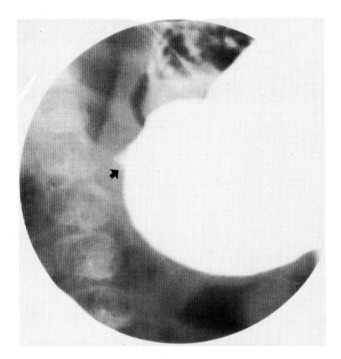

Figure 10–3. Hypertrophic pyloric stenosis. Spot film, showing antral beak.

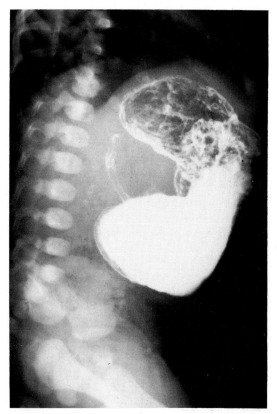

Figure 10–4. Hypertrophic pyloric stenosis. Elongated pyloric canal is shown as two lines of barium.

or barium produced by distention of the antrum by a peristaltic wave and the indentation formed by the hypertrophied pyloric muscle.

Many cases of pyloric stenosis show evidence of spasm of the distal end of the stomach following a peristaltic wave. If films are exposed during this contraction, the pyloric canal appears longer than it actually is (Figs. 10–7 and 10–8). Careful fluoroscopic examination is important because only by determining where a gastric peristaltic wave terminates can one identify the proximal portion of the pyloric canal accurately. Interval films of the abdomen usually show marked delay in gastric emptying, but this information is unimportant and only enhances the possibility of vomiting and aspiration.

After the diagnosis has been made, a catheter should be passed into the stomach and the gastric contents removed in an effort to avoid the complication of vomiting and tracheal aspiration.

Differentiation of pyloric stenosis and the usual type of pylorospasm should not cause confusion. Infants with pylorospasm have some delay in fill of the bulb, but the pyloric canal is of normal length and emptying of the stomach begins usually within

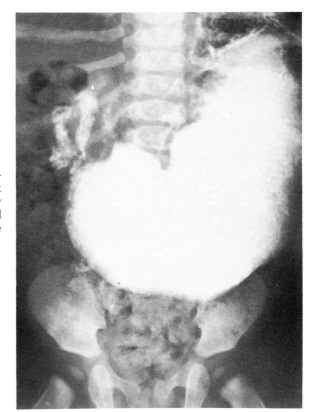

Figure 10-5. Hypertrophic pyloric stenosis. Infant, aged 5 months, with one-week history of vomiting. Stomach is extremely dilated and atonic. Pyloric canal is outlined as narrow band of barium rather than the usual string sign.

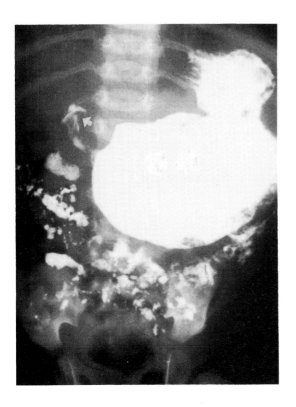

Figure 10-6. Hypertrophic stenosis, showing elongated pyloric canal, delayed gastric emptying, and compression by the enlarged muscle on duodenal bulb (arrow) and antrum.

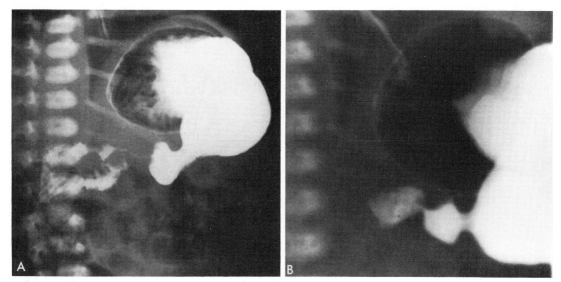

Figure 10–7. Pylorospasm in a 13-day-old infant. *A,* Antral contraction has produced a false string sign. *B,* Spot film made a few minutes later shows a distended prepyloric area with a normal pyloric canal.

ten minutes after ingestion of the barium. However, there is a less common form of pylorospasm which may simulate hypertrophic pyloric stenosis. The alleged relationship between this type of pylorospasm and adrenal cortical insufficiency has been dis-

cussed on page 126. In this condition there may be projectile vomiting and visible gastric peristaltic waves. However, differentiation between the conditions can usually be made fluoroscopically by detecting the end of a gastric peristaltic wave, this marking

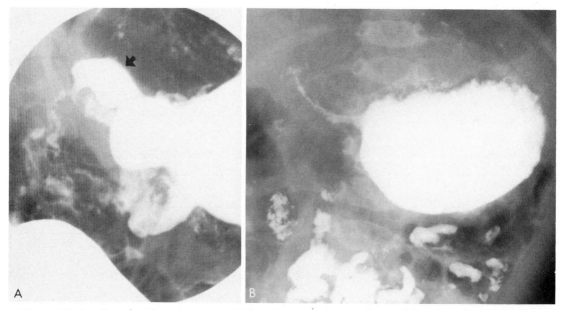

Figure 10–8. Pseudopyloric stenosis. Male infant, aged 6 weeks, with history of vomiting. *A,* At time of fluoroscopy, duodenal bulb (arrow) has filled promptly and pyloric canal is of normal length. *B,* Film of abdomen made one hour later, showing apparent elongation of pyloric canal as result of antral contraction.

the end of the stomach and the beginning of the pyloric canal. In pyloric stenosis the size of the constriction is constant and peristaltic waves stop abruptly at the proximal end of the narrowed pylorus. In addition, indentation of the base of the duodenum, although common in pyloric stenosis, is not present in pylorospasm.

The radiologic diagnosis of hypertrophic pyloric stenosis may be difficult in the early stages. Occasionally, clinical findings may be suggestive but the radiologic studies normal except for some delay in gastric emptying. Reexamination in two to three days has demonstrated classical x-ray findings of hypertrophic pyloric stenosis.

Treatment of hypertrophic pyloric stenosis in the Scandinavian countries has for many years been nonsurgical. The morbidity in such cases and the expense of long hospitalization have not seemed practical in this country, where equally satisfactory surgical results have been obtained. In patients treated medically, Runstrom described the characteristic roentgenographic findings in the acute or "manifest" stage of

the disease and in the recovery period. Following supportive therapy, and after cessation of vomiting, the roentgenographic findings remain essentially unchanged except for a slightly widened pyloric canal in which several longitudinal folds are to be seen, and the opening time of the stomach is normal or only slightly delayed, although the emptying time remains prolonged. These anatomic and physiologic changes may persist until the patient is several years old. Patients treated surgically by incision of the pyloric muscle have only a few days of hospitalization, and the extremely low mortality rate is as good as that of the conservative method of treatment.

According to Faber and Davis, immediately after pylorotomy there is a profound depression of gastric peristalsis which regularly lasts for 24 hours but may last several days. Following this initial period of inertia, gastric emptying time becomes normal, but persistent elongation of the pyloric canal may be noted for months and years (Fig. 10–9). However, there is prompt appearance of the contrast material in the

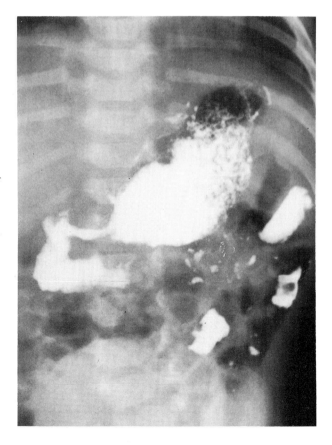

Figure 10–9. Postoperative study of pyloric stenosis. Infant with hypertrophic pyloric stenosis who became asymptomatic after pyloromyotomy. Repeat gastrointestinal examination two weeks after surgery, showing persistent elongation of pyloric canal but normal gastric emptying.

duodenum and the pyloric canal, although elongated and narrowed, is less stenotic than noted preoperatively. Among 16 infants who had a Fredet-Ramstedt operation for hypertrophic pyloric stenosis, Olnick and Weens found residual pyloric deformity in 15 from 5 months to 22 years afterward.

Infants who continue to vomit after surgery should be examined radiologically in order to evaluate the success of the operation. If the vomiting is due to inadequate incision of the pyloric muscle, changes similar to those described preoperatively will be found—e.g., antral beak, delayed gastric emptying, and a long stenotic pyloric canal. Vomiting after an adequate Ramstedt procedure may be due to chalasia, partial thoracic stomach, or associated duodenal obstruction.

INFLAMMATORY DISEASES

Gastric Ulcer

Ulceration of the stomach is uncommon in the pediatric patient. The neonatal group is more susceptible than older children and, in all probability, ulceration of the gastric mucosa in the newborn group is more common than realized, only those lesions complicated by bleeding or perforation being suspected or diagnosed, the others healing without incident. Ulceration of the stomach or duodenum in this age group apparently is always acute and does not become chronic, as in older children and adults.

The reason for development of gastric ulcer in the neonatal period is not definitely known. Historically there are several theories, some or all of which may be pertinent. Because of the relatively common development of gastric ulcers in older patients with central nervous system lesions, such as brain tumors, bulbar poliomyelitis, meningitis, and encephalitis, the neural mechanism of Cushing may be applicable in infants who have suffered brain injury. Another closely related theory is the humoral or "stress" theory, which presupposes that gastric ulceration is mediated through the hypothalmic-pituitary-adrenal cortical axis. A third but less plausible theory is that overdistention of the stomach

by swallowed air ruptures one or more of the small vessels in the mucous membrane, resulting in local necrosis and digestion of the altered mucosa by gastric juices.

The more current and accepted explanation of gastric ulceration in the neonate is similar to that already given in the section on esophageal ulceration—hypoxic changes secondary to the "dive reflex."

Regardless of the sequence of events leading to ulcer in the newborn, the gastric acidity undoubtedly plays a major role. It has been shown that within a few hours after birth there is a sharp increase in gastric acidity which reaches a maximum level in 24 hours. This sudden rise in acidity and its action on an unconditioned mucosa is probably important in neonatal gastric ulceration when associated with other conditions which may lower the resistance of the mucosa.

Gastric ulcers in older infants and children are uncommon, and are probably similar in etiology and development to gastric ulcer in the adult (see *duodenal ulcer*). The older child with a gastric ulcer is usually tense and overactive, and frequently has emotional problems.

Although the Zollinger-Ellison syndrome is rare in children, it should be considered in cases of chronic or recurrent gastric ulcer. The associated dilatation or "colonization" of the duodenum due to the abundant secretions is, as in the adult, a helpful diagnostic finding.

SYMPTOMS. Gastric ulceration in the neonatal infant is suspected only if hematemesis or perforation occurs. Hematemesis at this age is often the result of esophageal or gastric ulceration, and roentgenologic investigation is rarely performed.

Perforation of a gastric ulcer is usually found at surgery for investigation of pneumoperitoneum. An abdominal scout film will disclose the pneumoperitoneum, but radiographic demonstration of the gastrointestinal tract with positive contrast is contraindicated.

Abdominal pain is a more common symptom of gastric ulcer in older infants and children. The pain motivates a roentgenologic investigation of the upper gastrointestinal tract and a gastric ulcer may be discovered. Hematemesis and perforation may occur in the older group but apparently is less likely than in the newborn.

ROENTGENOLOGIC EXAMINATION. Recumbent and upright films of the abdomen should precede fluoroscopy. If pneumoperitoneum is present, causes other than perforated ulcer such as defects in the gastric musculature and other intrauterine stress or anoxia-produced ulcerations in other parts of the intestinal tract should be suspected. The administration of contrast material, as well as other radiologic procedures, is omitted if pneumoperitoneum is present, and the nature of the perforation determined during laparotomy. Pneumoperitoneum in the newborn period is often extensive, producing a more striking roentgenogram than usually seen in the adult. Occasionally, however, a small amount of air is present, and this is usually apparent on the upright film. A lateral film of the abdomen with the infant supine may at times be more helpful in demonstrating free air in the peritoneal cavity (Fig. 10–10). If there is no evidence of free peritoneal air, fluoroscopy of the infant's stomach is carried out in a manner described in Chapter 2.

Barium is administered through a bottle so that the esophagus also may be examined. Gastric ulcer in this age group is frequently impossible to detect because of its minute size. It is most often on the lesser curvature of the antrum and is identified as a small crater. Multiple ulcerations are apt to be present in the young infant. In the older child the crater is more easily identified. However, at any age a gastric ulcer may be overlooked unless the patient is positioned properly and adequate spot films are obtained (Fig. 10–11). A greater curvature ulcer in a child is extremely rare. We have seen one in a 10-year-old child which did not project beyond the boundary of the greater curvature and had the radiologic characteristics of a malignant ulcer seen in the adult (Fig. 10–12). The patient's gastric acidity was elevated and cytologic studies of the gastric secretions were negative. Although surgical investigation was advised, the patient was put on a medical regime, and subsequent studies made elsewhere several months later showed com-

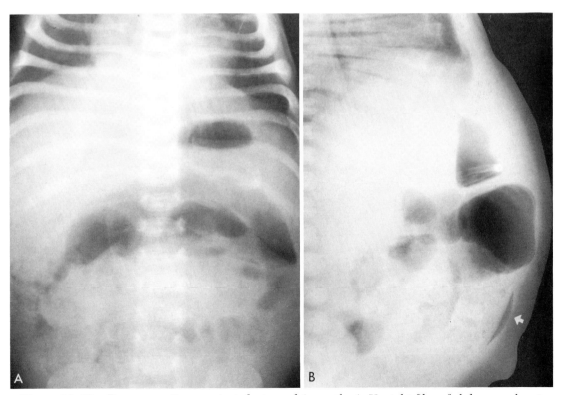

Figure 10–10. Pneumoperitoneum in infant, aged 1 month. *A*, Upright film of abdomen, showing no evidence of free air. *B*, Lateral supine film, showing small collection of free peritoneal air (arrow).

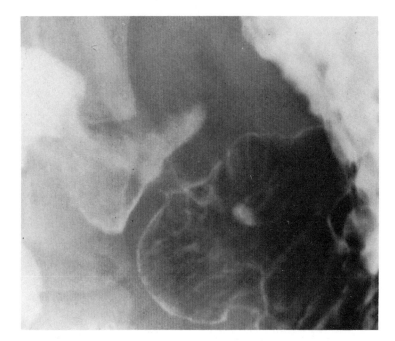

Figure 10–11. Small gastric ulcer in a 14-year-old girl seen only with the patient in the supine position, allowing the antrum to fill with air.

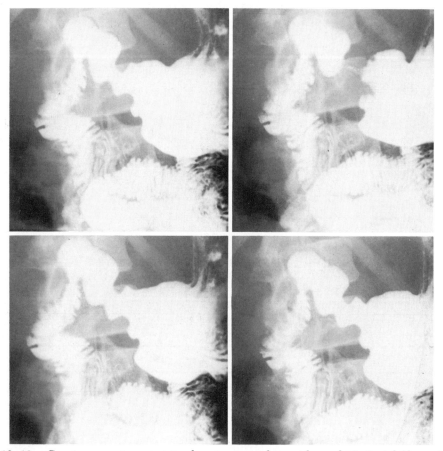

Figure 10–12. Greater curvature gastric ulcer in stomach in girl, aged 10. Serial films of the distal portion of the stomach show filling defect with associated ulcer on greater curvature of antrum. After a short period of medical therapy, the ulcer and associated filling defect disappeared completely.

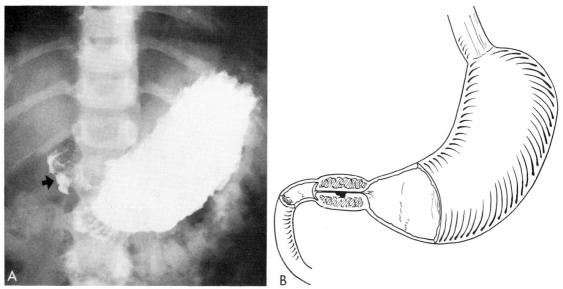

Figure 10–13. Hypertrophic pyloric stenosis with gastric ulcer. Girl, aged 2½, with history of repeated vomiting attacks. *A,* Upper gastrointestinal examination, showing elongated narrowed pyloric canal with compression of enlarged muscle on atrum and duodenal bulb as well as delayed gastric emptying. Irregular ulceration is identified on the greater curvature side of the elongated pylorus (arrow). *B,* Drawing showing surgical findings.

plete disappearance of the ulcer. We have seen also a 2½-year-old child with radiologic signs of hypertrophic pyloric stenosis and a gastric ulcer (Fig. 10–13).

Varicella gastritis with gastric ulceration is extremely rare but should be considered if ulcer symptoms develop in a patient with chickenpox (Fig. 10–14).

Most infants and children swallow a moderate amount of air during the inges-

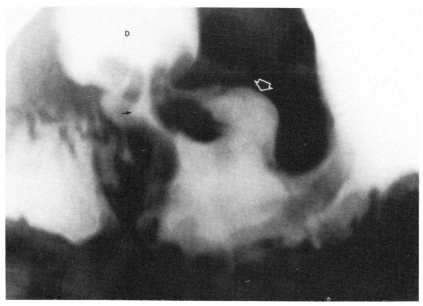

Figure 10–14. Probable varicella gastric ulcers (arrow) in an 8-year-old girl. The ulcers were persistent on numerous spot films (*D*, duodenum). (Courtesy of C. J. Baker et al., *South Med. J.,* **66**:539, 1973.)

tion of barium. This is utilized to obtain films with the child supine and the right side elevated. By this maneuver the air fills the antrum and produces a double contrast effect, making small defects in the mucous membrane of the antrum more discernible. A similar double contrast study of the body and fundus may be obtained by turning the patient to the prone position. If insufficient air is swallowed a small amount of carbonated beverage may be given to introduce gas into the stomach. Although the use of mineral oil is of value in obtaining a similar double contrast effect in the adult patient, its use in children is impractical because of their reluctance to swallow the substance.

In the infant and the older child there may be additional signs of gastric inflammatory disease, consisting of hyperperistalsis and increased prominence of the gastric rugae. The latter is not evident in the neonatal group because of the underdevelopment of the rugae at this age.

The roentgenologic identification of the small acute ulcer in the newborn is seldom repeated because of the rapidity with which it heals. However, follow-up examinations of the older child with a chronic ulcer are essential in evaluating the course of healing.

Eosinophilic Gastroenteritis

This is apparently an allergic condition which may affect the stomach of a child. It should not be confused with eosinophilic granuloma of the stomach. Epigastric pain and vomiting and occasionally gastrointestinal bleeding occur. There is usually a history of allergy and invariably a blood eosinophilia. Pathologically there is thickening of the bowel wall with extensive infiltration of inflammatory cells, predominately eosinophils.

Radiographically, hypertrophic rugal folds usually involve the pylorus and antral area with resulting narrowing and occasionally obstruction (Fig. 10–15). The roentgenologic changes are similar to those seen in lymphosarcoma. The condition is usually self-limiting and after a period of several weeks symptoms and radiologic abnormalities disappear.

Thickening of the gastral rugal folds and concentric narrowing of the gastric antrum may occur in chronic granulomatous disease of childhood and should be considered in the differential diagnosis of eosinophilic

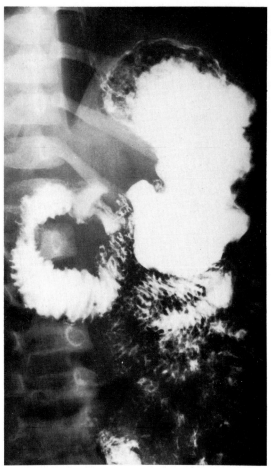

Figure 10–15. Eosinophilic gastroenteritis in a 5-year-old child. Gastrointestinal series shows marked coarsening of the rugal folds of the stomach, duodenum, and proximal jejunum. Surgical exploration provided the diagnosis. Reexamination two months later showed no abnormality of the stomach. (Reprinted with permission from *Semin. Roentgenol.*, **6**:233, 1971.)

gastroenteritis and Crohn's disease of the stomach.

Ménétrier's Disease

Ménétrier's disease is rare in the pediatric age group. The cause is unknown and radiographically differentiation from eosinophilic gastritis may be difficult, both conditions showing hypertrophy of the rugal folds (Fig. 10–16). However, in Ménétrier's disease loss of protein from the intestinal tract is common and consequently the clinical findings are usually those of other protein-losing enteropathies.

Other important features include anemia and diminished serum protein. The disease

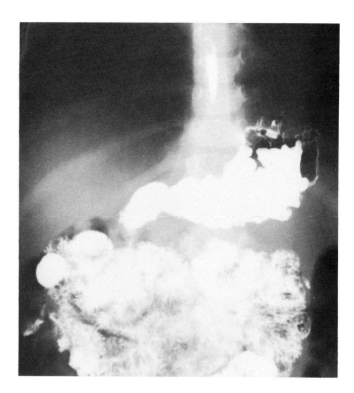

Figure 10–16. Ménétrier's disease in 2-year-old girl with anasarca and protein-losing enteropathy. Proved by peroral capsule biopsy.

may involve the small bowel as well as stomach; it is a reversible process, and is benign in the pediatric patient.

Gastric Syphilis and Tuberculosis

Gastric inflammatory disease caused by syphilis or tuberculosis is extremely uncommon in children but has been reported. Mendl described the radiographic appearance of syphilitic gastritis in a 10-year-old girl. The child's stomach was small, contracted, and tapered in the pyloric region, resembling linitis plastica (Fig. 10–17).

Gastric tuberculosis is always secondary to pulmonary tuberculosis. It is identified radiologically as a chronic ulcer, usually on the lesser curvature and indistinguishable from other, nontuberculous ulcers.

Emphysematous Gastritis

Emphysematous gastritis is most unusual in infants and children but may occur in pneumatosis intestinalis and may on rare occasions occur with severe gastric outlet obstruction such as duodenal atresia or severe pyloric stenosis (Fig. 10–18). We have

seen one case of emphysematous gastritis produced by *Clostridium* infection (Fig. 10–19). In all cases radiographs show gas outlining a portion of the gastric wall.

Corrosive Gastritis

Gastritis due to the ingestion of irritants is less common than esophagitis. Most of the caustic substances which may be accessible to the young child are alkalis which, when swallowed, severely damage the esophagus but are considerably neutralized by the acidity of the stomach contents. However, some of the newer liquid concentrated alkalis may produce severe gastritis and gangrene. Occasionally, concentrated acid compounds are ingested and cause severe damage to the stomach.

Symptoms consist of persistent vomiting, the vomitus containing varying amounts of blood ranging from mere streaking to frank hematemesis. Epigastric pain is present and increases in severity if perforation occurs.

ROENTGENOLOGIC EXAMINATION. In the acute stage radiographic study is unnecessary and ill-advised. After abdominal pain and vomiting have abated, fluorosco-

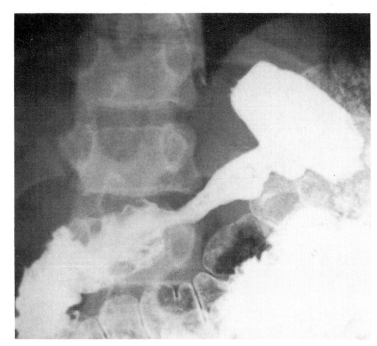

Figure 10-17. Syphilis of stomach in girl, aged 10. Distal two thirds of stomach are constricted as in radiographic picture of linitis plastica. (Courtesy of Dr. K. Mendl, Swansea, Wales. Reprinted from *Br. J. Radiol.*, **29**:48, 1956.)

Figure 10-18. Pneumatosis intestinalis involving the stomach in an infant with necrotizing enterocolitis. Proved at autopsy.

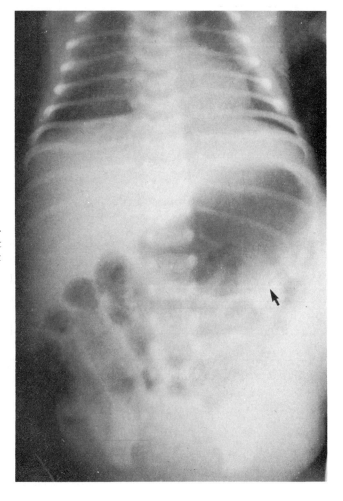

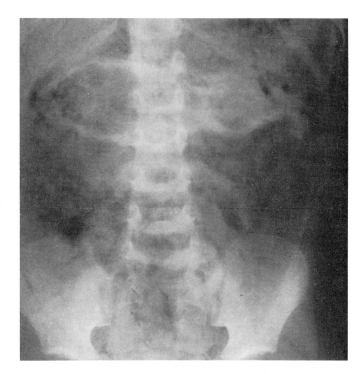

Figure 10-19. String bean bezoar causing emphysematous gastroenteritis in a hemophiliac with *Clostridium* infection of the gastric wall. (Courtesy of Dr. Alexander Margulis, Univ. of California.)

pic studies may be carefully performed. The peristaltic activity may be accentuated if the irritation has been mild, or atonic if severe. Multiple minute serrations may be present along the margins of the stomach; these represent multiple ulcerations in the mucosa. Larger, more definite ulcers may also be identified. Later, after cicatricial changes have occurred, the stomach is smaller and its contour distorted in the areas of greatest fibrosis. Scarring in the pyloric region may produce complete obstruction, and in such cases there are often distention of the esophagus and incompetence of the gastroesophageal junction.

The introduction of calcium chloride into the stomach of the newborn for treatment of neonatal tetany has led to severe necrotizing gastritis of the stomach and upper small bowel (Fig. 10–20). In such cases the concentration of the solution has always been greater than the recommended 2%. Similar severe gastritis may follow the ingestion of ferrous sulfate tablets (Fig. 10–21) and zinc chloride. In both situations, deformity of the stomach develops similar to other forms of corrosive gastritis. Early calcification of the necrotic mucosa has been reported following calcium chloride administration. The harmful effects of calcium

chloride on the infant's stomach are presumably due to hydrolysis and formation of hydrochloric acid which damages the gastric mucosa. The pathogenesis of the calcium deposition is probably similar to that of calcification of necrotic tissue, which may occur in any portion of the body.

FOREIGN BODIES

Radiographic examination of the chest and the abdomen to locate an ingested foreign body is one of the more common x-ray examinations in young children. It would appear that nearly any object the child is able to place in its mouth can be swallowed. Many of these objects lodge in the esophagus, but the majority pass into the stomach, where they remain for a varying length of time.

RADIOLOGIC EXAMINATION. Unless the object is metallic, it usually cannot be identified. Several views may be necessary to localize the object within the stomach accurately. Fluoroscopy will show movement of the foreign body in the confines of the stomach. When the patient lies supine, the object usually falls into the dependent fundus, and when the patient is turned on

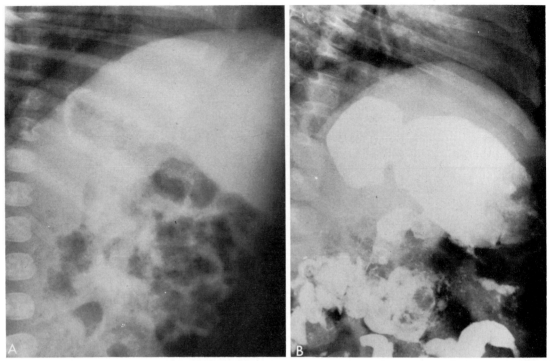

Figure 10-20. Necrotizing gastritis following gavage feeding of calcium chloride for treatment of neonatal tetany. *A*, Lateral view of abdomen two weeks later, showing calcification in fundus of stomach. *B*, Upper gastrointestinal examination made after recovery, showing persistent cicatricial deformity of stomach. (Courtesy of Dr. W. C. Hall. Reprinted from *Am. J. Roentgenol. Radium Ther. Nucl. Med.*, **66**:204, 1951.)

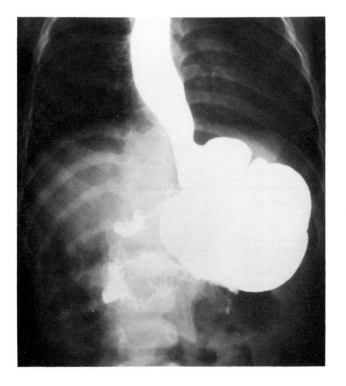

Figure 10-21. Caustic deformity of the distal stomach following ferrous sulfate tablet ingestion. (Reprinted with permission from *Semin. Roentgenol.*, 6:232, 1971.)

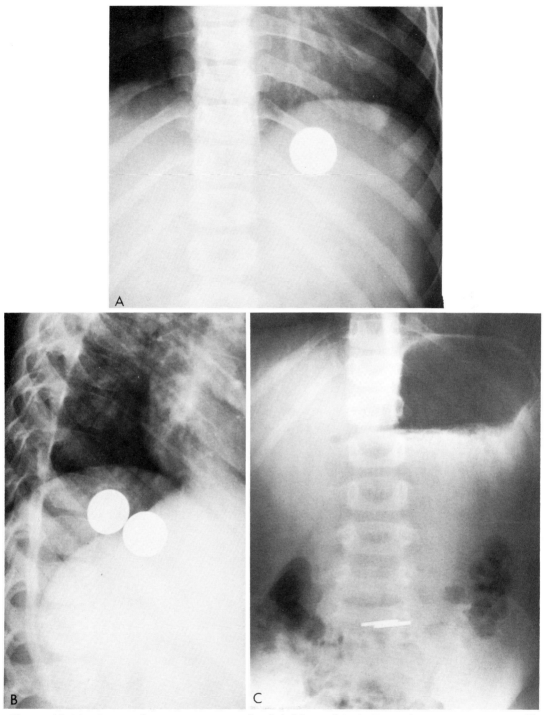

Figure 10–22. Ingested pennies in stomach of child, aged 3. *A*, Recumbent anteroposterior film of abdomen, showing what appears to be single coin in fundus. *B*, Lateral view, showing that there are actually two coins. *C*, Upright film showing shift of coins into antrum, thereby definitely localizing them in gastric lumen.

his right side or stands, it drops anteriorly into the antrum (Fig. 10–22). If after this maneuver the true location of the object is still indefinite, the patient is given a drink of barium; the object will then, if in the stomach, be confined within the barium silhouette. Nonopaque objects may be identified in this manner as filling defects in the stomach. The smaller objects pass within a few hours into the small intestine, but the larger ones may remain in the stomach for several days before passing into the duodenum. A watchful attitude is advisable when the objects are round and smooth-edged. However, because of the danger of elongated, sharp-pointed objects such as bobby pins and large needles or nails perforating the duodenum, they should be removed with an alnico magnet (Fig. 10–23). Unfortunately, present-day metallic objects are rarely magnetic and conse-

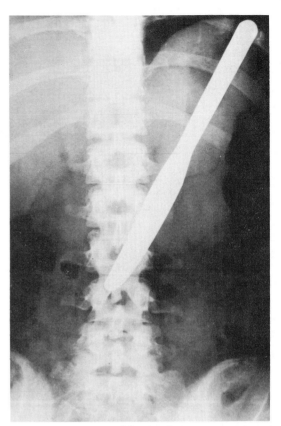

Figure 10–24. Table knife in stomach of psychopathic girl, aged 12. Removed surgically. (Courtesy of Dr. A. O. Singleton, Jr., Univ. of Texas.)

quently the use of this method of removal is rarely possible. If the object is not magnetic and is small enough to pass the duodenal loop, we allow it to pass into the jejunum where, if it lodges, it is promptly removed by surgery. The foreign body illustrated in Figure 10–24 naturally had to be removed by gastrostomy, whereas the earring seen in Figure 10–25 passed spontaneously.

BEZOARS

Indigestible organic material that accumulates in the stomach forms a ball-shaped mass, or bezoar. Hairballs, or trichobezoars, are the most common types and result from the ingestion of hair plucked from the head or less often from the swallowing of down from a blanket or furry toy. Trichobezoars are usually found in girls because of their

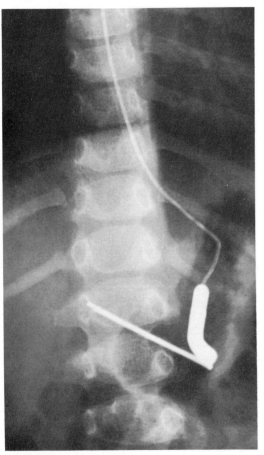

Figure 10–23. Bobby pin in stomach being removed by alnico magnet.

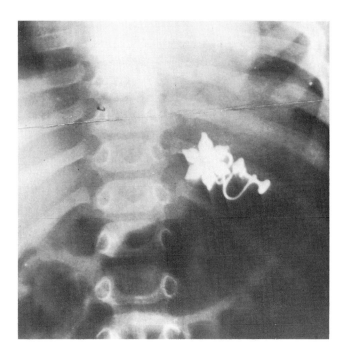

Figure 10-25. Ingested earring in the stomach of a young infant. The object passed without complication.

longer hair. The next most common type is the phytobezoar, which is composed of vegetable matter, usually persimmon seeds and skins. The hydrochloric acid of the stomach transforms a phlobatannin in the unripe fruit into a sticky coagulum, which remains in the stomach. Tar, shellac, and a variety of other bezoars have been reported.

Symptoms produced by the intragastric bezoar include anorexia, weakness, malaise, vague upper gastrointestinal complaints, hematemesis, and often a palpable epigastric mass. Occasionally, acute gastric obstruction ensues.

RADIOLOGIC EXAMINATION. A scout film of the abdomen may disclose the bezoar if there is sufficient air in the stomach. In such cases, the bezoar, if large enough, casts a silhouette of soft tissue density within the lumen of the stomach. After the ingestion of barium, the filling defect is obvious (Figs. 10–26 and 10–27). Fluoroscopically, the barium on reaching the stomach will, if the bezoar is large, hesitate at the cardia, then trickle down and around the mass. Smaller bezoars can be moved about in the stomach. After the barium has left the stomach, the bezoar remains impregnated with the contrast material and appears as a mottled, partially opaque, and radiolucent filling defect within the stomach. A segment of the bezoar, especially trichobezoar, may extend into the small intestine.

Lactobezoar is an uncommon form of bezoar seen within the first few months of life in infants whose formula consists of inadequately hydrated powdered milk or other highly concentrated milk substances. Symptoms consist of vomiting and diarrhea, and occasionally gastrointestinal bleeding. The bulky formula not only produces a coagulum within the stomach, but becomes even more inspissated as fluid is absorbed from the bezoar to compensate for the patient dehydration.

A varying sized movable mass is palpable in the left upper quadrant. It can often be outlined by air within the stomach or clearly confirmed with an upper gastrointestinal series. Therapy should be conservative and generally consists of intravenous medication. Spontaneous resolution of the bezoar will usually occur, but gastric obstruction and perforation can result.

VARICES

Gastric varices with severe portal hypertension develop as do esophageal varices. Because of the normally prominent gastric rugae, the radiologic detection of gastric

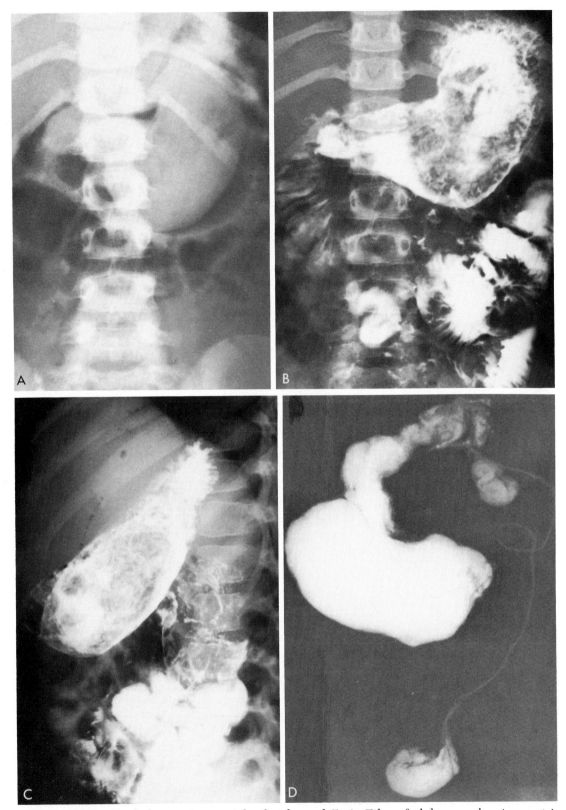

Figure 10–26. Trichobezoar in stomach of girl, aged 5. A, Film of abdomen, showing gastric intraluminal mass outlined by air in the stomach. B, Ingested barium, showing large filling defect which, on lateral view (C), is noted to extend into the duodenum. D, At gastrostomy large hair ball linked with a smaller hair ball in the duodenum by a slender twisted cord of hair was removed.

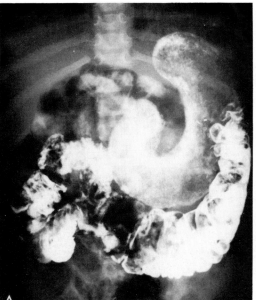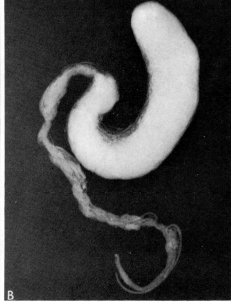

Figure 10–27. Trichobezoar in a 3-year-old child who habitually swallowed strings and her own hair. *A,* Barium outlines the large hair ball in the stomach. *B,* Removed hair ball specimen impregnated with barium.

varicosities is usually impossible. Occasionally, however, extensive varices may be detected (Fig. 10–28). A splenic venogram is useful in determining the extent of the involvement accurately.

EXTRINSIC PRESSURE

Extrinic pressure on the stomach can be detected only if the stomach is distended by air or contrast material. A pressure defect on the lesser curvature is usually due to enlargement of the left lobe of the liver. Distortion or medial displacement of the greater curvature results from splenomegaly. Occasionally, interposition of the enlarged spleen between the gastric fundus and left hemidiaphragm is observed. Anterior displacement of the stomach is usually due to a pancreatic cyst or retroperitoneal (often renal) mass. Mesenteric and omental cysts will displace the stomach posteriorly and often superiorly, producing an indentation in the inferior portion of the greater curvature.

NEOPLASMS

Benign neoplasms of the stomach, usually hamartomas, adenomas, myomas or teratomas may occur in the pediatric patient, but are extremely rare. They are identified only after contrast material is introduced into the stomach, where they appear as filling defects in the barium mixture. The usual symptom leading to radiologic investigation is gastrointestinal bleeding or intussusception. Gastric hamartomas may occur in the Peutz-Jeghers syndrome (Fig. 10–29) and although these are theoretically benign lesions, adenocarcinoma of the stomach has been reported in a child with this syndrome.

HEMANGIOMA

Hemangioma of the stomach as an isolated lesion is rare and is more commonly seen with multiple hemangiomas of other portions of the intestinal tract or other viscera, or with subcutaneous hemangiomas. Gastrointestinal bleeding is the usual symptom. Gastric hemangiomas are more easily identified by routine upper gastrointestinal tract studies, whereas small bowel lesions may require selective arteriographic studies for localization. Radiographically, the lesion may produce an irregular filling defect, depending upon its size (Fig. 10–30). It may also be part of the Osler-Weber-Rendu syndrome.

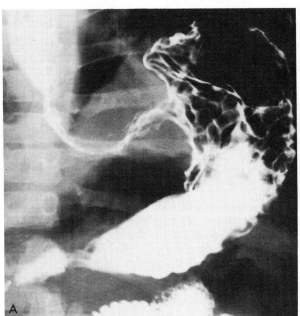
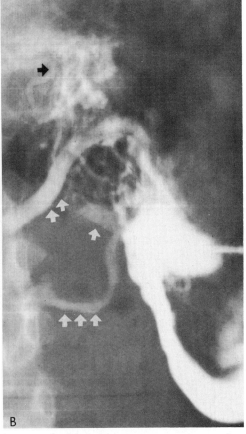

Figure 10-28. Gastric varices in child, aged 5, with portal hypertension. *A*, Stomach examination showing multiple filling defects most noticeable along lesser curvature and constricting cardia. Involvement of esophagus is also evident. *B*, Percutaneous splenic venogram, demonstrating extensive varicosities involving mainly the coronary veins and short gastric veins along lesser curvature (black arrow). *Single white arrow*—an obstructed splenic vein; *double white arrows*—gastroepiploic vein; *triple white arrows*—an aberrant vein extending between spleen and inferior vena cava.

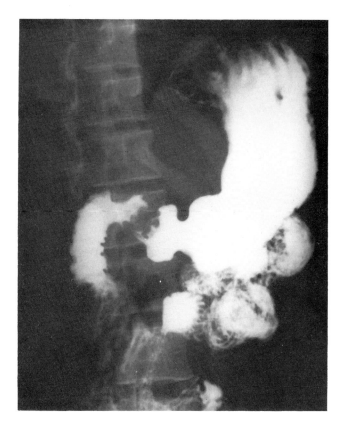

Figure 10–29. 17-year-old girl with Peutz-Jeghers syndrome. Filling defect in the prepyloric area was found at surgery to be a hamartoma.

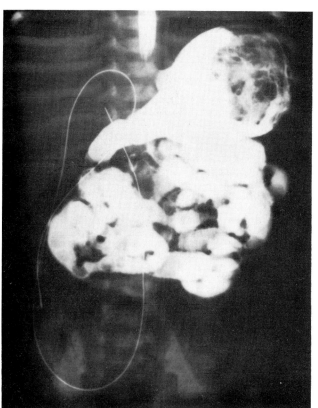

Figure 10–30. Young infant with hemangioma. Filling defect in the stomach was found at surgery to be a hemangioma.

REFERENCES

Hypertrophic Pyloric Stenosis

Belding, H. H., III, and Kernohan, J. W. Morphologic study of myenteric plexus and musculature of pylorus with special reference to changes in hypertrophic pyloric stenosis, Surg. Gynec. Obstet., 97:322, 1953.

Currarino, G. The value of double-contrast examination of the stomach with pressure "spots" in the diagnosis of infantile hypertrophic pyloric stenosis, Radiology, 83:873, 1964.

Faber, H. K., and Davis, J. H. Gastric peristalsis after pylorotomy in infants, J.A.M.A., 114:837, 1940.

Feinberg, S. B., Margulis, A. R., and Nice, C. M. Dehydration and deficiency of intestinal gas in infants with hypertrophic pyloric stenosis, Am. J. Roentgenol. Radium Ther. Nucl. Med., 76:551, 1956.

Haran, P. G., Darling, D. B., and Seiammas, F. F. The value of the double-track sign as a differentiating factor between pylorospasm and hypertrophic pyloric stenosis, Radiology, 86:723, 1966.

Laron, Z., and Horne, L. M. The incidence of infantile pyloric stenosis, Am. J. Dis. Child., 94:151, 1957.

LeWald, L. T. Roentgenologic examination of the digestive tract of infants and children, Radiology, 21:221, 1933.

Meuwissen, T., and Sloof, J. P. Roentgenologic diagnosis of congenital hypertrophic pyloric stenosis, Acta Paediatr., 14:19, 1932.

Morse, J. L., et al. Case of infantile pyloric stenosis with autopsy, Boston M. S. J., 158:480, 1908.

Olnick, II. M., and Weens, II. S. Roentgen manifestations of infantile hypertrophic pyloric stenosis, J. Pediatr., 34:720, 1949.

Riggs, W., and Long, L. The value of the plain film roentgenogram in pyloric stenosis. Am. J. Roentgenol. Radium Ther. Nucl. Med., 112:77, 1971.

Rintoul, J. R., and Kirkman, N. F. The myenteric plexus in infantile hypertrophic stenosis, Arch. Dis. Child., 36:474, 1961.

Runstrom, G. On roentgen-anatomical appearance of congenital pyloric stenosis during and after the manifest stage of the disease, Acta Paediatr., 26:383, 1939.

Seaman, W. B. Hypertrophy of the pyloric muscle in adults, Radiology, 80:753, 1963.

Shopfner, C. E. The pyloric tit in hypertrophic pyloric stenosis, Am. J. Roentgenol. Radium Ther. Nucl. Med., 91:674, 1964.

Shopfner, C. E., Kalmon, E. H., Jr., and Coin, C. G. The diagnosis of hypertrophic pyloric stenosis. Am. J. Roentgenol. Radium Ther. Nucl. Med., 91:796, 1964.

Shuman, F. I., Darling, D. B., Fisher, J. H. The radiographic diagnosis of congenital hypertrophic pyloric stenosis, J. Pediatr., 71:70, 1967.

Wallgren, A. Incidence of hypertrophic pyloric stenosis, Am. J. Dis. Child., 62:751, 1941.

Wallgren, A. Preclinical stage of infantile hypertrophic pyloric stenosis, Am. J. Dis. Child., 72:371, 1946.

Weens, H. S., and Golden, A. Adrenal cortical insufficiency in infants simulating high intestinal obstruction, Am. J. Roentgenol. Radium Ther. Nucl. Med., 74:213, 1955.

Woolley, M. M., Felsher, B. F., Asch, M. J., Carpio, N., and Isaacs, H. Jaundice, hypertrophic pyloric stenosis, and hepatic glucuronyl transferase, J. Pediatr. Surg., 9:359, 1974.

Inflammatory Diseases

Binder, I., et al. Tuberculosis of stomach with special reference to its incidence in children, Gastroenterology, 5:474, 1945.

Burns, B., and Gay, B. B., Jr. Menetrier's disease of the stomach in children, An. J. Roentgenol. Radium Ther. Nucl. Med. 103:300, 1968.

Ebers, D. W., Smith, D. I., and Gibbs, G. E. Gastric acidity on the first day of life, Pediatrics, 18:800, 1956.

Edelman, M. J., and March, T. L.: Eosinophilic gastroenteritis, Am. J. Roentgenol. Radium Ther. Nucl. Med., 91:773, 1964.

Griscom, N. T., Kirkpatrick, J. A., Girdany, B. R., Berdon, W. E., Grand, R. J., and Mackie, G. G. Gastral antral narrowing in chronic granulomatous disease of childhood, Pediatrics, 54:456, 1974.

Hall, W. C. Roentgen changes in upper intestinal tract following use of calcium chloride in neonatal tetany, Am. J. Roentgenol. Radium Ther. Nucl. Med., 66:204, 1951.

Henry, G. W.: Emphysematous gastritis, Am. J. Roentgenol. Radium Ther. Nucl. Med., 68:15, 1952.

Holgersen, L. O., Borns, P. F., and Srouji, M. N. Isolated gastric pneumatosis, J. Pediatr. Surg., 9:813, 1974.

Lachman, R. S., Martin, D. J., and Vawter, G. F. Thick gastric folds in childhood, Am. J. Roentgenol. Radium Ther. Nucl. Med., 112:83, 1971.

Lemak, L. L. Roentgenological manifestations of gastroduodenal ulceration (gastric ulcer) in the newborn, Am. J. Roentgenol. Radium Ther. Nucl. Med., 66:191, 1951.

Lloyd, J. R. The etiology of gastrointestinal perforation in the newborn, J. Pediatr. Surg., 4:77, 1969.

Martel, W. Radiologic features of esophagogastritis secondary to extremely caustic agents, Radiology, 103:31, 1972.

Mendl, K., Jenkins, R. T., and Hughes, J. R. Congenital and acquired syphilis of stomach: with special reference to gastric deformity in various stages, and a report of two cases, Br. J. Radiol., 29:48, 1956.

Mendl, K., Jenkins, R. T., and Penlington, E. R. Gastric ulcer in the newborn and its association with antral spasm resulting in hypertrophic pyloric stenosis, Br. J. Radiol., 35:831, 1962.

Miller, R. A. Observations on gastric acidity during first month of life, Arch. Dis. Child., 16:22, 1941.

Pinto, R. S., Zausner, J., and Beranbaum, E. R. Gastric tuberculosis: a report of a case with discussion of angiographic findings, Am. J. Roentgenol. Radium Ther. Nucl. Med., 110:808, 1970.

Robinson, A. E., Grossman, H., and Brumley, G. W. Pneumatosis intestinalis in the neonate, Am. J. Roentgenol. Radium Ther. Nucl. Med., 120:333, 1974.

Rosenlund, M. L. The Zollinger-Ellison syndrome in children; a review, Am. J. Med., 245:884, 1967.

Stevens, H., Guin, G. H., and Gilbert, E. F. Gastrointestinal ulceration in central nervous system lesions, Am. J. Dis. Child., 106:613, 1963.

Tudor, R. B. Peptic ulceration in childhood, Pediatr. Clin. North Am., 14:109, 1967.

Vuthibhagdee, A., and Harris, N. F. Antral stricture and the delayed complication of iron intoxication, Radiology, 103:163, 1972.

Wilmers, M. J., and Heriot, A. M. Pyloric stenosis complicating acute poisoning by ferrous sulphate, Lancet, 2:68, 1954.

Foreign Bodies

Alexander, W. J., Kadish, J. A., and Dunbar, J. S. Ingested foreign bodies in children, Progr. Pediatr. Radiol., 2:256, 1969.

Equen, M. *Magnetic Removal of Foreign Bodies* (Springfield, Ill.: Charles C Thomas, Publisher, 1957).

Laff, H. I., and Allen, R. P. Management of foreign objects in alimentary tract, J. Pediatr., 48:563, 1956.

Bezoars

Cremin, B. J., Fisher, R. M., Stockes, M. J., and Rabkin, J. Four cases of lactobezoar in neonates, Pediatr. Radiol., 2:107, 1974.

Cremin, B. J., Smythe, P. M., and Cywes, S. The radiologic appearance of the "inspissated milk syndrome"; a cause of intestinal obstruction in infants, Br. J. Radiol., 43:856, 1970.

DeBakey, M., and Ochsner, A. Bezoars and concretions: Comprehensive review of literature with analysis of 303 collected cases and presentation of eight additional cases, Surgery, 4:934, 1938.

Levkoff, A. H., Gadsden, R. H., Hennigar, G. R., and Webb, C. M. Lactobezoar and gastric perforation in a neonate, J. Pediatr., 77:875, 1970.

Wolf, R. S., and Davis, L. A. Lactobezoar, a foreign body formed by the use of undiluted powdered milk substance. J.A.M.A., 184:782, 1963.

Varices

Buonocore, E., Collmann, I. R., Kerley, H. A., and Lester, T. L. Massive upper gastrointestinal hemorrhage in children, Am. J. Roentgenol. Radium Ther. Nucl. Med., 115:289, 1972.

Evans, J. A., and Delany, F. Gastric varices, Radiology, 60:46, 1953.

Fleming, R. J., and Seaman, W. B. Roentgenographic demonstration of unusual extra-esophageal varices, Am. J. Roentgenol Radium Ther. Nucl. Med., 103:281, 1968.

Extrinsic Pressure

Grossman, H., and Redo, S. F. Unusual causes of gastric displacement in children, Radiology, 87:725, 1966.

Neoplasms

Atwell, J. B., Claireaux, A. E., and Nixon, H. H. Teratoma of the stomach in the newborn, J. Pediatr. Surg., 2:197, 1967.

Dozois, R. R., Judd, E. S., Dahlin, D. C., and Bartholomew, L. G. The Peutz-Jeghers syndrome. Is there a predisposition to the development of intestinal malignancy?, Arch. Surg., 98:509, 1969.

Jakubowski, A., Jakubowski, K., Naumik, A., and Pietron, K. Primary Tumors of the stomach in children, Ann. Radiol., 13:169, 1970.

Hemangioma

Halpern, M., Turner, A. F., and Citron, B. P. Hereditary hemorrhagic telangiectasia: An angiographic study of abdominal visceral angiodysplasias associated with gastrointestinal hemorrhage, Radiology, 90:1143, 1968.

Chapter 11

THE NORMAL SMALL INTESTINE

ROENTGENOLOGIC ANATOMY. The small intestine extends from the pyloric canal to the ileocecal junction. It consists of three parts, the duodenum, the jejunum, and the ileum. Each segment has rather distinctive radiologic characteristics, although the junction of one with the other is imperceptible. However, the anatomic position of the duodenojejunal junction is accurately identified posterior to the stomach at the suspensory attachment of the ligament of Treitz. The roentgenologic identification of the segments of small intestine depends on their location in the abdomen and the appearance of their mucosal folds, known as the valvulae conniventes or the plicae circularis. Occasionally the air content of the intestine outlines the folds of jejunal or ileal mucosa, but because of the relative absence of air in the small intestine of older children and the frequent overaccumulation of air in the infant's intestinal tract, the roentgenologic study of the mucosal pattern and the physiology of the small bowel is possible only when it contains opaque material.

The *duodenum*, which is the shortest segment, begins at the distal end of the pyloric canal and consists of a bulb or cap, a descending or vertical portion, and a distal segment which curves superiorly to the left, where it becomes continuous with the jejunum behind the stomach at the ligament of Treitz. In the older child and adult the duodenal bulb is cone-shaped, with a wide base. Variability in the width and length of the bulb is common at all ages. In the infant, the bulb is small and usually round or cylindrical, the cone configuration being less common (Fig. 11–1). Occasionally, however, a miniature replica of the adult bulb is encountered in the young infant. The duodenal bulb in the infant is usually directed more posteriorly than in the older child and adult. Consequently it often cannot be visualized in a direct frontal view but is identified with the infant in a lateral or extreme right anterior oblique position. Because of this posterior direction, the antrum often interferes with optimal visualization of the bulb, but by careful positioning of the patient at the time of fluoroscopy the bulb usually can be thrown clear of the antrum and, if not, can be seen through the gas-distended fundus. The less distended the stomach by contrast material, the more often the infant's bulb can be identified in a frontal view. This is evident from the greater frequency with which the bulb is seen in anteroposterior interval films made after most of the contrast material has left the stomach. The bulb of the older child has less of a posterior direction and extends more prominently to the right. The type of stomach seen in the older child determines to a great extent the form of the duodenal bulb. The child or adult with the J-shaped stomach usually has an elongated, vertical, cone-shaped bulb which extends cephalad to the right and terminates in a narrow apex. With the transverse-type stomach the bulb usually is less conical, shorter, and more horizontal, extending posteriorly and to the right without forming as abrupt an angulation with the second portion of the duodenum. The mucosa of the duodenal bulb is relatively flat, and the margins of the distended bulb are smooth. However, without adequate fill and distention, the contour is irregular.

The second or vertical portion of the duodenum is firmly fixed by its retroperitoneal location and is slightly concave on its medial surface where it curves around the head of the pancreas. The mucosal folds distal to the duodenal bulb are more prominent than those in the bulb, becoming progressively deeper and more closely spaced in the second and third portions of the duodenum. In the newborn and infant, the plicae are not as prominent or deep as in older children and adults. The ampulla

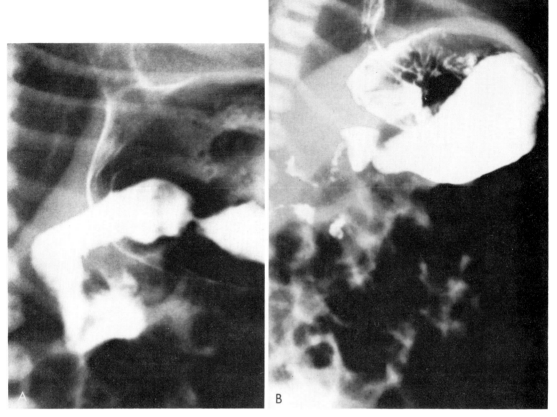

Figure 11–1. Normal duodenal bulb of the neonatal infant. *A*, Usual cylindrical bulb. *B*, Cone-shaped bulb occasionally seen in the young infant but more common in older infants and children.

of Vater is occasionally seen in the adult, but rarely visualized in children. The third portion of the duodenum passes anteriorly and cephalad to the left, crossing the spine and joining the jejunum behind the stomach at the duodenojejunal flexure (ligament of Treitz; Fig. 11–2). The upward oblique course of the superior mesenteric artery not infrequently indents the third portion of the duodenum in asthenic individuals and may cause obstruction in the acute form of the superior mesenteric artery syndrome. The valvulae conniventes in the distal portion are indistinguishable from the pattern of the jejunum. In the young infant, the folds in this area are usually identifiable but not prominent.

The *jejunum*, which consists of approximately three fifths of the jejuno-ilial segment, extends from the duodenojejunal junction at the ligament of Treitz to its junction with the ileum. The point of tran-sition between jejunum and ileum is ill-defined and consists of a gradual change in mucosal pattern. The proximal portion of the jejunum lies in the left upper quadrant of the abdomen, the middle and distal portions of the jejunum in the midabdomen, and the ileum in the lower abdomen and pelvis. The mucosal pattern of the upper jejunum consists of deeply serrated plicae which, when coated with barium, have a characteristic fine, feather, or lacelike pattern. The narrowness and closely packed arrangement of the plicae in the proximal jejunum may occasionally simulate the coiled-spring appearance of an intussusception (Fig. 11–3). After the barium has passed through the jejunum, the particles which remain adherent to the mucosa often produce a snowflake effect (Fig. 11–4). The jejunal plicae become gradually shorter and more widely spaced on progression toward the ileum. In the distal portion of

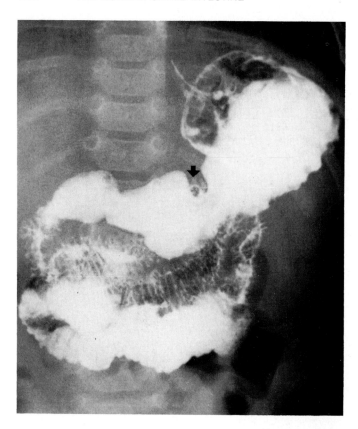

Figure 11-2. Mucosal pattern of duodenum and jejunum of child, aged 3. Plicae become progressively deeper in distal portion of duodenum and proximal jejunum. Duodenojejunal junction is posterior to stomach at ligament of Treitz (*arrow*).

Figure 11-3. Mucosal pattern of proximal jejunum of child, aged 1 year. Plicae are deep and arranged close together, suggesting the coiled-spring appearance of an intussusception.

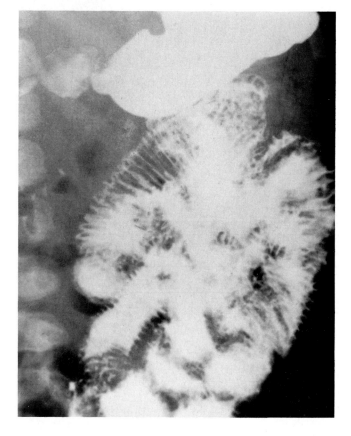

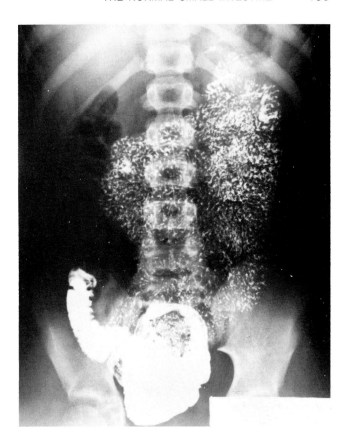

Figure 11-4. Barium which clings to the jejunal mucosa after passage into the terminal small bowel often produces a snowflake or feathery appearance. (Child aged 11.)

the jejunum and the proximal ileum, the folds are no longer feathery or lacelike, but are coarser and have a cog-wheel outline (Fig. 11-5). The mucosal folds become more widely spaced in the midportion of the ileum and, in the distal portion, the borders of the barium column are smooth and tubular. This typical radiographic pattern of the various segments of the small bowel is seldom, though occasionally, seen in the very young infant, but becomes increasingly evident after the fourth or fifth month. The explanation for absence of the characteristic pattern in the neonatal period is not clear, since the plicae are well developed. However, the crevices between the plicae are perhaps too small or blocked by mucus to allow complete filling by the contrast material.

In the ileum, the mucosal pattern of the terminal portion is not clearly identified unless pressure films are obtained or an exposure is made during contractions of this segment of bowel. In such instances three patterns may be encountered, transverse folds, longitudinal folds, or a cobblestone effect produced by the relative large lymphoid patches in children. Wells demonstrated the last pattern radiographically by coating postmortem specimens of normal ileum with contrast material. The resulting roentgenogram showed the multiple filling defects and the cobblestone effect to be due to the normally large Peyer's patches in children. In our experience the cobblestone pattern is most often encountered in children between 3 and 10 years of age (Fig. 11-6A). This is a normal finding and clinical significance should not be attributed to it. In the young infant no definite mucosal pattern is characteristic, but occasionally pressure films will show the longitudinal striations characteristic of the adult ileum, or at times transverse folds (Fig. 11-6B). Abdominal scout films of both the infant and older child occasionally show superior displacement of the terminal small bowel by a distended urinary bladder (Fig. 11-7).

ROENTGENOLOGIC PHYSIOLOGY. The duodenum is difficult to examine in the first few months of life. The transit time of barium through the duodenal loop is rapid, and full distention of the loop is difficult to obtain because of the relatively weak peristaltic action of the stomach and because normal fill of the duodenum by the palpating hand is usually ineffectual due to the high inaccessible position of the stomach. As the gastric activity becomes more prominent and the stomach position more vertical with growth of the child, the radiologic evaluation of the duodenal structures becomes more accurate. This is especially true of the duodenal bulb. In the young infant, the small size of the bulb, its rapid filling and emptying, and the usual lack of full distensibility make it nearly impossible to decide whether a small niche in the bulb is an ulcer or barium caught within the mucosal folds. The posterior position of the infant's bulb and the resulting difficulties in obtaining pressure films accentuate this problem. In older children and adults, there is often hold-up of barium in the bulb, allowing more thorough examination. This is especially true in the vertical-type bulb, due presumably to the angulation at the apex and descending or second portion of the duodenum. Similar hold-up is en-

countered at the duodenojejunal junction, again due to the angulation formed by the ligament of Treitz. As the rapidly propelled barium reaches this point of temporary delay, additional duodenal peristaltic contractions often force barium back into the bulb. This is more common in older children but may be seen in infants.

After barium enters the jejunum, the forward progress is slowed, the diminished activity being present at all ages. Progression in the small intestine consists of a churning, to-and-fro type of peristaltic activity which leads to an uneven but steady forward movement of the intestinal contents. The movements are less prominent and often slower in the young infant. There may be marked retardation of the progression of the meal when it reaches the ileum, where the peristalsis has a more kneading type of action. Entrance of food or additional barium into the stomach will reflexly increase the motility of the ileum and probably also relax the ileocecal valve, thereby allowing passage into the cecum. During peristaltic contractions, the mucosal markings become arranged longitudinally, paral-

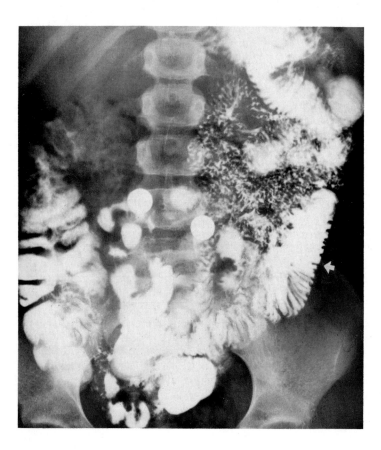

Figure 11–5. Plicae of distal portion of jejunum and proximal ileum are more widely spaced than above and a cog-wheel configuration (*arrow*). (Child aged 7.)

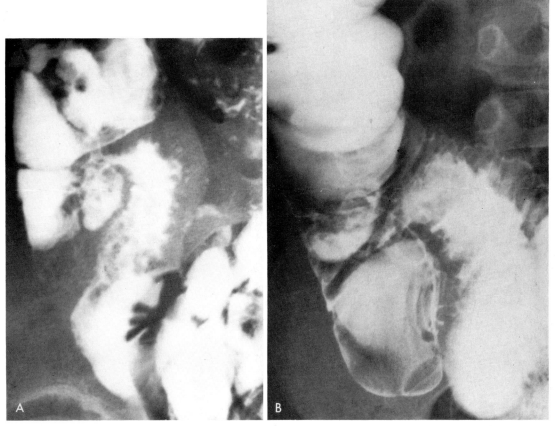

Figure 11-6. Normal ileum. A, Irregular filling defects in terminal ileum represent large lymphoid patches. (Child aged 7.) B, Transverse folds of normal ileum of infant.

lel to the long axis of the bowel (Fig. 11–8), and on relaxing resume their circular configuration. This change in mucosal pattern with peristalsis is usually not apparent during the first four or five months of life.

Because of the wide variation in peristaltic activity at different ages, the transit time of barium through the small intestine is also extremely variable. The position of the patient greatly affects this by delaying the emptying time of the stomach (see Chapter 8, The Normal Stomach). In normal infants and children, the head of the barium column reaches the cecum two to five hours after ingestion; the tail of the column usually passes through the ileocecal valve in seven to eight hours. In the neonatal period transit time is usually slower, the head of the meal reaching the cecum three to six hours after ingestion (Fig. 11–9). Commercially prepared barium products of micro-sized particles pass more rapidly through the intestinal tract of both infants and children. It is not unusual for barium to reach the terminal ileum and cecum in one and one half to two hours after ingestion. Consequently the evaluation of transit time as an index of altered small bowel motility is unreliable.

In the adult and older child the barium column in the small intestine is usually uniform and continuous, without significant gaps in its continuity. An interrupted column accompanied by variation in the width of the barium-filled segments and coarsening or loss of the normal mucosal pattern is known as clumping or segmentation, and is usually indicative of one of several malabsorption syndromes. However, in infants this pattern may be normal. Radiographically, the barium on reaching the small intestine becomes segmented and divided into multiple "puddles." The mucosal margins are ill-defined or coarse, and there is often a marked variation in the width of the scattered segments. The degree of clumping or segmentation is often greatest in the ileum (Fig. 11–10). Occa-

Text continued on page 160.

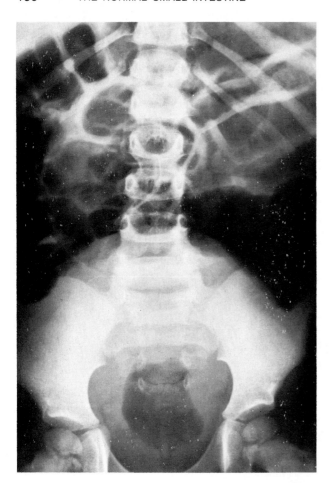

Figure 11-7. Distended urinary bladder causing superior displacement of distal loops of small intestine.

Figure 11-8. Constricted segments of small intestine (*arrows*) represent sites of active peristalsis. During these contractions, mucosal folds become arranged longitudinally, parallel to long axis of bowel.

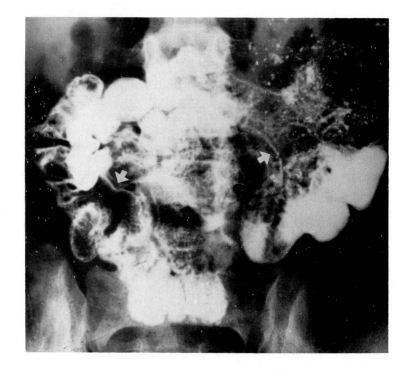

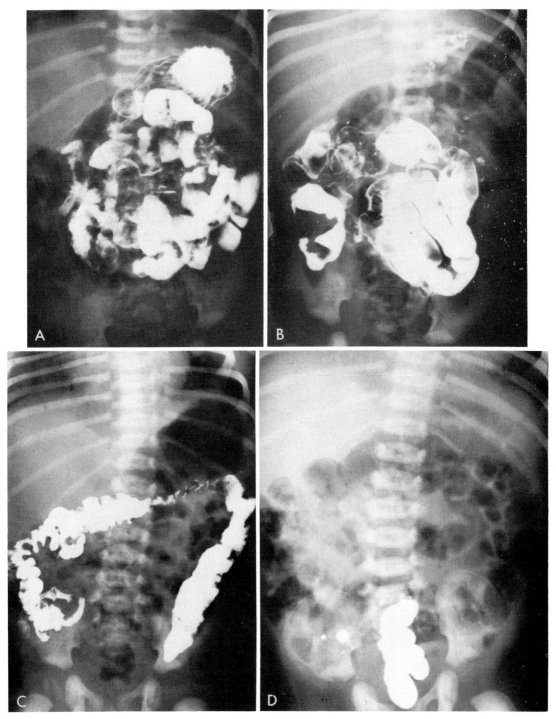

Figure 11-9. Normal passage of barium through gastrointestinal tract of infant, aged 2 weeks. *A*, Forty minutes after ingestion, head of contrast material has reached the ileum. Note smooth outline of mucosal pattern at this age. *B*, Two hours after ingestion head of barium column has reached terminal ileum and stomach is nearly empty. *C*, Eight hours after ingestion, head of barium column has reached sigmoid. *D*, At 24 hours, most of the barium has been expelled but a portion remains in rectum.

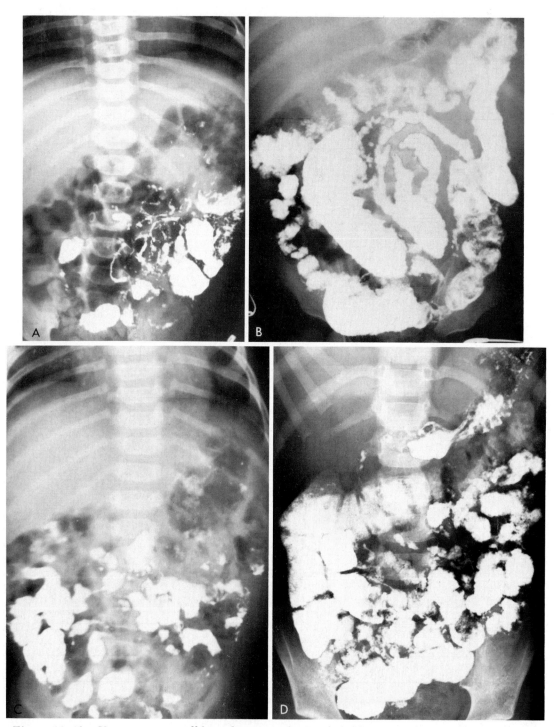

Figure 11–10. Variations in small bowel pattern of normal children. *A*, Infant, aged 3 months. Narrow linear columns of barium should not be mistaken for ascarids. *B*, Child, aged 2. Pronounced segmentation and variation of caliber of bowel. *C*, Infant, aged 2 months. Typical clumping of barium in small bowel. *D*, Child, aged 4. Segmentation in small bowel.

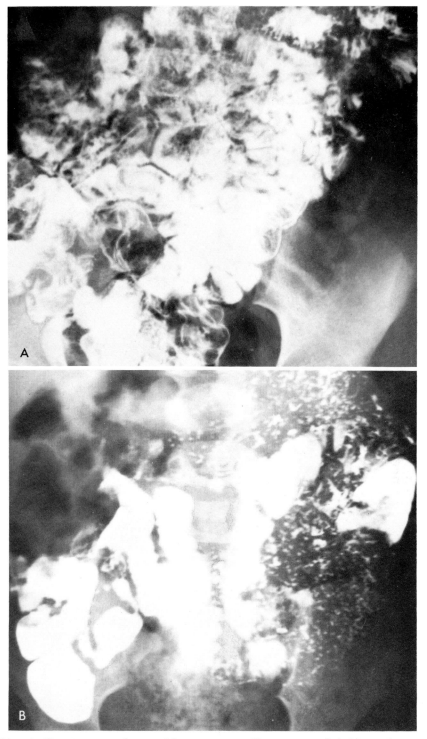

Figure 11–11. A, Continuous column of barium in small intestine of child, aged 2. B, Film exposed 30 minutes later shows marked segmentation of barium.

sionally, a continuous adult type of pattern will, between radiographs, become converted into a segmented clumped column (Fig. 11–11).

The clumped pattern of the small intestine observed with the barium meal in normal infants is apparently produced by mucus, which in turn suggests that there must be an excessive amount of mucus in the intestinal tract of infants and children. Support for this is found in the work of Frazer and Ravdin, who showed that fats, fatty acids, partially hydrolyzed fats, lactic acid, and acetic acid will induce flocculation of barium sulfate in the small intestine, apparently due to the formation of mucus produced by the stimulating effect of these substances. The abundance of lactobacilli in the intestinal tract of infants and children and the lactic acid formed by these organisms is possibly responsible for the mucus content of the child's intestinal tract and the consequent clumping of the barium. It is also possible that in the young infant there normally is an excessive amount of mucus independent of extraneous factors. Support for this belief is found in two newborn infants, reported by Astley, who received a suspension of barium sulfate in water at the first meal of life and who showed radiographic evidence of segmentation and clumping of the barium within the small intestine. If a colloidal barium suspension or commercial microsized barium solutions are used, the degree of segmentation is considerably reduced. However, even when a nonflocculent barium suspension is used, the depth of the folds in the infant jejunum still is not as great as in older children and adults, probably because the crevices between the plicae are so small that the suspension cannot enter or because mucus blocks the crevices. The role of emotional factors in producing the segmental pattern of barium in the small bowel of children is not known. It is our impression that an apprehensive child is more apt to have a segmented small bowel pattern than the calm, phlegmatic child. Whether this is the result of excess mucus formation in the intestinal tract, increased swallowing of salivary mucus, or altered neurologic impulses reaching the small bowel is not known.

Water-soluble iodide contrast materials have little use in the examination of the upper gastrointestinal tract of the pediatric patient. In special considerations they may be used advisedly, rather than barium, for examinations of esophageal and gastric or perhaps duodenal perforations. Although the problems of segmentation, flocculation, etc., are not encountered and the small intestine is opacified as an uninterrupted column, the irritating and hypertonic effects of the iodide compounds produce an increase in the transit time, diarrhea, and may produce severe hypovolemia. Several deaths have been reported following their use.

REFERENCES

Altman, D. H., and Puranik, S. Superior mesenteric artery syndrome in children, Am. J. Roentgenol. Radium Ther. Nucl. Med., 118:104, 1973.

Astley, R., and French, J. M. Small intestine pattern in normal children and in coeliac disease, Br. J. Radiol., 24:321, 1951.

Bouslog, J. S., et al. Roentgenologic studies of the infant's gastrointestinal tract, J. Pediatr., 6:234, 1935.

Chamberlin, G. W. Roentgen anatomy of the small intestine, J.A.M.A., 113:1537, 1939.

Davenport, H. W. *Physiology of the Digestive Tract* (3rd. ed.; Chicago: Year Book Medical Publishers, 1971).

Dillon, J. G. Respiratory function of the digestive tract as basis of roentgenographic life test, Am. J. Roentgenol. Radium Ther. Nucl. Med., 48:613, 1942.

Frazer, A. C., et al. Radiographic studies showing the induction of a segmentation pattern in the small intestine in normal human subjects, Br. J. Radiol., 22:123, 1949.

Henderson, S. G. Gastrointestinal tract in the healthy newborn infant, Am. J. Roentgenol. Radium Ther. Nucl. Med., 48:302, 1942.

Jorup, S. L., and Kjelberg, S. R. Radiologic studies of intestine in normal infants and in colonic hyperperistalsis in neurolabile infants, Acta Radiol., 41:109, 1954.

Kim, S. K. Small intestine transit time in the normal small bowel study, Am. J. Roentgenol. Radium Ther. Nucl. Med., 104:552, 1968.

Liu, H-Y., Whitehouse, W. M., and Giday, Z. Proximal small bowel transit pattern in patients with malabsorption induced by bovine milk protein ingestion, Radiology, 115:415, 1975.

Lönnerblad, L. Transit time through the small intestine. A roentgenologic study on normal variability, Acta Radiol., Stockholm, Suppl. 88, pp. 9–85, 1951.

Mattsson, O., Perman, G., and Lagerlöff, H. The small intestine transit time with a physiologic contrast media, Acta Radiol., 54:334, 1960.

Ravdin, I. S., et al. Effect of foodstuffs on the emptying of the normal and the operated stomach and small intestinal pattern, Am. J. Roentgenol. Radium Ther. Nucl. Med., 35:306, 1936.

Wells, J. Mucosal pattern of terminal ileum in children, Radiology, 51:305, 1948.

Zweiling, H., and Nelson, W. E. Roentgenologic pattern of small intestine in infants and children, Radiology, 40:277, 1943.

Chapter 12

CONGENITAL ABNORMALITIES OF THE SMALL BOWEL AND INTESTINAL OBSTRUCTION

GENERAL CONSIDERATIONS

The intimate association of congenital lesions of the gastrointestinal tract with neonatal intestinal obstruction makes it impossible to consider one without the other. Congenital abnormalities involving the stomach, small bowel, or colon are, with few exceptions, detected in the neonatal period only when they are the direct cause of obstruction. In addition, the clinical and radiologic signs of intestinal obstruction in the newborn are the result of a congenital abnormality which must be rectified surgically if the infant is to survive. In such cases, procrastination, other than for a very few hours to improve the infant's general condition, has no place in modern treatment. The rate of survival is closely related to the time of surgical intervention, the mortality rising sharply if surgery is postponed after the first two days of life. An attempt to get the infant "in shape" for laparotomy is of value up to a point, but repeated attempts to improve the infant's condition at the expense of prompt surgery denies the infant an optimal chance for recovery. Mortality in surgically untreated cases is 100%, and the sooner surgical treatment is undertaken, the greater the chance of survival.

The clinical features of abdominal distention, vomiting, obstipation, and frequently abdominal pain prompt the clinician to consult the radiologist, who, as the middleman, is faced with the difficult task of informing the waiting surgeon whether or not bowel obstruction is present. Much of the responsibility rests with the radiologist, who is relied upon to answer three major questions: Is the obstruction present? What is the location of the obstruction? What is the etiology?

The most valuable aid in determining whether or not obstruction is present is the abdominal scout film, the interpretation of which depends largely on a knowledge of the many variations in both the distribution and quantity of intestinal gas in infants.

With regard to intestinal gas, it is necessary to consider the time of appearance of gas in the various segments of the newborn's alimentary tract. By injection of Thorotrast into the amniotic fluid early investigators demonstrated that deglutition and peristaltic activity of the alimentary tract begin early in fetal life. The use of amniography preceding intrauterine transfusions also demonstrated the fetal ingestion of amniotic fluid. It is generally accepted that this activity of the alimentary tract in utero is important in regulating the amount of amniotic fluid, the swallowed fluid being eliminated by absorption into the fetal circulation and then transferred to the maternal blood and excreted through the maternal kidneys. Just as important is absorption of ingested fluid into the fetal circulation and its excretion as urine into the amniotic sac. Therefore, at the time of birth, the ability of the alimentary tract to propel either air or liquids from the mouth to the anus is well established. Air enters the intestinal tract as the result of swallowing and to a lesser extent as a result of respiratory movements of the thorax, by which a pressure gradient is set up between the esophagus and the environment, forcing air into the alimentary tract. There is no convincing evidence that the absorption of gas from the bloodstream causes intestinal gas, nor is a significant amount formed by the normal bacterial flora. The amount of air entering the alimentary tract by respiratory efforts is not definitely known. However, Maddock and other investigators have shown that air will regularly enter the esophagus and frequently the stomach during inspiratory movements against a closed glottis in individuals who, either consciously or not, relax the superior esophageal sphincter, which is the physiologic sphincter at the pharyngoesophageal junction. This perhaps explains the rapid accumulation of gas in the stomach and intestinal tract of the hiccupping or crying child whose many inspiratory sobs are frequently made on a closed glottis (Fig. 12–1). Increased swallowing undoubtedly also adds to the gaseous content of the crying child, but this does not explain as satisfactorily the extremely rapid accumulation of intestinal gas which occasionally occurs. Passive respiratory movements produced by vigorous but unsuccessful attempts to resuscitate a stillborn infant may draw air into the stomach, where it is identified radiographically (Fig. 12–2). Therefore, air in the stomach should not in itself be considered reliable evidence that life was momentarily present before death. However, under ordinary conditions the gas in the alimentary tract is swallowed air, and respiratory movements play a minor part in the transference of air into the stomach, the small amount which may enter the esophagus being promptly eructated.

Air usually appears in the alimentary tract immediately after birth. Occasionally, however, in babies born of overly sedated mothers, in brain-damaged babies, or in babies with low Apgar evaluation, the appearance of gas in the stomach and its progression through the small bowel may be delayed (Fig. 12–3). A deficiency in small bowel gas is also expected in infants with gastrostomies because of the absence of oral intake of food and escape of ingested air from the gastrostomy site. The absence of gas in the stomach of the newborn should therefore suggest one of these

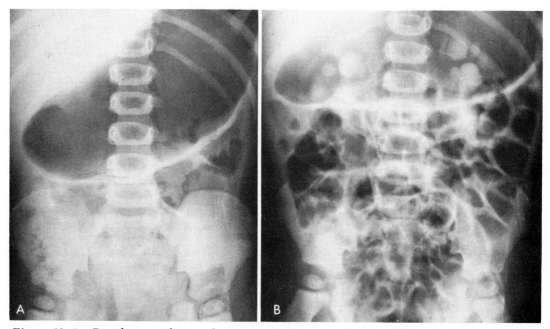

Figure 12–1. Rapid accumulation of gas in intestinal tract of 3 year old crying child having intravenous pyelogram. *A,* Initial scout film made before excretory pyelography, showing excess accumulation of gas in stomach. *B,* Five minutes later, gas is scattered throughout intestinal tract. Bilateral hydronephrosis is present.

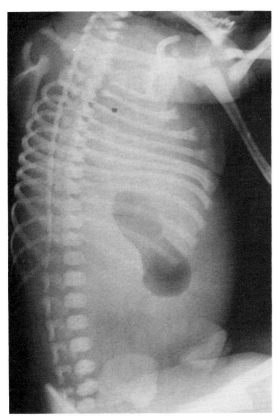

Figure 12-2. Radiograph of stillborn infant after unsuccessful attempt at resuscitation. Note air in stomach and absence of pulmonary aeration. (Courtesy of Dr. W. Whitehouse, University of Michigan.)

conditions, or esophageal atresia. An excess amount of gas in the stomach should alert one to the possibility of tracheoesophageal fistula or respiratory distress of many causes. On the other hand, infants with respiratory distress who have an intratracheal tube are NPO and may show a decrease in intestinal gas.

In the normal infant air is usually identified in the stomach within minutes after birth. Air progresses from the stomach into the small intestine within five to 30 minutes and reaches the proximal portion of the small bowel during the first hours of life. By three hours the entire small bowel usually contains gas. Podolsky and Jester, in serial roentgen studies of 35 newborn infants, found gas in the stomach and proximal small bowel of each infant on the initial roentgenogram. Between the third and fourth hour after birth, 93% had air in the cecum or ascending colon, and at five to six

hours gas in the transverse and descending portions of the colon could be identified. At eight to nine hours all subjects showed sigmoid gas. The presence of air in the rectum was exceedingly variable, probably due to its repeated accumulation and passage between examinations. On the basis of these figures, it seems that in the evaluation of suspected intestinal obstruction the presence of air in the transverse and descending portions of the colon five to six hours after birth, or in all segments of the intestinal tract eight to eleven hours after birth, would exclude an obstructive lesion. There are, of course, exceptions to this time sequence, one of which has been given (Fig. 12-3).

The scout film of the normal neonate as well as of the older infant shows gas distributed throughout stomach, small bowel, and colon. Typically, the small bowel gas pattern appears as multiple ill-defined areas of radiolucency having a honeycombed pattern and confined for the most part to the left side of the abdomen, the right half being occupied in its upper portion by the relatively large liver of this age group and inferiorly by the cecum and terminal ileum. The bowel is not distended, and definite continuity of loops is undetectable. Such a picture is unequivocally normal (Fig. 12-4). However, many different gas patterns are observed, many of which, if they were to be seen in the older child or adult patient, would suggest an obstructive lesion. Distention of the bowel, continuity of loops, hairpin turns, the stepladder formation of parallel segments of bowel, and the air-fluid levels which constitute the cardinal radiographic signs of intestinal obstruction in the adult patient are not always applicable in the infant age group.

Abundant accumulation of gas in the intestinal tract of a healthy infant, even accompanied by clinical evidence of distention, is not unusual. The amount of crying and the number of hours spent in the supine position are largely responsible. In such cases gas is also found in the stomach and colon, presenting an appearance which may simulate exactly an early low mechanical obstruction or paralytic ileus (Fig. 12-5). Follow-up films may be necessary to determine if the distention is progressing before an obstructive lesion can be definitely excluded. The same situation may

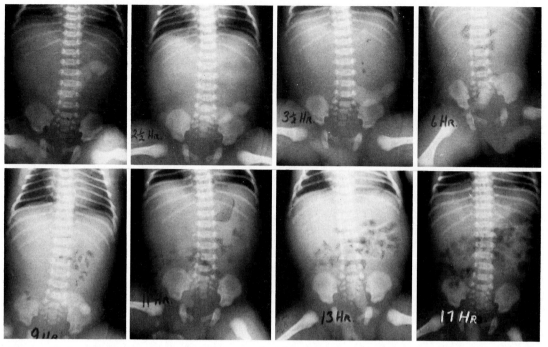

Figure 12–3. Multiple radiographs of over-sedated newborn for 17 hours after birth. First evidence of air entering alimentary tract is at 3½ hours, and it is not until after the first feeding at 10 hours that a normal gas pattern develops.

occur in older debilitated children who spend long periods in the recumbent position.

Considerable distention of bowel may be seen in the newborn if passage of mecon-

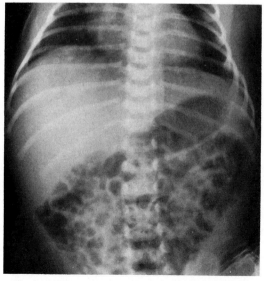

Figure 12–4. Normal distribution of intestinal gas in the young infant.

ium is delayed by a meconium plug in the rectum. This may account for clinical evidence of mild distention. Meconium is usually passed during the first 12 to 24 hours of life. If this is delayed, digital rectal examination will often dislodge the plug. Information regarding the passage of meconium is therefore of value to the radiologist in deciding whether the mild distention of bowel often noted in the first few hours of life is significant.

Fluid levels in the small bowel are not rare in unobstructed infants when films are taken with the patient in an upright position. Air-fluid levels in the small bowel and colon are especially noticeable in infants, as well as older children, with diarrhea which, if not obvious clinically, will be forthcoming a short time after the examination (Fig. 12–6). Severe gastroenteritis in infants and children commonly causes radiographic signs which simulate low colonic obstruction. The history of sudden onset of diarrhea unaccompanied by prior evidence of colonic abnormality provides a clue to the true nature of the condition. In such cases there is an increase in the amount of intestinal fluid associated with

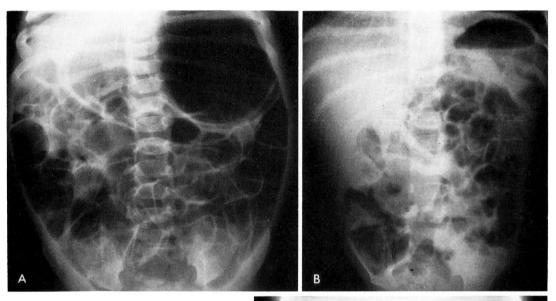

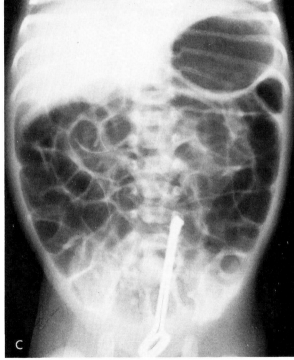

Figure 12–5. Excessive gas in intestinal tract of normal infants. *A*, Child, aged 2, with febrile convulsion. Abdomen became distended, probably as a result of excessive air swallowing. *B*, 24 hours later, gas distribution is not unusual. *C*, Newborn with abundance of gas in all portions of gastrointestinal tract.

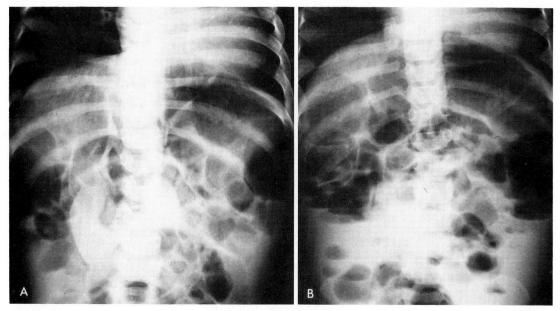

Figure 12–6. Normal child, aged 16 months. Quantity of intestinal gas, although excessive, is not unusual. Multiple fluid levels, present in *B*, should not be mistaken for evidence of an obstructive lesion. Patient began to have diarrhea shortly after examination. *A*, Recumbent, and *B*, upright view.

increased air swallowing. A prone radiograph of the abdomen may be helpful in the diagnosis of gastroenteritis by showing gas filling the rectum (Fig. 12–7).

Another variation, although rare, is a decrease in the amount of intestinal gas which is apparently associated with dehydration in the infant. The dehydration may be the result of sepsis, vomiting, or diarrhea, or may be associated with adrenal cortical insufficiency secondary to congenital adrenal hyperplasia. The radiologic appearance may mimic hypertrophic pyloric stenosis or consist simply of a decrease or absence of gas distal to the stomach. The cause of the deficiency in the gas pattern is unknown. Consequently, the factor of dehydration should be considered in any infant having an apparent pyloric or duodenal obstruction. In such cases a small amount of contrast material introduced into the stomach usually passes slowly but without interruption through the small bowel (Fig. 12–8).

A deficient gas pattern may also occur in brain-damaged infants whose general debility and inactivity decreases the amount of ingested air and crying efforts. Infants who are on parenteral feedings may also show a deficiency in the normal intestinal gas pattern.

These examples of the wide variations in the appearance of the abdominal scout films in the infant age group are given to emphasize the fact that before a diagnosis of intestinal obstruction is made it is imperative that there be accurate correlation of the radiographic signs with the clinical picture. Unless this is done, the radiologist may be led astray by the variable and often equivocal scout film.

After the infant age is passed and the child spends less time in the recumbent position, the distribution of intestinal gas becomes similar to that seen in the adult; that is, gas collects for the most part in the stomach and colon. The pattern of intestinal gas is less variable and the collection of gas in small bowel, air-fluid levels, and so on, become in themselves more significant.

Having established the fact that an obstructive lesion is present, the radiologist is faced with the additional problem of determining its location and etiology. Both of these decisions are usually more difficult; nevertheless, an attempt should be made to determine whether the obstruction is in the colon, low small bowel, or high small bowel, or at the gastric outlet. Once this is established, a reasonable differential diagnosis can be considered. Obstruction involving

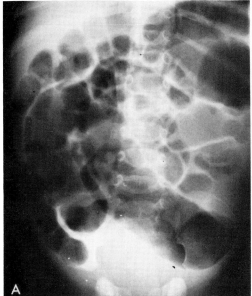

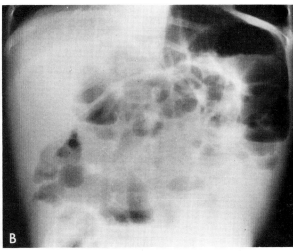

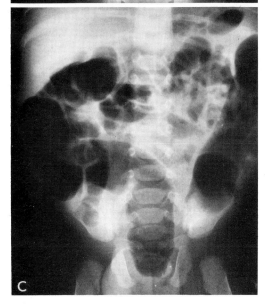

Figure 12-7. Severe gastroenteritis in 5 month old infant. *A*, Supine film shows accumulation of gas within small bowel and colon. *B*, Upright film shows multiple air-fluid levels throughout the intestinal tract. *C*, Prone film results in filling of the rectosigmoid area with gas, thereby excluding an obstructive lesion in this area.

the gastric outlet or duodenum usually offers no problem. The confusing fortuitous gas patterns of distended gut encountered with low obstructive lesions are not present, and it is the conspicuous absence or decrease of gas in the abdomen which leads to the diagnosis. Frequently, the stomach and that part of the duodenum proximal to the obstruction are distended. Examination with contrast material is usually unnecessary, the gas in the distended bowel providing accurate localiza-

tion of the lesion. Clinically, vomiting is severe but distention is not a conspicuous feature. If the vomitus is bile-stained, one may assume that the obstruction is below the ampulla of Vater. This combination of roentgenographic and clinical findings in a newborn infant is indicative of a congenital obstructive lesion of the duodenum. The lesion may be atresia, stenosis, peritoneal band, annular pancreas, or volvulus. The congenital obstructive abnormalities of the stomach are discussed in Chapter 9.

The lower the obstructive lesion in the small bowel, the more difficult is the accurate localization of the site of obstruction. As intestinal loops become distended with air, they are displaced from their normal position so that identification of segments of bowel on the basis of their position in the abdomen becomes impossible. However, in cases of obstruction involving the jejunum, an upright film may be helpful by showing the gas-filled loops confined to the upper portion of the abdominal cavity (Fig. 12–9). As the obstructive lesion persists, fluid collects in many of the loops, obliterating them as identifiable segments of bowel and giving the impression that the lesion is higher than is actually the case. In early obstruction the pattern of the bowel may be helpful in locating the site of the obstruction, the prominent plicae of the jejunal mucosa being differentiated from the smoother mucosa of the ileum. Unfortu-

nately, with increasing distention the folds become effaced, producing a smooth outline in all segments of the small bowel. If the colon cannot be identified with certainty, barium enema studies should be carried out. Then, if the colon is normal, the obstruction must be in the small intestine. A small amount of contrast substance may then be given by mouth to determine the exact site of the obstruction. This, however, only serves to satisfy the academic mind, enhances the danger of vomiting and aspiration, and unnecessarily delays the surgery. With obstructive lesions of the ileum, if seen in the early stages, the abdomen is filled with gas-distended loops of intestine. Consequently, it is often impossible to outline the colon accurately, and what may appear to be colon is actually distended ileum. This mimicry is especially noticeable in the lateral view, in which the distended ileum is seen to lie parallel to

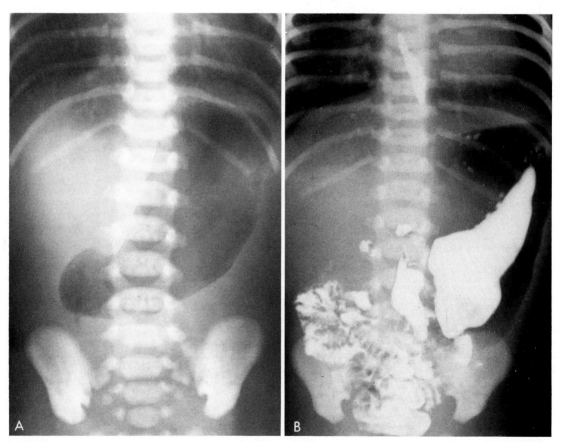

Figure 12–8. Deficiency gas pattern of 2 day old infant with dehydration. *A,* Abdominal scout film showing gas in stomach but none in small intestine and colon. *B,* Upper gastrointestinal tract examination showing no evidence of obstruction at gastric outlet.

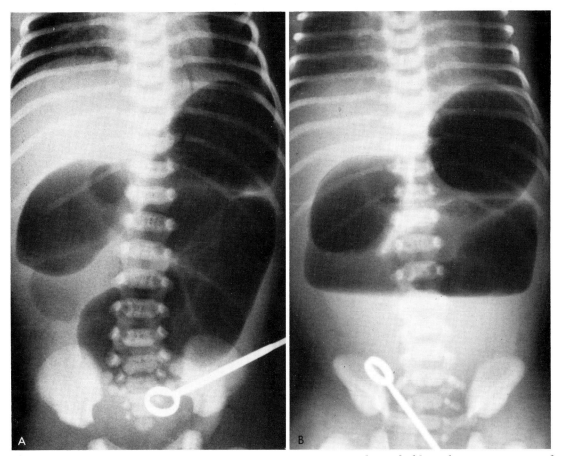

Figure 12–9. Jejunal atresia. *A*, Recumbent film, showing gas-distended bowel occupying most of abdominal cavity. *B*, Upright film, identifying obstruction in proximal jejunum.

the anterior abdominal wall (Fig. 12–10). Again, barium enema will serve to locate the colon, thereby identifying the lesion in the distal small bowel.

Etiologic possibilities to be considered in mid and low small bowel obstruction are as numerous as the causes already mentioned. Atresia and stenosis should always be considered. Herniation of the small intestine through mesenteric defects and resulting strangulation of the gut is an uncommon cause of obstruction and usually is diagnosed only at the time of surgery. A duplicated segment of ileum may, if distended by secretions, obstruct the adjacent normal segment and even, by virtue of its weight, form a volvulus. Meconium ileus and aganglionosis, should also be considered in all cases of low small bowel obstruction.

Anomalies of the colon which produce

complete obstruction lead to marked abdominal distention. Scout films show the abdominal cavity to be filled with gas-distended loops of bowel, and many fluid levels are seen in upright films. Barium enema studies will disclose the exact site of these obstructive lesions (see Chapter 16).

When reviewing the discussion of congenital lesions of the small intestine which follows, one should keep in mind the fact that congenital defects may also be responsible for intestinal obstruction in older infants and children; that is, the obstructive manifestation of the abnormality is not always present at birth. Of course, the atresias of bowel, meconium ileus, and imperforate anus are always evident in the immediate neonatal period, but other malformations, such as the stenoses, duplications, annular pancreas, malrotation, peritoneal bands, and aganglionosis, although occasionally responsible for obstruction in the newborn period, may not become manifest until later in life. Therefore, when intestinal obstruction is encountered in the older infant and child or even in the adult, the possibility that the underlying cause is a congenital anomaly should be considered. These conditions, and other congenital lesions not causing obstruction, are considered in the following pages.

ATRESIA AND STENOSIS

The most common location of small bowel atresia is the distal portion of the ileum, usually near the level of the omphalomesenteric duct; the second most common site is the duodenum, usually slightly distal to the ampulla of Vater. Atretic lesions are often multiple, estimates ranging as high as 15 to 25%. Stenosis of the diaphragm type is more common in the duodenum, and multiple areas of involvement are rare. Either atresia or stenosis may involve any portion of the small intestine.

DEVELOPMENTAL ANATOMY. The nor-mal embryonic and fetal development of the alimentary tract is given in Chapter 3 and a thorough understanding of the normal development is necessary to appreciate the various anomalies which may occur. Early theories indicated that during the fifth week of fetal life rapid proliferation of the epithelial lining of the digestive tract occurred, occluding the lumen and converting the hollow structure into a solid cord of epithelial cells. Later, at about the tenth fetal week, vacuoles formed within the cells, enlarged, and coalesced until the lumen was reestablished, probably at the twelfth week. If coalescence was incomplete, so that the continuity of the re-formed lumen was interrupted, atresia would result. This concept has largely been replaced by a completely different pathogenesis based on intrauterine vascular compromise to the developing gut. A number of investigators have produced atresias, stenoses, duplications, and mesenteric cysts by focal interruption of the intestinal blood supply in experimental animals. Consequently, the current popular explanation of the pathogenesis of bowel atresia is based upon focal vascular changes

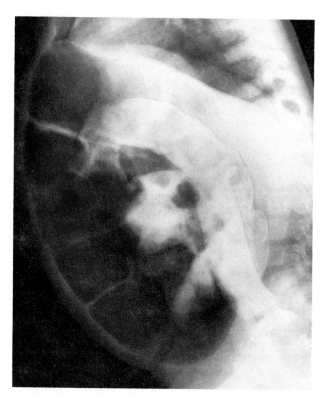

Figure 12–10. Obstruction at terminal ileum (aganglionosis) of infant. Lateral view. The gas-distended bowel along the anterior abdominal wall is the ileum; colon is of normal size, as outlined by contrast material. (Courtesy of Dr. J. F. Holt, University of Michigan.)

accompanying intrauterine stress or hypoxia. In these conditions there is vascular constriction produced by splanchnic stimulation, with resulting decrease in perfusion of the intraabdominal organs and resulting increase in cerebral blood flow. In such circumstances of clinically unrecognized fetal stress, the intestinal tract, including the esophagus and stomach, may suffer focal areas of necrosis which in the process of repair and cicatrization become atretic. If the condition occurs early in fetal life (before the twelfth week) meconium distal to the obstruction will not contain bile and the other normal constituents of meconium. If it occurs later, meconium distal to the obstruction may be normal. If the vascular insult occurs shortly before birth and is associated with perforation, pneumoperitoneum may be the presenting finding. This will be discussed more completely in the section on necrotizing enterocolitis.

An unusual accompaniment in a few cases of jejunal atresia is agenesis of the dorsal mesentery. The etiology is presumably an intrauterine occlusion of the superior mesenteric artery which produces not only aseptic necrosis and resorption of small bowel supplied by the affected artery but also resolution of the involved mesentery. The proximal segment derives its blood supply from small jejunal arcades, while the distal small bowel is supplied by minute ileal branches, as well as by the ileocolic artery. The remaining small bowel grows at a faster rate than its blood supply, producing a spiraling of the distal small bowel around the residual mesentery and small vascular pedicle. This anomaly has been called the "apple-peel small bowel" or "Christmas tree mesentery." The radiographic features are no different from those in the usual cases of jejunal atresia. At surgery the distal spiraled segment is noted to lie free in the peritoneal cavity. The significance of this lesion lies in the surgical resection of sufficient bowel at each end of the atresia to the point where the vascular supply appears satisfactory. Failure to do this results in devitalized bowel with resulting peritonitis and death. Malabsorption with diarrhea and failure to thrive are common postoperative complications.

SYMPTOMS. All cases of atresia of the intestinal tract are characterized clinically by vomiting early in the newborn period. The vomiting is usually delayed until after the first feeding, but increases progressively thereafter. Because most atresias are below the ampulla of Vater, the vomitus usually contains bile. However, in the rare cases in which the atresia is proximal to the ampulla, bile is naturally absent from the vomitus. Duodenal atresia at the level of the ampulla is rare but should be suspected if jaundice accompanies clinical and radiographic evidence of duodenal obstruction. A significant percentage of patients who survive surgical treatment of duodenal atresia are found later to be mongoloid. This incidence has been estimated to be as great as 1:3. The radiologic signs of the Down syndrome, abnormally shallow acetabula, wide ilia, and tapering ischia, should be considered in the radiologic evaluation of all cases of duodenal atresia. Atresias of the lower small intestine and colon apparently are not significantly associated with mongolism. The presence of one or more meconium stools does not exclude intestinal atresia. The presence of bile, amniotic cells, lanugo hairs, etc., in meconium does not exclude atresia as was formerly believed (Farber's test), but instead indicates that the obstruction developed later in intrauterine life.

Severe congenital stenosis of the small bowel is usually accompanied by vomiting and abdominal distention, identical in severity to that seen in atresia. In less severe cases, these symptoms may be mild or even delayed for several days or weeks. When the lumen is only slightly narrowed, only vague episodes of abdominal pain and distention with or without vomiting may occur, the condition not being discovered until much later in life, if ever. Occasionally intestinal stenosis is unsuspected until an ingested foreign body becomes lodged at the narrowed segment.

ROENTGENOLOGIC EXAMINATION. The radiologic evaluation should begin with supine and upright films of the infant's abdomen. Often these clinch the diagnosis, and additional examinations are unnecessary. In cases of duodenal atresia the stomach and duodenal bulb are markedly distended, and there is no gas in other portions of the intestinal tract. Exceptions to this may be seen if the infant has been given an enema with introduction of air

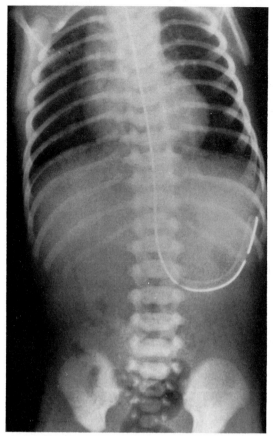

Figure 12-11. Newborn with duodenal atresia. Nasogastric tube is coiled within the deflated stomach. Air is present within the rectum and portions of the colon as a result of digital examination and repeated enemas. Subsequent radiographs made after inflation of the stomach demonstrated duodenal atresia.

into the colon (Fig. 12-11). The distention of the duodenal bulb is often relatively greater than that of the stomach (Fig. 12-12). This has also been referred to as the double-bubble sign and may be seen in any severe upper duodenal obstruction. Atresias located more distally in the duodenum naturally have a longer segment of dilatation. It may be impossible to differentiate radiologically between atresia of the proximal portion of the duodenum and complete obstruction produced by such extrinsic factors as volvulus of the midgut, annular pancreas, and peritoneal band. However, partial differentiation is frequently possible. In both duodenal atresia and annular pancreas the bulb and usually the stomach are enormously distended, whereas in complete obstruction produced by a peritoneal band and/or volvulus the bulb is less distended and the obstruction is usually lower than in atresia and annular pancreas. Therefore, if the obstruction is in the proximal portion of the duodenum, just distal to an enormously distended bulb, the lesion is probably atresia or possibly, but statistically less likely, annular pancreas. Obstructions involving the third portion of the duodenum are more likely to be the result of an anomalous band (Ladd-Waugh syndrome) or volvulus of the midgut.

In complete or severe obstruction of the upper small bowel, regardless of the etiology, the air within the stomach and duodenum is the only contrast material needed, the introduction of opaque contrast material into the stomach being completely unnecessary and hazardous. If there is insufficient air, a catheter should be passed into the stomach and air injected. Radiographs made in an inverted position will show the continuity of antrum and duodenal bulb (Fig. 12-12B). The presence of a small amount of gas distal to the area of dilatation usually excludes atresia and indicates that the obstruction results from duodenal stenosis or one of the extrinsic types of obstruction (Figs. 12-13 and 12-14). Rare cases of an anomalous pancreatic duct bridging the atretic segment and allowing air distal to the obstruction have been reported. Occasionally, obstruction is not severe enough to decrease significantly the amount of small bowel gas; the use of a small amount of constrast material is then warranted (Fig. 12-15).

The lower the atresia, the more difficult it becomes to locate definitely the site of obstruction. Instead of the normal honeycomb pattern of gas, there are only a few markedly distended loops which pass horizontally across the abdomen. Multiple air-fluid levels are always present. There is no gas in the lower portion of the abdomen; this is observed to best advantage in the upright film. The colon cannot be identified and gas is not found in the rectum. These signs indicate an obstructive lesion in the small intestine, and immediate surgery is mandatory. Here also when the obstruction can be definitely identified in the small intestine, there is no need to delay surgery to give contrast material by mouth. On the few occasions we have used barium orally in small bowel obstruction, considerable flocculation and dispersion of the medium have occurred, due

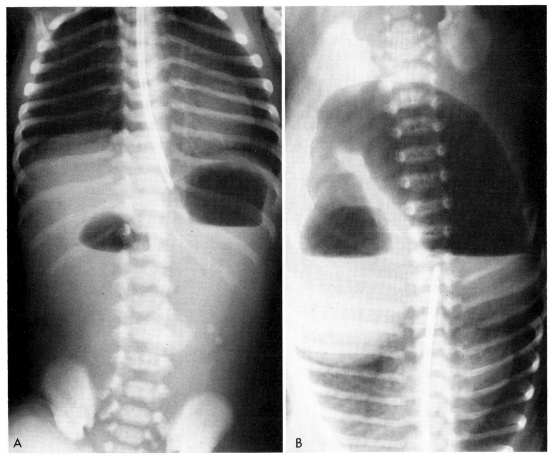

Figure 12-12. Duodenal atresia. *A*, Abdominal scout film, showing air in markedly distended duodenal bulb and stomach without gas distal to the bulb, the double-bubble sign. *B*, Inverted film, demonstrating continuity of stomach and duodenum. Similar appearance may be produced by annular pancreas.

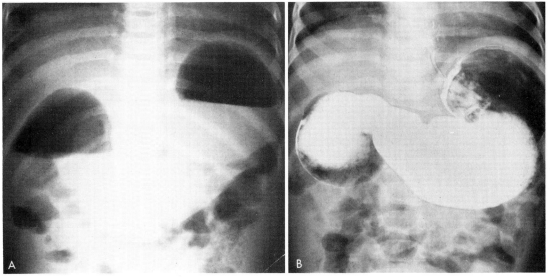

Figure 12-13. Duodenal stenosis. Infant, aged 6 months, had been vomiting sporadically since birth but progressively more often since solid foods had been given. *A*, Abdominal scout film with the infant upright, showing markedly dilated duodenal bulb and fluid levels in stomach and duodenum. Gas in distal portions of intestinal tract excludes complete obstruction. *B*, Contrast material in stomach is unnecessary for the diagnosis but shows the obstruction in vertical portion of duodenum.

173

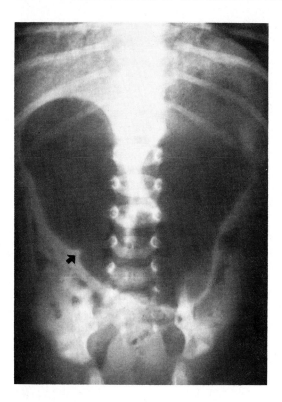

Figure 12–14. Duodenal stenosis. Newborn with abdominal distention and vomiting. Scout film, showing marked distention of duodenum and stomach and gas in distal portions of bowel, thereby excluding duodenal atresia. Constriction (*arrow*) marks pyloric canal. Surgery revealed a duodenal diaphragm with small central opening.

probably to the high mucus content of the distended segment, and little information has been gained. The use of water-soluble iodide media is contraindicated. The hypertonic properties of these substances may produce severe hypovolemia and, in addition, are irritating to the tracheobronchial tree if aspirated. The increase in fluid content associated with their high osmolarity also enhances the possibility of vomiting and aspiration pneumonia.

If the obstruction involves the terminal ileum, the resulting distention of the longer segment of bowel may occupy the entire abdominal cavity, including the pelvic portion (Fig. 12–16). When this degree of distention is reached the mucosal pattern of small bowel is effaced and it may be impossible to differentiate small bowel from colon. Examination of the colon, both fluoroscopically and radiographically, is then warranted and will disclose the presence or absence of a colonic lesion (Fig. 12–17). If there is no evidence of colon obstruction one may assume that the obstruction is in the terminal ileum and so advise the surgeon. In complete obstruction of the terminal ileum such as occurs in atresia and meconium ileus, the barium-filled colon is often of minute caliber, the so-called microcolon. In such cases the colon has never served as a passageway for normal amounts of fetal meconium. Normally, meconium reaches the cecum in the fourth month of intrauterine life and is in the rectum by the fifth month. The development of obstruction at an early period will consequently prohibit the passage of meconium into the colon, leaving this structure collapsed and narrowed, although still potentially distensible. The degree of microcolon in complete obstruction varies. Presumably this is due to the variable amount of meconium formed by internal secretions below the obstruction. In our experience, the higher the obstruction in the small intestine, the greater the caliber of colonic lumen, probably due to a larger quantity of succus entericus formed below the lesion. In fact, the demonstration of an abnormally small colon in the presence of a high atretic lesion suggests that multiple or lower areas of atresia are also present. Consequently, the preoperative evaluation of the colon, even in obvious high obstructive lesions, is advocated to alert the surgeon to the possibility of additional lower obstructive lesions. The scattered soap-bubble pattern of

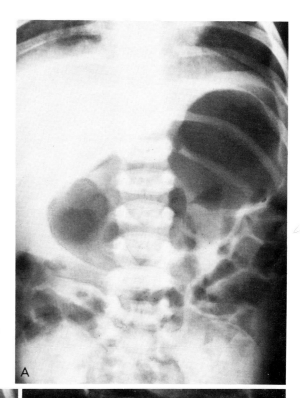

Figure 12–15. Obstruction by peritoneal band. Infant, aged 18 days, with vomiting. *A*, Supine film, showing mild gaseous distention of stomach and normal quantity of small bowel gas. *B*, Upright film, showing air-fluid level in stomach extending into duodenum (*arrow*), suggesting possibility of partial duodenal obstruction. *C*, After ingestion of contrast material, obstruction visualized in third portion of duodenum. At operation a peritoneal band was found obstructing duodenum proximal to ligament of Treitz.

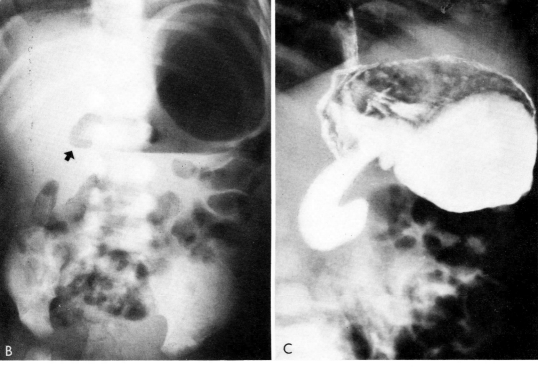

feces and gas in the small bowel seen in meconium ileus is occasionally noted in ileal atresia (Fig. 12–16A) and in colonic aganglionosis.

The scout film of low intestinal obstruction may disclose intraperitoneal fluid, evident from separation of the loops and increased density of the abdomen, especially in its lower portion on the upright film. This is not necessarily indicative of peritonitis, since the fluid may form secondary to the obstruction alone. The presence of pneumoperitoneum indicates that perforation has occurred, and colon examination, as well as the oral administration of a small amount of contrast material, is contraindicated.

Intraperitoneal calcifications, indicative of meconium peritonitis, are not uncommon in ileal atresia. (This subject is discussed later in this chapter under meconium peritonitis.) Intramural calcification is a rare complication of intestinal atresia and presumably is the result of intrauterine calcification of necrotic bowel (Fig. 12–18).

In stenosis of the terminal ileum, the appearance may be indistinguishable from atresia or show no evidence of obstruction, depending entirely on the degree of constriction. In partial obstruction, examination with contrast material is necessary if the site of involvement is to be demonstrated. Colon examination should be performed first and, if the caliber is normal, barium introduced into the stomach. The area of transition from dilated to normal-sized bowel determines the site of the partial obstruction.

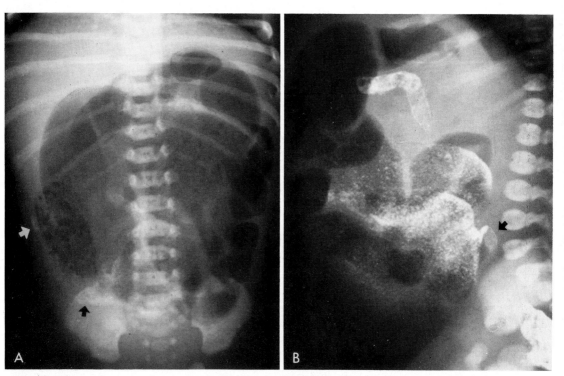

Figure 12–16. Low ileal atresia. A, Abdominal scout film showing extreme gaseous distention of small bowel, making it impossible to distinguish between dilated small intestine and colon. In this patient barium enema studies showed an unusually small colon, thereby locating obstruction in terminal ileum. Meconium peritonitis, identified from scattered areas of calcification, also present (*black arrow*). Note also mottled densities representing mixture of air and meconium (*white arrow*). B, Contrast material given through intestinal decompression tube, although finely dispersed, identifies point of obstruction (*arrow*). This procedure is unnecessary. Residual barium of the enema is present in small colon and rectum. Ileal atresia was found at operation.

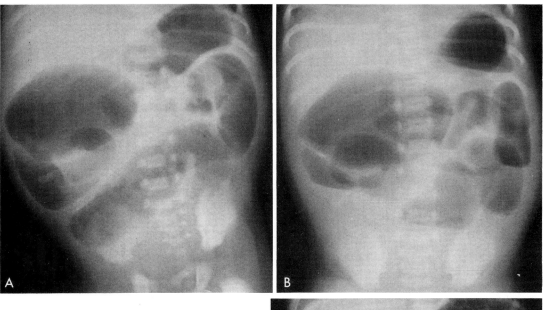

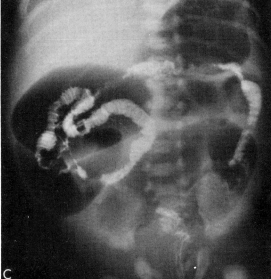

Figure 12–17. Ileal atresia in newborn. *A,* Radiograph of abdomen shows multiple distended loops of bowel, the differentiation between small bowel and colon being impossible. *B,* Upright film shows multiple air-fluid levels within small bowel and possibly colon, the distended loop in the right upper quadrant having the appearance of hepatic flexure. *C,* Barium enema examination shows a small unused colon, indicating that the obstruction is in the terminal ileum.

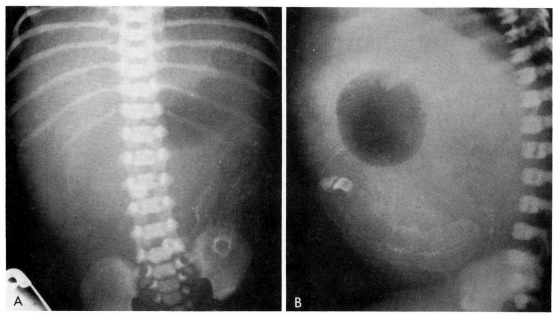

Figure 12–18. Supine (A) and lateral (B) views of the abdomen show tubular calcification of bowel as well as linear calcification within the peritoneal cavity. At autopsy calcification was seen within the wall of the atretic bowel, the entire small bowel from the duodenum to the terminal ileum being involved. (Courtesy of Dr. John R. Steinfeld and Dr. R. Brent Harrison. Reprinted from *Radiology, 107*:405, 1973).

ANNULAR PANCREAS

Annular pancreas is an anomalous band of pancreatic tissue which arises from the head of the pancreas and encircles the second portion of the duodenum. If it forms a complete ring, there may be partial or complete obstruction of the duodenum at the time of birth. If incomplete, obstruction may occur later in life or may never be responsible for symptoms.

PATHOGENESIS. The pancreas develops early in embryonic life (fourth week) from ventral and dorsal outgrowths of the distal portion of the foregut at the level of the future duodenum. A description of the normal development is given in Chapter 3.

Annular pancreas apparently results from failure of the distal portion of the ventral pancreas to rotate dorsally with the proximal portion of its duct. This in turn leaves the ventral pancreas in its original anterior position closely adherent to the duodenum and forming a ring with its duct and the dorsal pancreas constricting the duodenum.

SYMPTOMS. In complete or nearly complete duodenal obstruction produced by an annular pancreas, the clinical picture is identical to that of other forms of congenital duodenal obstruction. Vomiting follows the first feeding attempts and becomes increasingly severe. The vomitus may or may not contain bile, depending on the relation of the constricted segment to the common bile duct. Jaundice may be present if the constriction involves the common duct. Associated congenital anomalies, especially duodenal atresia, are common.

If the encircling band is not complete, symptoms may be delayed until childhood or adulthood, or may never appear, the condition being discovered only as an incidental finding at autopsy. When symptoms do occur in the child or adult, they consist of intermittent bouts of vomiting and upper abdominal pain due to partial obstruction. The pain may be secondary to associated pancreatitis, the resulting edema of the head of the pancreas probably explaining the onset of the obstruction at this later stage of life.

ROENTGENOLOGIC EVALUATION. Duodenal obstruction by annular pancreas in neonatal life causes a radiographic picture similar to that of duodenal atresia or diaphragm. If the obstruction is complete or if there is underlying duodenal atresia, there is gaseous distention of the duodenal bulb and stomach and absence of gas in other portions of the alimentary tract (Fig. 12–19). The duodenal distention is often extreme and out of proportion to the gastric distention.

Incomplete obstruction also causes considerable dilatation of the duodenum and stomach, but there is a small amount of gas distal to the obstruction (Fig. 12–20). Hope called attention to the double-bubble sign, which, when present, is highly suggestive of annular pancreas. This sign results from the absence of gas in the constricted second portion of the duodenum and the collection of gas proximal and distal to the constriction. The double-bubble sign of annular pancreas should not be confused with the identical descriptive term used by others when referring to gas in the duodenum and stomach with obstructive lesions of the duodenum due to any congenital anomaly. The constriction produced by an annular pancreas may be either concentric or an indentation on the right side of

the duodenal loop. But, wherever there is radiologic evidence of obstruction of the second portion of the duodenum, either partial or complete, annular pancreas should be considered and mentioned in the radiologist's report. Although contrast material in the stomach and duodenum will confirm the presence of duodenal obstruction and perhaps delineate the configuration of the obstruction more accurately than air, its use is usually unnecessary and may be harmful by increasing the frequency of vomiting and the hazard of aspiration.

It is often impossible to differentiate complete obstruction due to annular pancreas from duodenal atresia. In both conditions the duodenal bulb is markedly dilated. In obstruction by midgut volvulus or peritoneal bands the duodenum is usually less distended and the obstruction is more common in the third portion of the duodenum.

Duodenal obstruction by annular pan-

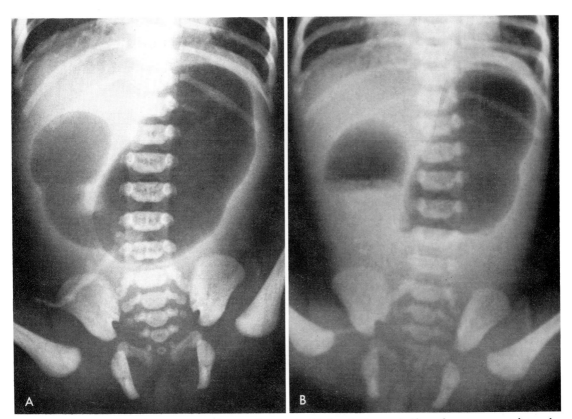

Figure 12–19. Annular pancreas in newborn. *A,* Abdominal scout film, showing complete obstruction at duodenal level. *B,* Upright film, showing double-bubble sign identical to that seen in duodenal atresia.

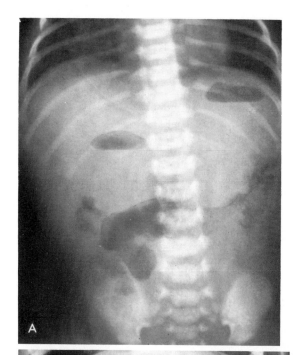

Figure 12-20. Annular pancreas in infant, aged 3 days, who had been vomiting since first feeding. *A*, Abdominal scout film, showing gas in stomach and distended duodenal bulb, but gas also distal to this. *B* and *C*, Contrast material, showing site of partial obstruction in second portion of duodenum.

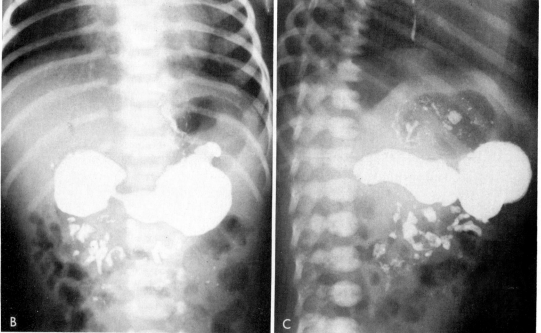

creas in the older infant or child is usually partial. Scout films of the abdomen show mild dilatation of the duodenum and stomach but not to the degree noted in the newborn group (Fig. 12–21). Contrast material may be used with greater safety at this age and, in the fluoroscopic examination of the duodenum, careful attention should be given to the configuration and distention of its second portion. Concentric constriction

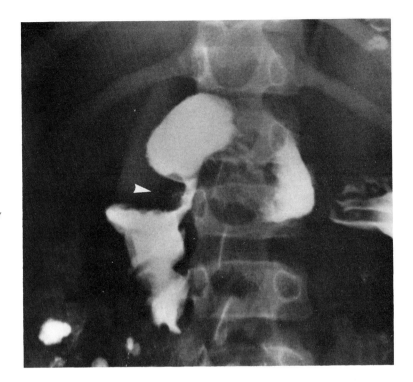

Figure 12–21. Annular pancreas in 8 year old boy. Extrinsic defect on second portion of the duodenum (*arrow*) was found at surgery to be annular pancreas.

or compression of the duodenum should be regarded as presumptive evidence of an annular pancreas.

ANOMALIES OF ROTATION

The process by which the primitive position of the alimentary tract is converted to that present at birth is called intestinal rotation. Disturbances of the normal orderly process of the return of the intestine from the umbilical cord into the abdomen and the accompanying errors of mesenteric-peritoneal attachment account for many congenital intestinal tract abnormalities. Patients having disorders of intestinal rotation usually come to the attention of the radiologist because of obstructive symptoms, or unsuspected cases are discovered during examination of the upper gastrointestinal tract or colon for other reasons. Many varieties of this anomaly may be met, and just as it is necessary for the surgeon to understand the mechanism of intestinal rotation in order to repair the defect, it is essential that the radiologist have this knowledge in order to evaluate accurately the radiologic findings.

PATHOGENESIS. The process of alimentary tract growth, herniation into the umbilical cord, and rotational return into the abdominal cavity is extremely complex and is described in detail in Chapter 3 (Fig. 12–22). The earliest descriptions of the process of intestinal rotation were given in 1817 by Meckel, who described the passage of the midgut loop into the umbilical cord, and by Mall, in 1898, who described its return. Since then additional observations have emphasized the remarkable phenomena of normal intestinal tract development.

The intestinal tract is originally a straight, tubular structure suspended on a common dorsal mesentery and divided into a foregut which extends from the mouth to the duodenojejunal junction, a midgut which extends from the duodenojejunal junction to the midtransverse colon and is supplied by the superior mesenteric artery, and a hindgut which extends from the midtransverse colon to the anus.

It is obvious that during such an intricate process many vagaries of rotation and fixation may occur, with many resulting anomalies. The most common of these, and the ones most important radiologically, are omphalocele, nonrotation, malrotation, reversed rotation, and normal rotation with inadequate mesenteric-peritoneal fusion. Any of these conditions may be complicated by volvulus of the midgut or obstruction by peritoneal bands.

Omphalocele (exomphalos, amniotic hernia) results from failure of rotation beyond the first stage and failure of the midgut to return from the umbilical stalk.

In *nonrotation,* the midgut returns to the peritoneal cavity without having rotated more than the initial 90 degrees, i.e., beyond the horizontal plane. The prearterial segment which lies to the right of the superior mesenteric artery at this stage of rotation returns to the right side of the abdomen, and the postarterial segment, consisting of the lower ileum and the right half of the colon, returns to the left side. Therefore in nonrotation the small intestine lies on the right side of the abdomen and the colon and cecum on the left, the ileum crossing the midline to enter the cecum from right to left.

Malrotation implies that rotation occurs but is incomplete, the intestine occupying an intermediate position between that of nonrotation and the normal postnatal disposition. In such cases the prearterial segment, which returns to the abdomen first, is usually in a normal position and the degree of malrotation is detected by the position of the cecum—the more complete the process, the more normal the position of the cecum. It may be on the left side, higher than normal on the right side, or in an intermediate position.

Reversed rotation occurs when the postarterial segment of the midgut returns to the abdomen first. The cecum begins the migration and passes to the right behind the superior mesenteric artery. This reversed process of migration unwinds the normal counterclockwise rotation which occurred during the first stage and substitutes a final clockwise rotation of 90 degrees, the transverse colon coming to lie behind the duodenum and separated from it by the superior mesenteric artery.

Volvulus of the small intestine often accompanies malrotation and is due to the short mesenteric-peritoneal attachment. In normal complete rotation the duodenocolic isthmus becomes widely separated by the returning loops of midgut, so that mesenteric fusion with the posterior parietes occurs along a broad base extending from duodenum to cecum. However, if rotation is incomplete, the duodenocolic isthmus maintains a more primitive, unseparated relationship and the resulting mesenteric-peritoneal attachment is narrow, allowing abnormal motility of the midgut and predisposing it to volvulus formation. In addition, the mesenteric-parietal attachments are often incomplete, further increasing the potentiality for volvulus.

Peritoneal bands are another complication of abnormal rotation. They consist of adhesions or cords of peritoneal tissue which presumably represent distorted attempts at fusion in an effort to compensate for the inadequate mesenteric fixation. Although these bands are frequently present in malrotation, they are also found in complete rotation but with abnormal fixation and fusion of the mesentery and peritoneum. They may be anywhere in the peritoneal cavity and become clinically significant when they produce pressure on a portion of the bowel. More commonly, they overlie the duodenum or terminal ileum, causing obstruction at these points. Sometimes a single band extends from the region of the cecum to its peritoneal attachment high in the posterior abdominal wall, obstructing both terminal ileum and duo-

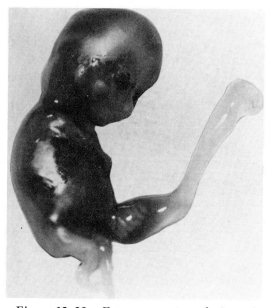

Figure 12-22. Fetus, approximately 9 weeks old, with coils of small intestine in umbilical cord.

denum. Duodenal obstruction by such a band is particularly common in malrotation when the cecum lies high in the right upper quadrant. Adhesion-like bands also occur in other areas of the abdomen, binding down and obstructing adjacent loops of bowel.

Mesenteric defects represent congenital malformations of the mesentery and become clinically significant when small bowel becomes incarcerated in the defect and thereby obstructed. Mesenteric pouches and peritoneal tunnels are similar examples of mesenteric abnormalities which are potential sites of obstruction of the bowel.

SYMPTOMS. In general, the symptoms of anomalies of rotation are those of obstruction. The obstruction may be partial or complete and results from volvulus of the midgut and compression by either peritoneal bands or continuous strictures. In the newborn, complete obstruction is the rule and is usually due to volvulus of the midgut or to extrinsic pressure by a peritoneal band, or a combination of the two. Vomiting is the presenting symptom. If the obstruction is caused by a band obstructing the lower portion of the small intestine, there is associated abdominal distention. In the older child, the obstruction is usually partial, with recurrent attacks of vomiting and occasionally distention. Such cases are easily mistaken for gastrointestinal allergy, cyclic vomiting, or celiac disease. The last condition deserves special mention because of the occasional similarity of its symptoms and those of malrotation. These children have persistent or recurrent abdominal distention, malnutrition, intolerance of certain foods, and either constipation or diarrhea. Presumably these complaints result from torsion of the midgut in such a way as to obstruct the terminal ileum partially, or else there are chronic edema and congestion of the bowel wall due to partial obstruction of the superior mesenteric vein. Consequently, any child suspected of having celiac disease should have a gastrointestinal examination to exclude malrotation as the cause of the celiac syndrome. Other patients may exhibit symptoms of recurrent partial obstruction for a long time and then become suddenly and acutely obstructed. Obstruction of the superior mesenteric vessels by volvulus of the midgut may cause melena, hematochezia and, less often, hematemesis.

ROENTGENOLOGIC EXAMINATION. Radiographic examination of an *omphalocele* is seldom performed, the diagnosis being apparent from direct inspection. When radiographs are obtained, the gas-filled loops of bowel, occasionally with air-fluid levels, are visualized. The size of the hernia varies according to the amount of bowel as well as solid viscus within the sac. If the communication between the omphalocele and abdominal cavity is relatively small, there may be moderate distention of the herniated loops. There is naturally, in such an anomaly, very little gas-filled bowel in the abdominal cavity (Fig. 12-23). Rarely, an omphalocele contains only the liver, the bowel having migrated back into the abdomen (Fig. 12-24). Gastroschisis is similar to omphalocele but is a herniation of abdominal contents through a congenitally weakened area of the upper abdominal wall. The defect is in a paramedian location rather than in the midline (Fig. 12-25). Radiologic differentiation is usually not possible. There is no parietal peritoneum covering a gastroschisis but it usually is present with omphalocele.

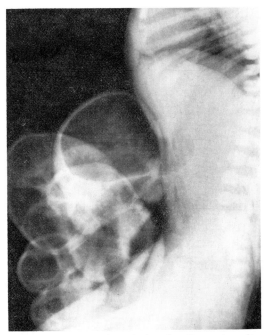

Figure 12-23. Omphalocele. Lateral radiograph of abdomen, showing practically the entire intestinal tract outside the abdomen.

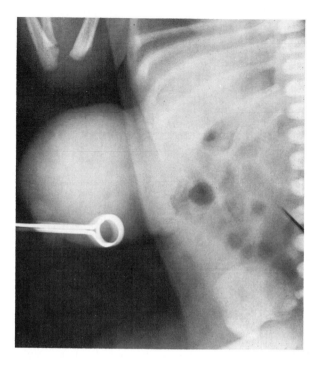

Figure 12-24. Omphalocele. Intestinal tract is in the abdomen, the omphalocele containing only liver.

Malrotation of bowel is inevitable in both conditions.

The chief value of radiologic identification of abnormal rotation of the intestinal tract is in determining the etiology of an intestinal obstruction for which there is no apparent clinical cause. This is particularly true with partial or recurrent obstruction. But whether the obstruction is acute, partial, or recurrent, if there is x-ray evidence of nonrotation, malrotation, or reversed rotation, the obstruction is probably due to volvulus of the midgut, peritoneal adhesions, or a combination of the two. The

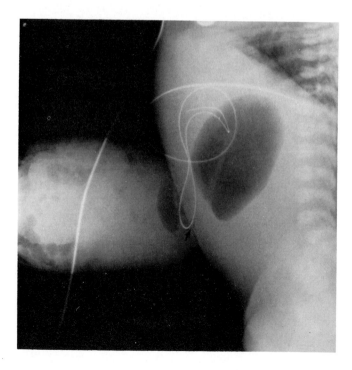

Figure 12-25. Gastroschisis. Bowel containing gas is identified in the extruded gut. Arrow denotes entrance of umbilical vein catheter.

diagnosis of abnormal rotation in such conditions is most easily and rapidly made by barium enema studies. If the cecum is on the left side, in the epigastrium, or high on the right side, some degree of malrotation is present and either volvulus or peritoneal band is probably causing the obstruction. If the cecum is in a normal position but freely movable, normal peritoneal fixation has not occurred and again volvulus or peritoneal adhesions are probably responsible for the symptoms. With these facts in mind, we can consider in more detail the radiologic features of the different types of abnormal rotation.

Nonrotation is characterized by the intestinal tract being in the same position as it was in the umbilical cord after the first stage of rotation. The condition may be suspected when scout films of the abdomen show the small bowel occupying the right portion of the abdomen and the colon is on the left. With barium studies, the malposition of the bowel is accurately revealed and the diagnosis made. Upper gastrointestinal tract examination in such cases shows the duodenum extending to the right, the duodenojejunal junction and upper jejunum being in the right hypochondrium. Studies of the colon show it to occupy the left side of the abdomen (Fig. 12–26). Nonrotation is often an incidental finding in older children and adults during routine examination. If volvulus or peritoneal bands are also present, there is additional evidence of intestinal obstruction, with dilatation of bowel proximal to the obstruction.

Malrotation with volvulus of the midgut may occur at any age but is most common in the neonatal period. The abdominal scout film shows evidence of obstruction, usually in the third portion of the duodenum (Fig. 12–27) but occasionally higher or even lower. The stomach and

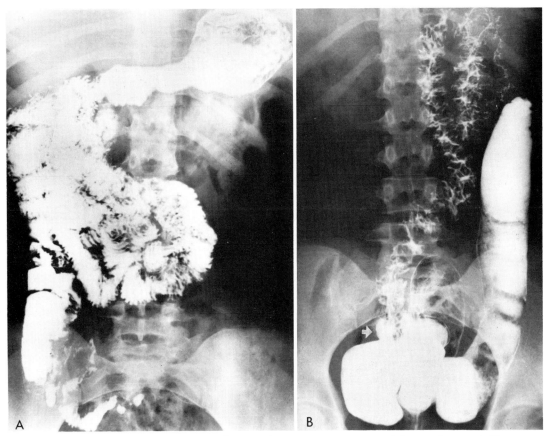

Figure 12–26. Nonrotation. Girl, aged 12, with vague intermittent abdominal pain. *A*, Upper gastrointestinal examination, showing small intestine to occupy right side of abdomen. *B*, Colon examination (postevacuation film), showing colon crowded into left side of abdomen. Note medial position of cecum (*arrow*).

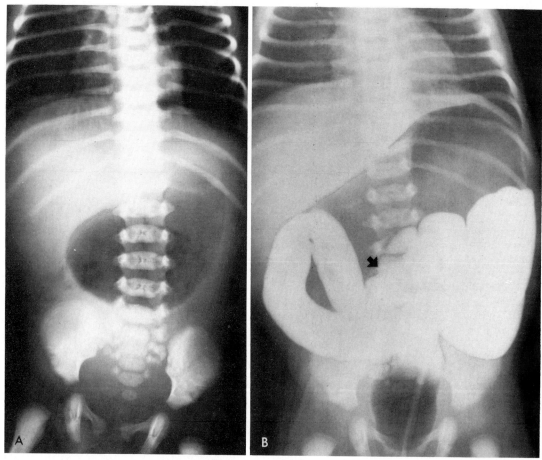

Figure 12-27. Volvulus with malrotation in 5 day old infant. *A,* Abdominal scout film showing air in stomach but absence of gas distal to it. *B,* Colon examination showing cecum in midportion of abdomen (*arrow*), indicating malrotation and suggesting that obstruction is due either to volvulus or to a peritoneal band. Redundant sigmoid occupies the right flank and should not be mistaken for proximal colon. Surgery disclosed volvulus of the midgut.

proximal portion of the duodenum are dilated, and if the obstruction is complete, there is no gas in the small intestine and colon. The appearance in such cases is usually indistinguishable from that of other congenital obstructions of the duodenum. There is radiologic and experimental evidence to suggest that the relatively gasless abdomen associated with midgut volvulus denotes patency of the venous drainage of the affected bowel, while the pattern of low small bowel obstruction signifies venous obstruction and infarction. Presumably a patent superior mesenteric vein allows resorption of intestinal gas while venous occlusion is associated with stagnation (Fig. 12–28). Incomplete obstructions, by either volvulus or peritoneal bands, usually show gas in the jejunum and ileum but associated dilatation of the duodenum. These cases are frequently identical in appearance to duodenal stenosis and other incomplete congenital duodenal obstructions.

Contrast material given by mouth will demonstrate the point of blockage more accurately. Also, barium enema studies will indicate the nature of the obstruction by showing a malpositioned or abnormally mobile cecum, indicating that the obstruction is the result of volvulus or a peritoneal band (Figs. 12–29 and 12–30). But because the acute obstructions in the young infant are surgical emergencies, the diagnosis of malrotation by radiologic procedures does not justify a delay in surgical intervention. However, in the infant with partial obstruction as determined by gas in the distal portions of the intestinal tract, or in the older

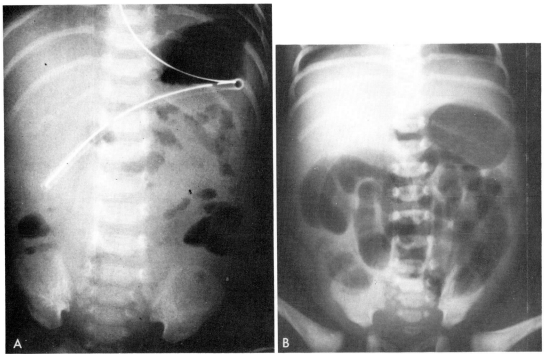

Figure 12-28. Volvulus of the midgut in two young infants. *A*, Deficient gas pattern suggests patency of the superior mesenteric vein and viability of the bowel. *B*, Obstructed distended gas pattern suggests devitalized bowel.

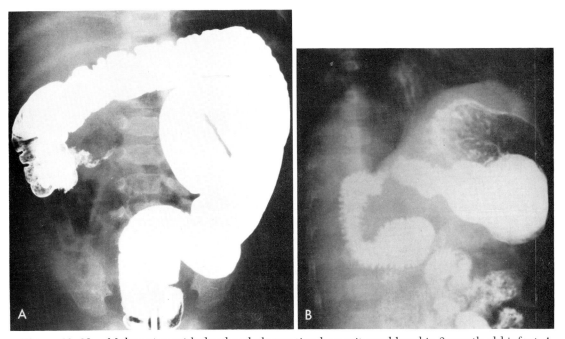

Figure 12-29. Malrotation with duodenal obstruction by peritoneal band in 3 month old infant. *A*, Barium enema examination shows high position of the cecum. *B*, Upper gastrointestinal study shows partial obstruction at the third portion of the duodenum. At surgery a peritoneal band was found to be responsible for the duodenal obstruction and the high position of the cecum.

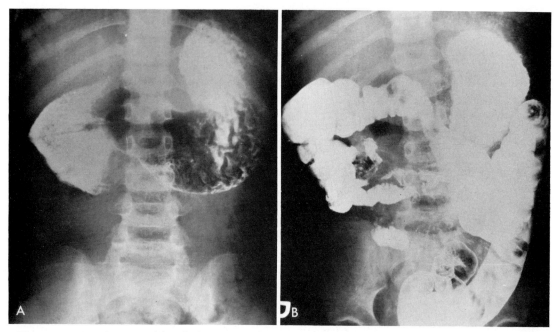

Figure 12–30. Peritoneal band obstructing duodenum in 4 year old boy. *A*, Upper gastrointestinal examination shows duodenal obstruction with dilatation of the duodenum proximal to the obstruction. *B*, Delayed film shows residual barium in the stomach and passage of contrast media to the colon. Cecum is in an abnormally high position. At surgery a peritoneal band was found extending from the cecum to the posterior portion of the diaphragm with obstruction of the duodenum. (Courtesy of Dr. William S. Conkling, Navasota, Texas.)

child with recurrent attacks of obstruction or with the celiac syndrome, barium enema studies should be performed to discover whether malrotation is present.

The collection of barium in several loops of small bowel crowded together in a localized area of the abdomen with delayed passage past this part should be considered herniation of bowel through a *mesenteric defect*. If herniation through such a defect produces complete obstruction, the appearance is indistinguishable from other forms of complete obstruction involving small bowel.

Volvulus of the cecum and ascending portion of the colon is extremely rare in children, but may occur as an isolated lesion, and is due to inadequate peritoneal fixation of these structures. The scout film shows gaseous distention of the cecum, usually out of proportion to the distention by gas of small bowel proximal to the lesion. The enlarged cecum may reach tremendous proportions and extend medially and superiorly past the midline.

In *reversed rotation* of the bowel, the relation of duodenum and colon is opposite

that of the normal, the duodenum overlying the transverse colon and being separated from it by the superior mesenteric artery. Adhesive bands or volvulus of the midgut may produce small bowel obstruction in these cases as in other forms of abnormal rotation. In addition, the pressure of the transverse colon on the duodenum may cause duodenal obstruction. Colon examination in such cases shows a filling defect in the transverse colon at the point of contact with the duodenum.

MECONIUM ILEUS

Meconium ileus is a form of intestinal obstruction seen in the newborn and represents the earliest clinical manifestation of cystic fibrosis of the pancreas. The condition was first described in 1905 by Landsteiner, who related the abnormal meconium to pancreatic disease. In 1944 Farber demonstrated that fibrocystic disease of the pancreas is a generalized condition affecting both the pancreas and the mucus-secreting cells of the alimentary tract and tracheobronchial tree. The term mucoviscidosis which became popular following this recognition is no longer adequate because the sweat glands are also involved. Consequently there has been a reversion to the term cystic fibrosis of the pancreas to describe the underlying condition. The increased concentration of sodium and chloride in the sweat of these patients has within recent years become the most reliable diagnostic test. Neonatal small bowel obstruction by inspissated meconium has been reported in patients who do not have cystic fibrosis. Consequently, definitive parental counseling should be delayed until an accurate sweat test can be obtained.

The etiology of cystic fibrosis is unknown, but in all instances there are fibrosis and atrophy of the pancreas with obstruction of the ducts by inspissated material and a generalized abnormality of the mucous glands of the intestinal tract, resulting in scanty and mucilaginous secretions. Genetically, fibrocystic disease is inherited as a simple autosomal recessive. Many parents who clinically do not have the disease do have duodenal secretions of increased viscosity, and Harrison has demonstrated abnormal salt concentrations in the sweat of a significant number of parents. Theories regarding altered autonomic innervation or dissociation between glandular elements of the intestinal tract and vagus innervation have not been substantiated.

The time of development of the pancreatic achylia determines the clinical form of the disease. If the pancreas is severely involved in intrauterine life, the resulting deficiency in pancreatic exocrine enzymes leads to abnormal tenacious meconium which cannot be propelled caudally by intestinal peristalsis, resulting in meconium ileus. More often, the pancreatic deficiency does not become manifest until after birth and then appears clinically as a malabsorption syndrome consisting of poor nutrition and steatorrhea. Although frequent bulky stools are characteristic, we have seen a few patients with sudden onset of constipation and bowel obstruction caused by fecal blockage that required surgical removal of the impaction. All patients eventually have pulmonary complications which usually appear during the first few months of life, although the onset of pulmonary disease

may be postponed for several years. Repeated attacks of "bronchiolitis or asthma" in young children may be early pulmonary manifestations of fibrocystic disease. The thick mucoid secretions of the tracheobronchial tree produce multiple areas of obstructive emphysema and atelectasis followed by progressive chronic bronchiectasis. Although early and intensive antibiotic and inhalation therapy has greatly prolonged the life of these individuals, the majority die of the pulmonary complications. The prognosis of all forms of cystic fibrosis of the pancreas, even the cases of meconium ileus successfully corrected by surgery, depends on the severity and rate of progression of the pulmonary involvement.

SYMPTOMS. The predominant symptom of meconium ileus, as in other forms of intestinal obstruction in the newborn period, is vomiting. Because the obstruction is low in the intestinal tract, abdominal distention is a prominent feature. Occasionally the hard meconium masses may be palpated through the abdominal wall. Obstructive obstipation is usual, although there are reports of the passage of a small amount of meconium. The diagnosis is made at the time of laparotomy, the thick tenacious meconium being characteristic of the disease.

RADIOLOGIC FEATURES. The abdominal scout film is often the only radiologic study necessary. The abdomen is filled with gas-distended loops of small bowel and the mucosal pattern is usually unrecognizable due to the effacement produced by the distention. The colon cannot be identified, and gas within the rectum is rare. Gross called attention to the variability in size of the intestinal loops, some being enormously ballooned out, others only moderately distended, and others of relatively normal size (Fig. 12–31). Generally speaking, however, the distribution and appearance of the dilated loops are similar to other forms of low small bowel obstruction. Neuhauser emphasized the importance of the soap-bubble pattern of the meconium content of the bowel. This is the result of the mixture of air with the viscid meconium, giving it a radiographic appearance similar to the fecal pattern of the colon in older patients. A similar fecal pattern may be seen in the small intestine of infants with ileal atresia and aganglionosis of the

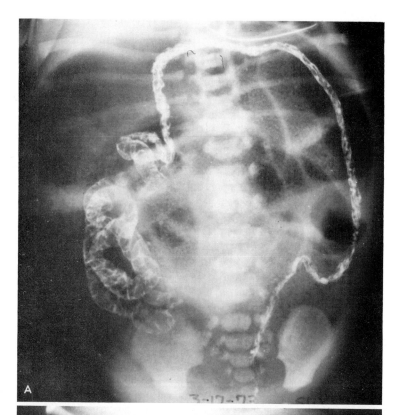

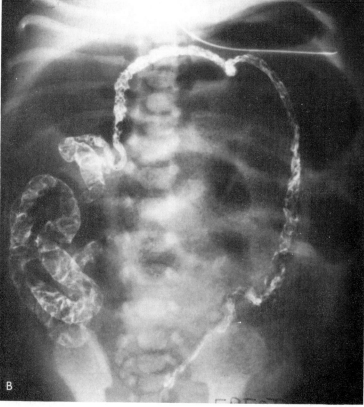

Figure 12–31. Meconium ileus. *A,* Recumbent film shows considerable gaseous distention of multiple loops of small bowel. Barium outlines an unused colon. Reflux into the terminal ileum shows meconium filling defects. *B,* Upright film shows absence of air-fluid levels in the distended small bowel.

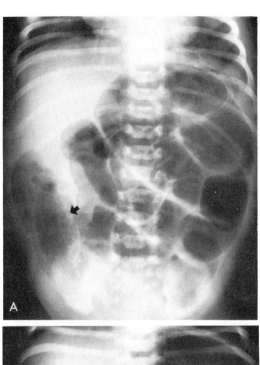

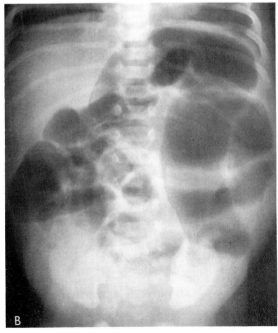

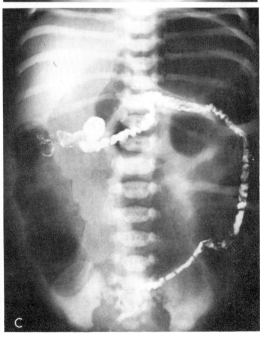

terminal ileum. The absence of air-fluid levels in the upright films in cases of meconium ileus is an important differential consideration and is the result of failure of the thick, tenacious meconium to shift and form an air-fluid level in the obstructed bowel. The absence of air-fluid levels in the upright films is presumptive evidence of meconium ileus but the presence of fluid levels does not exclude this condition.

Contrast material should never be given by mouth in suspected cases of meconium ileus. Barium enema studies are frequently helpful in identifying the site of obstruction and will demonstrate the abnormally small size of the colon, an indication that it has not served as a passageway for meconium (Figs. 12–32 and 12–33). In less severe cases in which meconium has passed to the rectum, the colon is of more normal size.

Hypertonic water-soluble iodide contrast

Figure 12–32. Meconium ileus. *A*, Abdominal scout film showing marked distention of small bowel with suggestive evidence of mottled air and feces in ascending colon and terminal ileum (*arrow*). *B*, Upright film showing absence of well-defined air-fluid levels. *C*, Colon examination demonstrating minute size of colon and intraluminal obstruction at hepatic flexure.

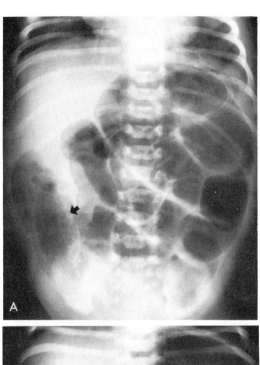

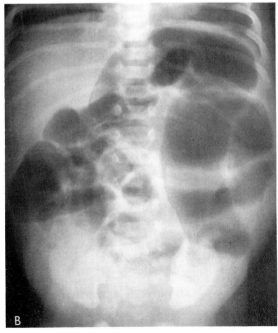

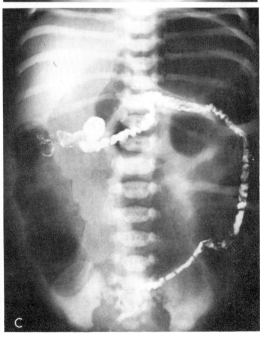

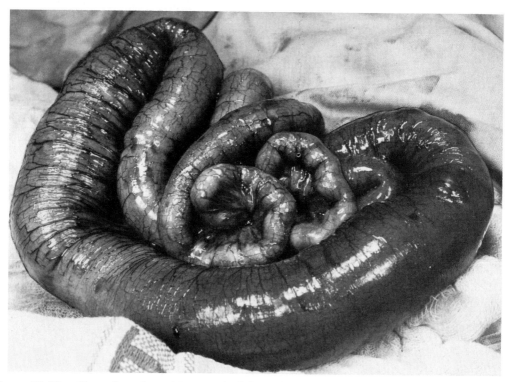

Figure 12–33. Meconium ileus. Note marked distention of ileum and the small collapsed colon.

enemas may be tried if the obstruction is in the colon but are more effective in the meconium plug syndrome. The osmotic properties of these solutions distend the colon with fluid and may dislodge the obstructing meconium. Careful evaluation of the serum electrolytes is mandatory to avoid hypovolemia.

Microcolon is also encountered in other forms of complete small bowel obstruction, but in our experience the smallest colons are found with meconium ileus, probably because in the other obstructive conditions more abundant mucoid secretions are formed below the obstruction. Although the soap-bubble sign, the presence or absence of air-fluid levels, and microcolon are helpful guides to the diagnosis of meconium ileus, the final diagnosis usually depends on direct inspection at the time of laparotomy. The complications of volvulus and ileal atresia are usually unsuspected until surgical exploration. Volvulus of the small bowel in these cases is due to the torsion effect of the heavy mass of inspissated meconium.

Ileal atresia is not uncommon with meconium ileus, and some authors have suggested that the atresia in such cases results from cicatricial changes in the bowel following trauma produced by peristaltic action on the hard tenacious meconium.

In some cases the inspissated meconium can be identified in the cecum and ascending colon by barium enema studies. The subjects of aganglionosis, meconium plug syndrome, and small left colon syndrome are discussed in Chapter 16, and should not be confused with obstruction due to meconium ileus.

MECONIUM PERITONITIS

Meconium in the peritoneal cavity may be definitely identified radiographically if it has been present long enough to become calcified, or its presence may be inferred without calcification if there are clinical and radiographic signs of bowel perforation at birth. Meconium is a sterile mixture of desquamated epithelial cells, vernix, lanugo, cholesterol, and mucopolysaccharide.

In the peritoneal cavity it acts as an irritant, promotes the formation of adhesions, and becomes calcified rather quickly, probably in some cases as early as 24 hours after it leaves the intestinal lumen. Neuhauser first associated meconium peritonitis with intraabdominal calcification but it may occur in any type of intrauterine bowel perforation. Calcification of meconium within the intestinal lumen in cases of congenital intestinal atresia has also been reported. An unusual form of meconium calcification is seen within the lumen of the colon in infants with imperforate anus and associated rectovesical or rectourethral fistulae (see Chapter 16).

Obviously, meconium peritonitis in the newborn indicates that there is or has been in prenatal life perforation of the bowel wall. Rarely the reason for this is never known, the finding of calcified meconium within the peritoneal cavity being incidental and clinically unimportant. Presumably in such instances there is extrusion of meconium into the peritoneal cavity through a perforation produced by intrauterine necrotizing enterocolitis, the perforation being completely repaired before birth. Meconium peritonitis resulting from a perforation of the intestinal tract which is present at birth or occurs immediately after birth signifies a grave situation, the initial sterile peritonitis becoming quickly converted into a bacterial infection. Although the perforation of bowel responsible for this may be independent of other abnormalities, the great majority are associated with some form of congenital intestinal obstruction such as atresia or stenosis, volvulus, obstructing peritoneal bands, incarcerated hernia, or meconium ileus.

SYMPTOMS. Infants in whom the passage of meconium into the peritoneal cavity occurred in utero independent of intestinal obstruction, with closure of the defect in the bowel wall before birth, are asymptomatic, and the abnormality is discovered only by chance if films of the abdomen are obtained. Otherwise, meconium peritonitis is an associated finding on abdominal films of a newborn who has intestinal obstruction. In such cases the symptoms are those of the obstruction, namely, vomiting and abdominal distention. If there is also pneumoperitoneum the distention may be extreme.

RADIOLOGIC EVALUATION. Meconium peritonitis is frequently noted in the newborn period as an incidental finding and is identified by its calcium content. In such cases, the meconium was extruded into the peritoneal cavity in utero and the defect in the bowel wall repaired before birth. The calcification may consist of a few irregular scattered areas or may be more extensive, consisting of continuous linear depositions of calcium localized usually in the peripheral portions of the peritoneum — in other words, underlying the anterior or posterior abdominal walls, in the flanks, or beneath the diaphragm (Figs. 12–34 and 12–35). This distribution is helpful in differentiating the occasional case of intestinal atresia in which the calcified meconium lies within the lumen of the bowel rather than in the peritoneal cavity. Meconium calcification in the scrotum may occur as a result of spillage of meconium into the peritoneal cavity early in fetal life when there was communication between the peritoneal cavity and the processus vaginalis of the scrotum (Fig. 12–36).

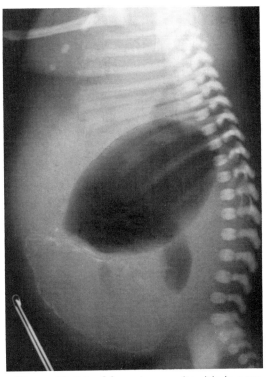

Figure 12–34. Meconium peritonitis in newborn with duodenal obstruction by peritoneal band. Calcified meconium appears as linear calcifications in peritoneal cavity.

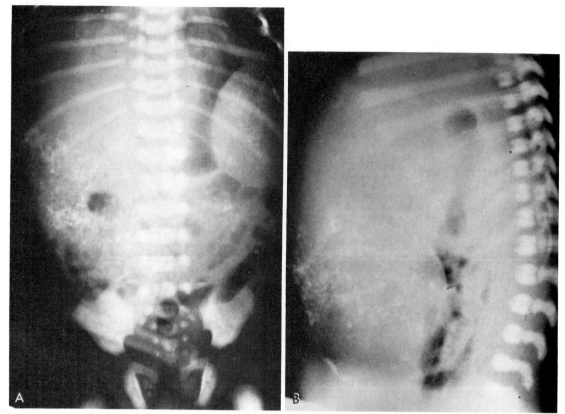

Figure 12–35. Meconium peritonitis in infant with ileal atresia and intrauterine volvulus. *A,* Anteroposterior film of the abdomen shows linear and flocculent areas of calcification within the peritoneal cavity. *B,* Lateral view shows the distribution of the calcified meconium within the peritoneal cavity.

The identification of meconium peritonitis may rarely be made on radiographs of the maternal abdomen (Fig. 12–37).

If pneumoperitoneum is evident at birth, meconium peritonitis with or without visible calcification is usually present. Regardless of whether intestinal obstruction is present or not, pneumoperitoneum in the newborn should be regarded as a surgical emergency and laparotomy performed in an attempt to locate and seal the defect before bacterial peritonitis has time to supervene.

Radiolucent bands paralleling the growth plates of the long bones and ilia may be seen in infants with meconium peritonitis but are nonspecific reflections of intrauterine growth disturbance.

AGANGLIONOSIS

Congenital deficiency in the number of ganglion cells of the myenteric plexus of the small intestine is an infrequent cause of intestinal obstruction in the infant. The condition is similar to Hirschsprung's disease except for the location of the aganglionosis. In 1948 Zuelzer and Wilson first described the condition as functional intestinal obstruction, but aganglionosis is a preferable description not only because the term "functional" implies an absence of organic abnormality but because it has also been used to describe another condition in which there is immaturity of the neural plexuses. The abnormality in these cases is a congenital absence of the ganglion cells, and the level of the obstruction corresponds to the level of the ganglion agenesis. The absence of these cells deprives the affected segment of both parasympathetic and local reflex innervation and results in absence of peristalsis. This acts as an effective obstruction even though a definite mechanical barrier is not present. The distal portion of the ileum is most often in-

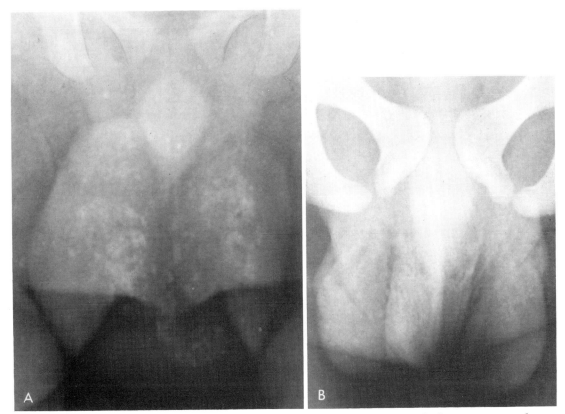

Figure 12–36. Calcified meconium in scrotum. *A*, Roentgenogram at birth showing scattered areas of calcification in scrotum. *B*, Five years later there is nearly complete disappearance of calcification. (*A*, Courtesy of H. M. Olnick, Atlanta, Ga., and M. B. Hatcher. Reprinted from *J.A.M.A.*, 152:582, 1953.)

volved, although cases affecting the jejunum have also been reported. Whatever the level, the deficiency of innervation usually extends caudad to involve the rest of the small bowel, colon, and rectum (Fig. 12–38).

SYMPTOMS. Abdominal distention, constipation, and vomiting are the predominant symptoms. The signs of obstruction appear within a few days after birth and unlike many cases of distal colon aganglionosis become increasingly severe during the first few days of life. The prognosis in all cases of small bowel and colonic aganglionosis is extremely poor, treatment consisting of enterostomy proximal to the aganglionic area.

RADIOLOGIC EVALUATION. The abdominal scout film of infants with this condition is similar to that of other forms of low small bowel obstruction. The abdomen is filled with several distended loops of small intestine whose type, as a rule, cannot be accurately identified because of the mucosal effacement. Air-fluid levels are promi-

nent in films made with the infant in an upright position. The colon usually is difficult to identify accurately, and what may appear to be colon lying parallel to the anterior abdominal wall in lateral views is actually distended ileum (Fig. 12–10). Barium enema studies demonstrate patency of the colon, which in such cases is short but usually of normal caliber (Fig. 12–39). With barium enema studies, considerable small bowel reflux is common. Differentiation of aganglionosis from meconium ileus and ileal atresia may be impossible, but in aganglionosis the colon is usually of more normal size. The soap-bubble pattern of meconium and gas which one thinks of in association with meconium ileus may also be present in aganglionosis. In the rare cases in which the neuromuscular dysfunction extends cephalad to the more proximal portions of small bowel, the distention is confined to the upper portions of the abdomen as in other forms of mid or high small bowel obstruction.

Oral administration of contrast material is

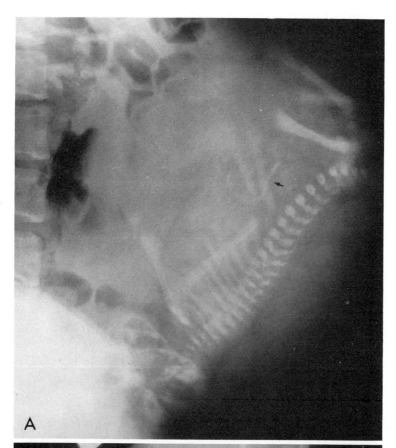

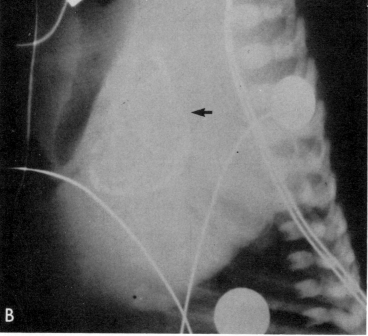

Figure 12–37. Intrauterine meconium peritonitis secondary to malrotation with volvulus. *A*, Fetogram shows the fetus in a vertex position. Calcification is identified within the fetal abdominal cavity (*arrow*). *B*, Lateral radiograph of the infant made following birth confirms the presence of meconium peritonitis (*arrow*). (Courtesy of Dr. Lee Rogers, Northwestern Univ.)

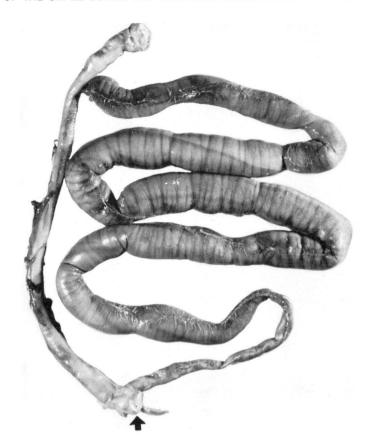

Figure 12–38. Aganglionosis of terminal ileum and colon. Note small size of colon and distal ileum and dilated ileum proximal to this. Arrow denotes cecum. (Courtesy of Dr. H. Rosenberg, Texas Children's Hospital, Houston, Texas.)

usually unnecessary, the identification of small bowel obstruction by abdominal scout films and, if needed, barium enema studies being all that is necessary.

In all infants with small bowel or colonic obstruction, the radiologist should consider the possibility of aganglionosis and include this condition in his report of the possible etiologic factors. The recognition that aganglionosis is a form of intestinal obstruction in which no mechanical barrier is grossly identified is imperative if the operable patients are to be saved. The transition zone between the distended and narrowed bowel seen at laparotomy will identify the proximal level of the aganglionosis. The level of extension must usually be determined by biopsy and histologic examination for ganglion cells. Only in this way can the patients having a localized and a resectable aganglionotic segment be distinguished. However, localized aganglionosis is extremely rare and in our experience all cases of small bowel aganglionosis have associated aganglionosis of

the entire caudal segment. More common forms of aganglionosis of the colon are discussed in Chapter 16.

DUPLICATIONS

This anomaly has many synonyms, including enteric cyst, gastroenterogenous cyst, enterogenous cyst, reduplication, giant diverticulum, and ileum duplex. Duplication is a simpler and more accurate description of the abnormality and may involve any portion of the alimentary tract. Esophageal duplications are considered in Chapter 6 and are more accurately described as neurenteric cysts. The majority of small bowel duplications are located in the ileum near or at the ileocecal junction. The second most common site involves the vertical portion of the duodenum.

PATHOGENESIS. The most acceptable previous hypothesis of alimentary tract duplications was based on the concept of recanalization of the intestinal tract following the proliferation of epithelial cells lining the primitive gut and obliterating its lumen, this being completed about the twelfth week. If one vacuole fails to blend completely with the re-formed lumen, it persists as a duplication, usually having the same muscular wall, blood supply, and mesentery as the parent structure. This process of development explains why some duplications connect with the adjacent lumen and others do not, depending on the completeness of the coalescence. Bremer has shown that variations in this process may result in the duplication having a separate muscular coat and even a separate mesentery. The mucosa of the duplicated segment may contain any type of alimentary tract musoca, most frequently gastric mucosa. However, the gradual discrediting of this theory suggests that duplication as well as atresia and stenosis is secondary to focal areas of vascular insufficiency sec-ondary to fetal stress and anoxia. It is conceivable that such circumstances developing in early fetal life (sixth through twelfth week) may be associated with an epithelial growth response which forms a diverticulum or duplication.

One variation of intestinal tract duplication is noteworthy regarding its development. This is the duplication which arises from the small intestine and extends as a tubular pouch through the diaphragm into the thorax. The tubular configuration and the great frequency with which anomalies of the cervical or upper thoracic spine accompany this abnormality support the theory that this type of duplication results from the persistence of an accessory neurenteric canal. The growth of the gut carries the base of the duplication caudally, leaving the distal portion which is attached to the notochord in the thorax.

SYMPTOMS. The symptoms of duplica-

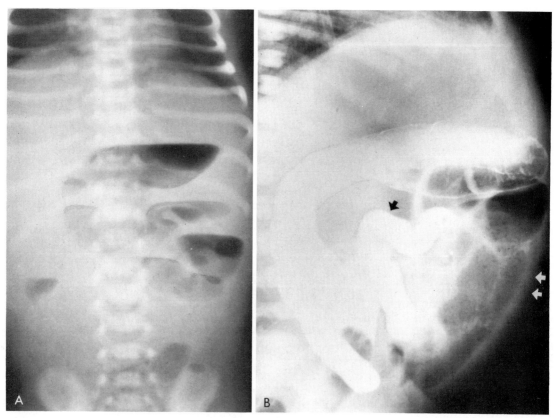

Figure 12–39. Aganglionosis of ileum in 5 day old infant with intestinal obstruction. *A*, Upright film of abdomen showing multiple fluid levels in moderately distended small bowel and absence of gas in colon. *B*, Colon examination showing no abnormality of this structure. A short segment of terminal ileum is also filled with contrast material (*arrow*) and appears to be normal, indicating that obstruction is proximal to this. Note mottled appearance of gas and feces in distended ileum (*double arrows*).

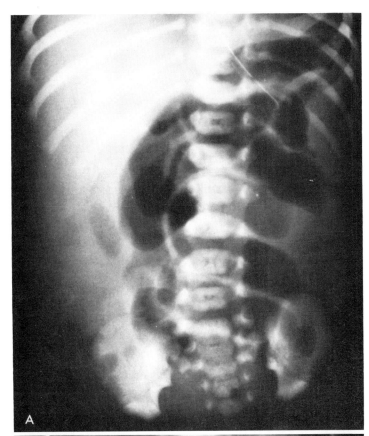

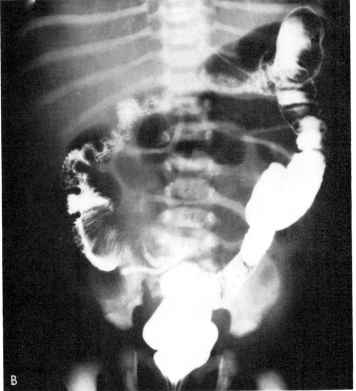

Figure 12–40. Duplication of terminal ileum in 3 day old infant. *A*, Scout film of abdomen shows multiple distended loops of small bowel without appreciable gas in the colon. *B*, Colon examination shows filling defect in the ileocecal area which at surgery was found to be extrinsic pressure by duplication of the terminal ileum.

tion of the small bowel are usually due to encroachment of the duplication on the adjacent bowel, causing either partial or complete intestinal obstruction. Consequently, vomiting and abdominal pain are predominant clinical findings. This is especially true of the majority of duplications which do not communicate with the adjoining bowel. The accumulation of secretions in the closed lumen leads to distention and consequent obstruction of the normal neighboring bowel. Occasionally the torsion produced by the weight of the duplication leads to small bowel volvulus. If the duplication contains gastric mucosa, pain secondary to peptic ulceration either of the duplicated portion or of the communicating segment frequently occurs, associated with intestinal bleeding which may be exsanguinating. These symptoms may occur at any age but are usually not evident until late infancy or early childhood. However, if the duplication is situated at a point where the bowel is relatively fixed in position and consequently easily obstructed by an adjacent mass, as in the second portion of the duodenum or in the region of the ileocecal valve, symptoms may develop in early infancy.

Duplications which arise from the upper small intestine and extend into the thorax cause, in addition, symptoms of cardiorespiratory distress and chest pain.

ROENTGENOLOGIC EXAMINATION. Because most duplications do not connect with the adjacent bowel, they are seldom identified radiographically but should always be considered in the differential diagnosis of small bowel obstruction in infants and children. With complete obstruction there is distention of loops of bowel above the lesion and absence of gas in the lower abdomen, the distribution depending on the level of the obstruction. In such cases it is usually impossible to identify the cause of the obstruction until laparotomy. If it cannot be determined whether obstruction is in the small bowel or in the colon, barium enema studies should be performed (Fig. 12–40), and if the colon is normal, contrast material may be given by mouth. Intussusception may be induced by an ileal duplication, but the duplication is discovered only during surgical reduction. If obstruction is not present but such other signs of duplication

as gastrointestinal tract hemorrhage, unexplained abdominal pain, and palpable abdominal mass are present, contrast material should be given by mouth; this will opacify the duplicated segment if there is sufficient communication between it and the adjacent bowel. In such cases, if the mass is in the lower abdomen the roentgen appearance is indistinguishable from Meckel's diverticulum (Fig. 12–41).

Duplications of the duodenum, if large enough, cause either partial or complete obstruction and resulting distention of the duodenal bulb and stomach (Fig. 12–42). This lesion is to be differentiated from a choledochal cyst which displaces the gastric antrum and duodenal bulb downward and medially. If the duplication communicates with the adjacent duodenum, it may fill with air or the ingested contrast material and thereby be demonstrated, appearing in such instances as a large duodenal diverticulum producing pressure or obstruction of the second portion of the duodenum. Figure 12–43 is a postmortem specimen of a duodenal duplication in a 3 week old infant who had had recurrent vomiting since the first week of life. Unfortunately, radiologic studies were not performed and the infant died suddenly after aspiration of vomitus. At autopsy, the distended duplication was found to be obstructing the duodenum.

The duplication which arises from the small bowel and enters the thorax is identified as a mass, usually tubular but occasionally spherical, paralleling the right side of the mediastinum and located posteriorly in the lateral projection. Anomalies of the lower cervical and upper thoracic vertebra are usually present. Additional loops of small bowel may accompany the duplication in the right hemithorax, thereby masking the duplication and exhibiting typical features of diaphragmatic hernia. Ingested contrast material may enter the duplication and be identified in the thorax. Its communication with the small intestine may also be localized in this manner. The transdiaphragmatic type of duplication usually originates in the jejunum near the ligament of Treitz but may arise from the duodenum or even the ileum.

Differentiation between a duplication
Text continued on page 204.

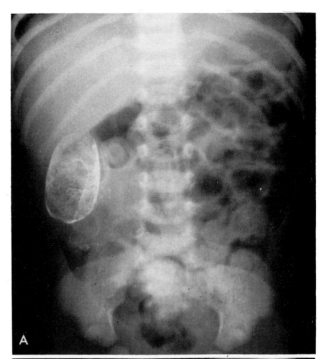

Figure 12–41. Duplication of the ileum in a 2 month old infant with melena. *A,* Residual barium is seen in a cystic structure following upper gastrointestinal tract examination. *B,* Colon examination shows terminal ileum which is obstructed by the extraluminal cyst. Laparotomy disclosed duplication of the ileum. (Reprinted from Margulis, A. R., and Burhenne, H. J., editors: *Alimentary Tract Roentgenology,* Vol. 2. St. Louis: C. V. Mosby Co., 1967, p. 1086.)

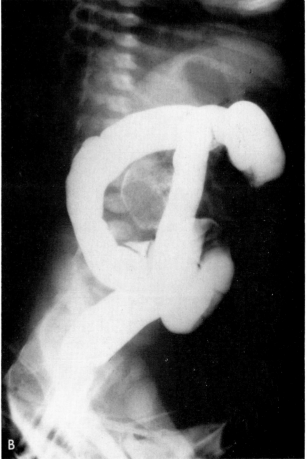

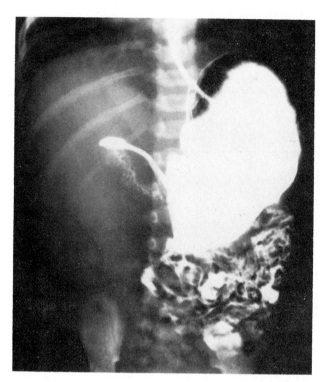

Figure 12-42. Duplication of duodenum in 6 day old jaundiced infant. There is upper displacement of the antrum and duodenal bulb by a large mass. At surgery duplication of the second portion of the duodenum was found.

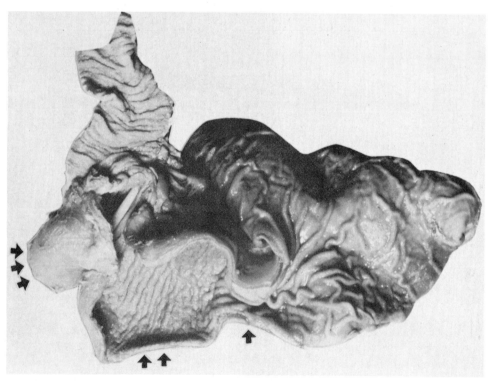

Figure 12-43. Duodenal duplication. Three week old infant with history of vomiting. Death followed aspiration of vomitus. Single arrow points to pyloric canal; double arrows, to a large dilated duodenal bulb; triple arrows, to duplication which compresses second portion of duodenum. Duplication was lined with gastric mucosa.

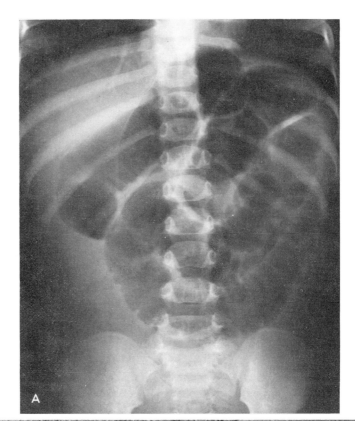

Figure 12-44. Mesenteric cyst obstructing terminal ileum of 3 year old child. *A*, Abdominal scout film showing gaseous distention of small bowel, absence of gas in colon, and displacement of small bowel away from right lower quadrant. *B*, Specimen at operation showing loculated mesenteric cyst surrounding and obstructing terminal ileum. (Courtesy of Dr. L. Able, Houston, Texas.)

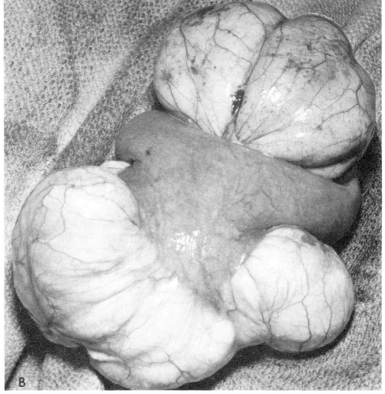

and mesenteric cyst in the ileocecal region with associated obstruction of the terminal ileum is usually impossible, both being capable of producing intestinal obstruction and displacing adjacent loops of bowel (Fig. 12–44). At surgery, the mesenteric cyst is found to have a thin wall composed of connective tissue without a muscular coat or mucosal lining. Surgical removal of a duplication necessitates removal of the adjacent bowel because of the common blood supply. This fact should be appreciated by radiologist and surgeon alike, as illustrated in Figure 12–45. This patient had a duplication of the ileum removed without removal of the adjoining ileum. Postoperatively, abdominal distention became severe and barium enema studies resulted in perforation of the devitalized, gangrenous terminal ileum and in barium peritonitis. Fortunately, the child survived the infection and a second operation.

Meckel's diverticulum also is usually impossible to differentiate from ileal duplex by radiologic means. Both conditions may cause obstruction, intestinal hemorrhage, and abdominal pain. Radiologically, either the duplication or the diverticulum may be identified by displacement of adjacent loops of bowel or by collection of air or contrast material within the pouch. Differentiation is made surgically, Meckel's diverticulum being on the antemesenteric side of the ileum and duplication on the mesenteric side.

MECKEL'S DIVERTICULUM

This structure arises from the ileum a short distance proximal to the ileocecal valve and is present in 2 to 3% of the population. It has clinical significance only when involved in an inflammatory or obstructive process.

DEVELOPMENTAL ANATOMY. In early embryonic life there is a wide anterior

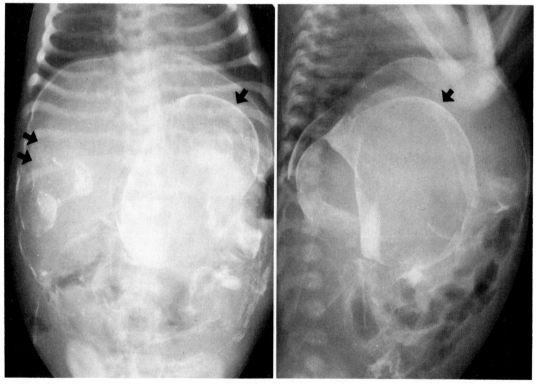

Figure 12–45. Barium peritonitis followint barium enema. Removal of duplication of ileum compromised the blood supply to the adjacent normal ileum. Postoperative barium enema caused leakage of contrast material from the gangrenous ileum into greater (*double arrows*) and lesser (*arrow*) peritoneal cavities. (Courtesy of Dr. L. Able, Houston, Texas.)

communication between the primitive intestine and the yolk sac. With development of the embryo, this communication becomes reduced in size, incorporated within the umbilical cord, and converted into the omphalomesenteric vitelline duct. It continues to diminish and at the 7-mm stage of the embryo is completely obliterated and loses its connection with the midgut. Meckel's diverticulum is formed if obliteration of the duct is incomplete at its attachment with the ileum. Failure of obliteration of the duct over its entire length produces a patent omphalomesenteric duct, leaving an open communication between ileum and umbilicus. Occasionally a vestigial band representing the obliterated duct extends between the ileum and the umbilicus and may cause intestinal obstruction if a loop of bowel becomes stretched over it.

The lining of Meckel's diverticulum may contain any type of mucosa of the gastrointestinal tract. Of 130 cases reported by Gross, 53 contained a mixture of gastric and ileal mucosa, 45 only ileal mucosa, 14 only gastric mucosa, and the rest, various combinations of ileal, gastric, colonic, or duodenal mucosa. One diverticulum contained pancreatic tissue.

SYMPTOMS. The clinical manifestations of Meckel's diverticulum usually appear during infancy and early childhood. Of Gross's patients, 45% came to the hospital within the first two years of life. The symptoms may be extremely variable, depending on the nature of the complications. If the diverticulum lining contains gastric mucosa, symptoms are most likely to develop because of irritation by the acid secretions. Hemorrhage is a common complication and is often profuse, with grossly bloody bowel movements. Less often, melena may occur, but in young infants hematochezia is more common. The amount of bleeding is usually greater than that seen with colonic polyps or anal fissures, and the relative lack of severity of the abdominal pain helps to differentiate a diverticulum from intussusception. The pain which accompanies Meckel's diverticulum is usually indistinguishable from that of acute appendicitis, there being right lower quadrant pain, fever, and leukocytosis. If the diverticulum causes an intussusception

or volvulus, the symptoms and signs of an obstructive lesion develop. It is impossible to differentiate between an intussusception that has Meckel's diverticulum as the cause and one that does not.

RADIOLOGIC EVALUATION. Only rarely does roentgenographic examination aid in the diagnosis of Meckel's diverticulum, and then it is more apt to be discovered as an incidental finding rather than during examination of a patient suspected of having this condition. Rarely, the diverticulum perforates and is responsible for extensive pneumoperitoneum (Fig. 12–46). The identification of a diverticulum by its gas content is exceptional (Fig. 12–47). The difficulty in identifying Meckel's diverticulum by radiologic methods is due to similarity of its appearance to that of the adjacent loops of bowel. The ostium is usually wide, so that barium empties from it as quickly as from the adjacent ileum. Frequently, the radiologist is asked to give a barium enema and retrogradely fill the ileum in a child with suspected Meckel's diverticulum. This is virtually impossible to do, and if the child has a competent ileocecal valve it will be painful and may be dangerous, especially if unsuspected appendicitis is present. Examination of the ileum fluoroscopically and radiographically following oral ingestion of barium is a more likely method of demonstrating the diverticulum, but success even with this is extremely rare (Fig. 12–48). Occasionally, if the diverticulum is distended or has a globular configuration with a narrow ostium, it can be identified on the scout film as a round collection of gas in the lower abdomen with displacement of adjacent loops of bowel. After administration of a barium meal, this type of diverticulum may become opacified. In such instances it is impossible to differentiate the diverticulum from a duplication of the ileum. Careful small bowel fluoroscopy is important in the identification of either condition. The differentiation is made at laparotomy by identifying Meckel's diverticulum on the antemesenteric side of the ileum or a duplication on the mesenteric side.

If the diverticulum becomes twisted, it may also involve the adjacent ileum and produce volvulus of this structure. If so, there will be radiographic signs of obstruc-

Text continued on page 210.

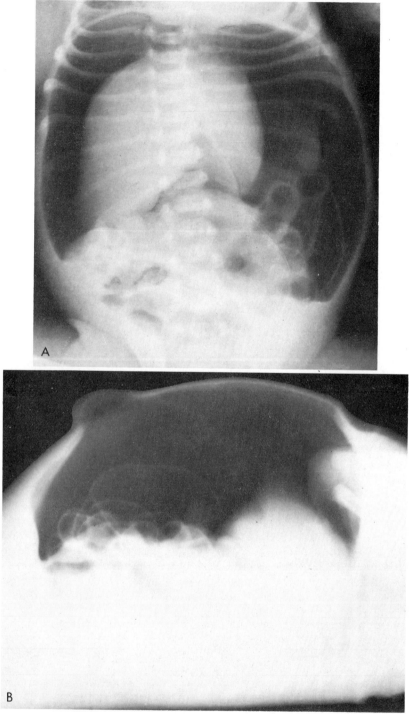

Figure 12–46. Pneumoperitoneum following perforation of Meckel's diverticulum in 5 day old infant. *A*, Anteroposterior film of abdomen showing abdominal viscera outlined by extensive pneumoperitoneum. *B*, Lateral supine film emphasizing enormous quantity of air collected in the peritoneal cavity. Perforated Meckel's diverticulum found at laparotomy.

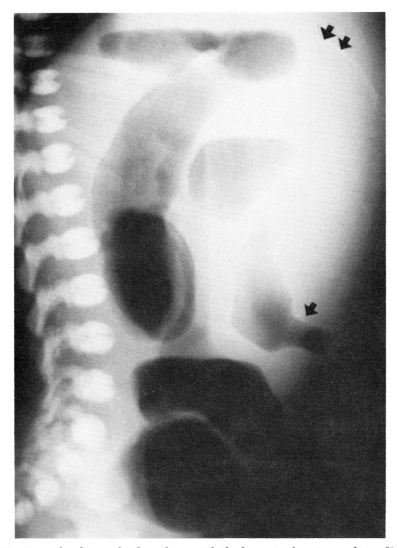

Figure 12–47. Lateral radiograph of newborn with ileal atresia showing outline of Meckel's diverticulum (*arrow*), proved at operation. Note also calcified meconium peritonitis (*double arrows*).

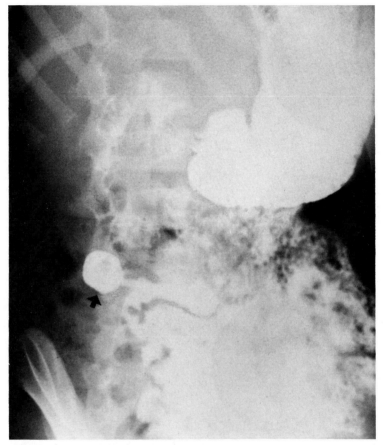

Figure 12–48. Meckel's diverticulum in 4 year old child. Diverticulum and connecting stalk indicated by arrow (unproved since the child was not operated on).

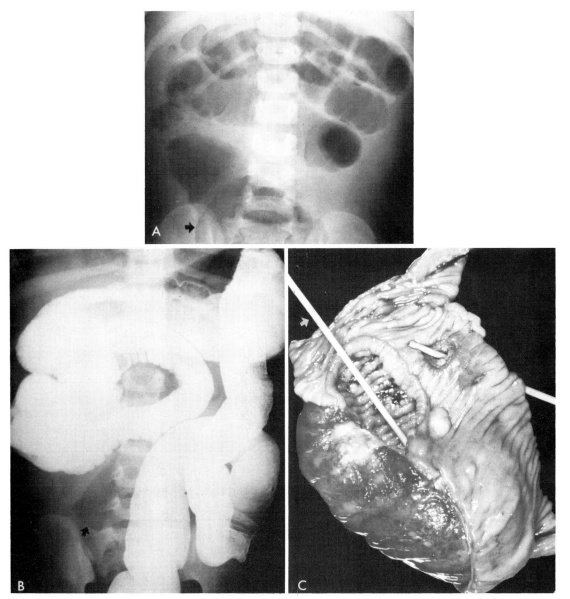

Figure 12–49. Meckel's diverticulum and volvulus in 4 year old child. *A*, Abdominal scout film showing distention of small intestine and distended segment of bowel in right lower quadrant (*arrow*). *B*, Colon examination showing upward displacement of cecum by persistent distended pouch (*arrow*). *C*, At operation, obstruction was found to be due to volvulus produced by large distended Meckel's diverticulum. Surgical specimen shows ileum opened, one probe (*arrow*) extending into diverticulum lined with gastric mucosa, and other probe through an ulceration of ileum. (Courtesy of Dr. J. F. Holt, University of Michigan.)

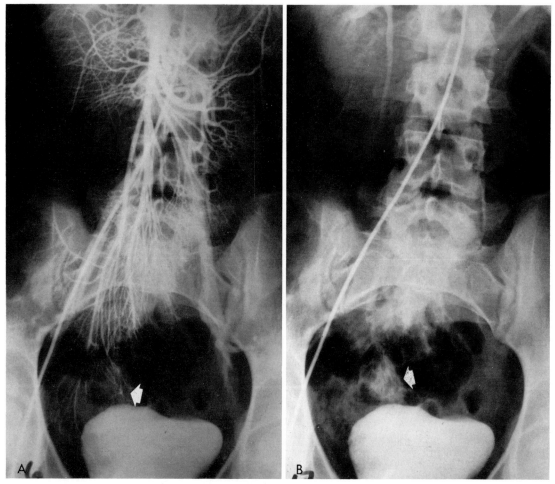

Figure 12–50. Meckel's diverticulum in child with intestinal bleeding. *A*, Superior mesenteric arteriogram shows small terminal branches in the wall of the diverticulum (*arrow*). *B*, Later radiograph demonstrates contrast medium within its lumen (*arrow*). An ulceration in a Meckel's diverticulum was found at surgery. (From Singleton, E. B., and Wagner, M. L.: The acute abdomen in the pediatric age group, *Semin. Roentgenol.*, 8(3):339, 1973. Reprinted by permission.)

tion with distention of small bowel, air-fluid levels, etc. Meckel's diverticulum associated with volvulus may be suspected in an obstructed patient whose scout film shows persistence of a distended loop of gut in the lower abdomen (Fig. 12–49).

Selective arteriography of the superior mesenteric artery performed while the patient is bleeding offers the best radiologic opportunity for making the diagnosis, but should be done by a radiologist experienced in vascular catheterization (Fig. 12–50).

The most accurate method of identifying a Meckel's diverticulum preoperatively is an abdominal scan utilizing technetium-99m. This isotope is picked up by the gastric

mucosa which is commonly present in both Meckel's diverticulum and duplication of the ileum.

DIVERTICULOSIS OF SMALL BOWEL

Diverticulosis of small bowel is a rare condition, the etiology of which is unknown. We saw persistence of such diverticula at autopsy in a mature infant who became obstructed two weeks after birth. Death was sudden, and postmortem examination revealed the obstruction to be secondary to distended diverticula in the ter-

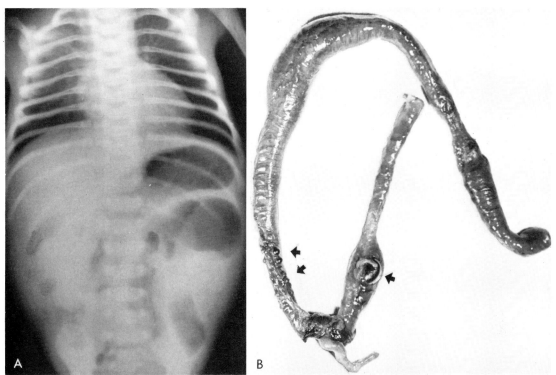

Figure 12–51. Diverticulosis of ileum and colon in 2 week old infant. *A*, Abdominal scout film showing loop of distended bowel in midabdomen. Infant died before further x-ray studies could be made. *B*, Postmortem specimen showing multiple diverticula in ileum and single large diverticulum in colon which had produced obstruction at this point. (Courtesy of Dr. H. Rosenberg, Texas Children's Hospital, Houston, Texas.)

minal ileum (Fig. 12–51). An older patient is seen in Figure 12–52.

PERSISTENT VITELLINE DUCT

The developmental anatomy of the vitelline or omphalomesenteric duct is described in Chapter 3. If this duct fails to close, it persists after birth as a sinus between the umbilicus and the ileum. Fecal material may drain from the sinus or if the tract should become infected the drainage may be of a purulent nature.

RADIOLOGIC EVALUATION. By careful probing the umbilical opening of the duct can be located and a polyethylene catheter of small caliber passed into the sinus. If possible, the catheter should be passed for a distance of several centimeters, at which point it should be within the ileum. Then, under fluoroscopy with the patient in a lateral position, a small amount of contrast material of thin viscosity (30% Renografin) is injected into the catheter and its passage into the ileum observed and recorded on spot films (Fig. 12–53). The catheter is then withdrawn nearly to the umbilical opening and additional contrast material injected. In this way, the size and configuration of the tract are most accurately determined.

If the catheter meets obstruction to its passage through the sinus, the injection of contrast material may demonstrate directly a small tract which was too small for the passage of the catheter or show contrast material in the ileum, thereby signifying the patency of the duct.

If the ileal communication of the duct is closed, there may be cyst formation within the tract. The injection of contrast material in such instances demonstrates the cyst and fails to show evidence of communication with the ileum.

Lateral supine radiographs of the abdomen made after installation of the peritoneal cavity with carbon dioxide or air may be of value in demonstrating a vitelline duct or Meckel's diverticulum.

INGUINAL HERNIA

Inguinal hernia in the infant and child is usually of the indirect type, occurs more commonly on the right than on the left, and is a potential site of intestinal obstruction.

DEVELOPMENTAL ANATOMY. The gonads of the male embryo are originally located high on the posterior wall of the abdominal cavity. As development progresses they gradually descend and at about the seventh month are drawn or led into the inguinal canal and scrotum by the gubernaculum, a mass of tissue attached to the lower pole of the testis. The descending gonad carries with it through the canal and into the scrotum a peritoneal pouch, the processus vaginalis, which communicates

with the peritoneal cavity. As the position in the scrotum becomes established, each testis becomes partially enveloped by the processus vaginalis, forming the tunica vaginalis of the testes, and the communicating portion of the processus vaginalis atrophies and closes. If this peritoneal stalk does not close, the sac remains as a congenital indirect inguinal hernia. The closure of the right processus vaginalis lags behind the left because of the normally slower descent of the right testis into the scrotum than of the left. This delayed series of events probably explains the greater frequency of right inguinal hernia. Even with normal closure, the inguinal canal remains a structurally weak spot which may at any time of life under excessive pressure become distended and permit heriation of intestine into it.

Most inguinal hernias are discovered after the neonatal period when the infant has gained sufficient strength to increase

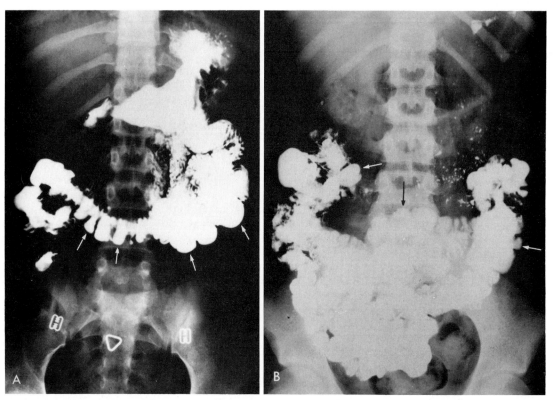

Figure 12–52. Diverticulosis of small bowel in 15 year old girl with chronic megaloblastic anemia. *A,* Upper gastrointestinal study shows collection of contrast media in proximal jejunum filling multiple diverticula in this structure (arrows outline only a few of the larger diverticula). *B,* Delayed film shows collection of barium in the terminal ileum also outlining multiple diverticula (*arrows*). Subsequent studies showed no abnormality of the colon.

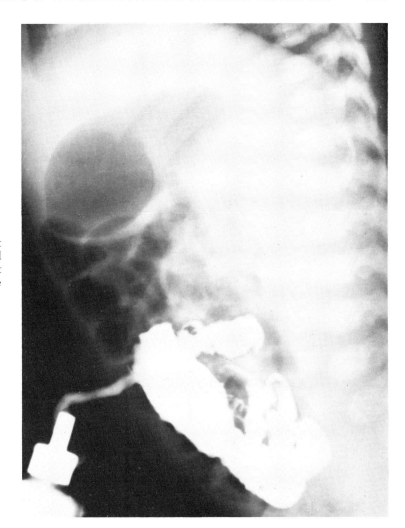

Figure 12–53. Persistent vitelline duct in a 3 week old infant. Large size of this duct allowed injection without use of catheter.

his intraabdominal pressure to a degree necessary to force bowel into the sac. Frequently, however, even large inguinal hernias are present at birth.

SYMPTOMS. Except for some local tenderness, inguinal hernia in infancy or childhood is usually asymptomatic until the herniated bowel becomes obstructed. Then tenderness of the herniated area increases and is followed by vomiting and abdominal distention, the severity depending on the degree of the obstruction and its duration.

RADIOLOGIC EVALUATION. The patient with an inguinal hernia is seldom examined by radiologic methods, even when obstruction is present, because the cause is readily apparent on physical examination. If gas-containing bowel is present in the scrotum, it may be identified on films of the lower abdomen (Figs. 12–54 and 12–55). Most hernias in infancy contain only small bowel, but in older children the omentum is longer and often projects into the hernial sac. Similarly, ingested contrast material will pass through the herniated bowel and be identified radiographically. With obstruction the abdominal cavity contains gas-distended loops of small bowel with decreased gas contents of the colon, the degree depending on the completeness of the obstruction. If the hernia is reduced and the obstruction relieved, there is a decrease in distention of the small bowel and gradual return of the normal bowel pattern (Fig. 12–56). An irreducible inguinal hernia with obstruction causes progressive clinical signs of intestinal obstruction accompanied

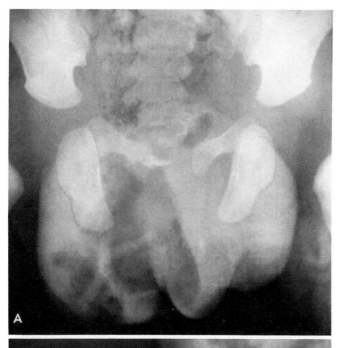

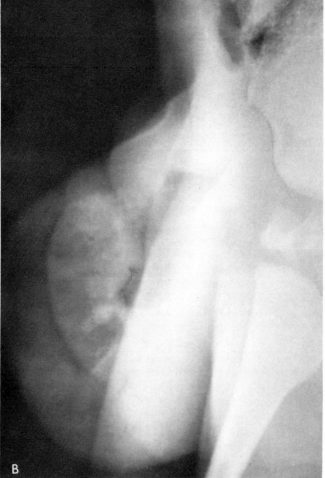

Figure 12-54. Large inguinal hernia in infant of 2 months, showing bowel in scrotum.

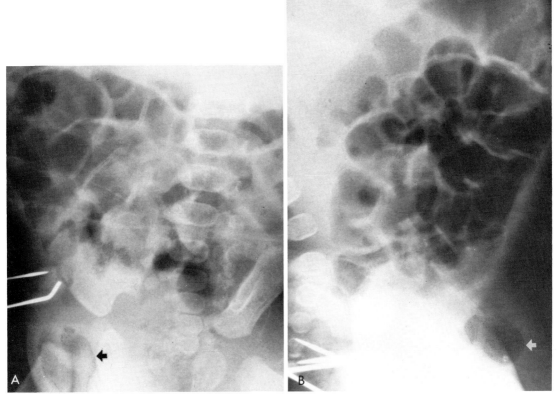

Figure 12–55. Inguinal hernia in child aged 6 months, identified on chest roentgenogram. (To improve clarity of the prints, only the pelvic portion of the original radiograph is reproduced.) Inguinal hernia is identified as collection of gas in right inguinal region in both anteroposterior (A) and lateral (B) views.

by radiographic evidence of bowel obstruction—small bowel distention, air-fluid levels, etc. Devitalization of the bowel is followed by peritonitis, which is characterized by further distention of bowel and separation of loops of dilated bowel by peritoneal exudate.

Inguinal hernia without air-containing bowel may be suspected by increased thickness of soft tissues in the inguinal area (Fig. 12–57).

Inguinal hernias may be demonstrated by the peritoneal injection of water-soluble iodide contrast medium. With the patient in an upright position the contrast material gravitates into the herniated peritoneal sac. This procedure has been successfully utilized in demonstrating unsuspected hernias on the side opposite the clinically identifiable site.

UMBILICAL HERNIA

Umbilical hernias are extremely common and occur as the result of muscular and fascial defects of the abdominal wall at the site of passage of the blood vessels of the umbilical cord. An increased incidence is known to occur in premature and black infants. Also, cretinism, gargoylism, the Down syndrome, and the Beckwith-Wiedermann syndrome are associated with an increase in umbilical hernia or omphalocele. The condition is obvious on direct inspection and when the infant cries becomes more prominent because of the increased intra-abdominal pressure. The condition may be responsible for abdominal pain if a knuckle of bowel becomes caught in the hernia. The incarceration of bowel within the defect is, however, very unusual.

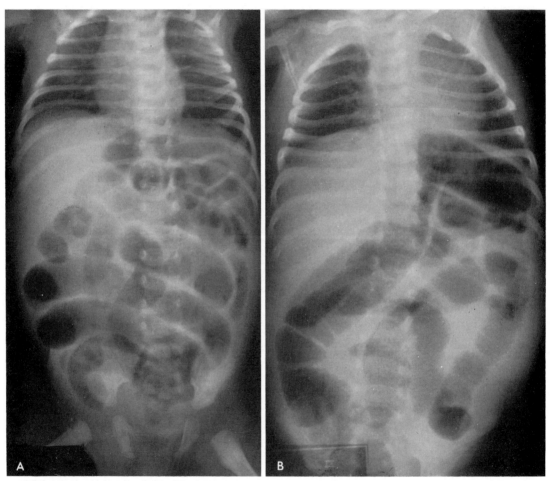

Figure 12–56. Obstructed inguinal hernia in 6 month old child. *A,* Abdominal radiograph exposed before external reduction of hernia showing evidence of low small bowel obstruction. *B,* Radiograph made shortly after reduction showing gas in colon and normal distribution of intestinal gas.

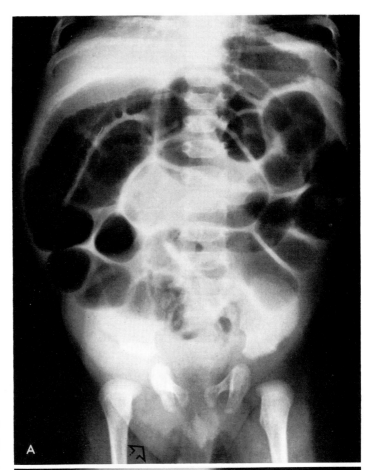

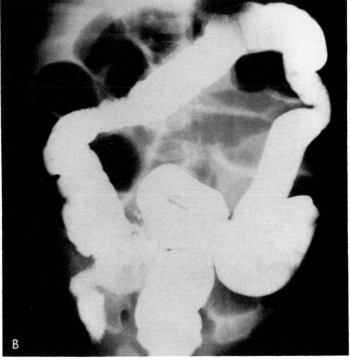

Figure 12–57. Incarcerated inguinal hernia in a 7 month old male infant. *A,* Radiograph of the abdomen shows marked distention of multiple loops of small bowel. Arrow denotes fullness in the right inguinal area. *B,* Barium enema examination shows extension of terminal ileum into the inguinal canal.

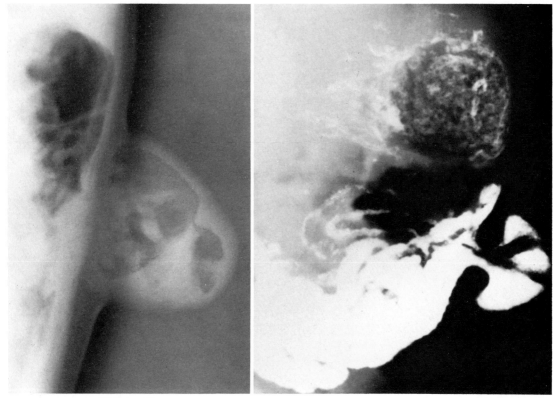

Fig. 12–58   Fig. 12–59

Figure 12–58. Umbilical hernia in 3 year old child.

Figure 12–59. Umbilical hernia in 6 month old infant with intermittent abdominal pain. Small intestine containing contrast material is identified in umbilicus.

Radiologic studies are rarely indicated but will often show the extension of bowel into hernial sac (Fig. 12–58). Contrast studies are unnecessary but will also disclose bowel within the umbilicus (Fig. 12–59). Kinking of a knuckle of small intestine in the hernia may be responsible for partial obstruction, and in such cases there will be mild dilatation of the bowel.

REFERENCES

General Considerations

Boreadis, A. G., and Gershon-Cohen, J. Aeration of respiratory and gastrointestinal tracts during first minute of neonatal life, Radiology, 67:407, 1956.

Burko, H. Toxic depression of the newborn causing deficient intestinal gas pattern, Am. J. Roentgenol. Radium Ther. Nucl. Med., 88:575, 1962.

Capitanio, M. A., and Kirkpatrick, J. A. The roentgenographic evaluation of intestinal obstruction in the newborn infant, Pediatr. Clin. North Am., 17:983, 1970.

Clatsworthy, H. W., Jr., et al. The meconium plug syndrome, Surgery, 39:131, 1956.

Davis, M. E., and Potter, E. L. Intrauterine respiration of human fetus, J.A.M.A., 131:1194, 1946.

Feinberg, S. B., et al. Dehydration and deficiency of intestinal gas in infants, Am. J. Roentgenol. Radium Ther. Nucl. Med., 76:551, 1956.

Frimann-Dahl, J., Lind, J., and Wegelius, C. Roentgen investigations of neonatal gaseous content of intestinal tract, Acta Radiol., 41:256, 1954.

Kassner, E. B., Koo, E. L., Harper, R. G., and Rose, J. S. Gasless abdomen in neonates with orotracheal tubes, Radiology, 112:659, 1974.

Liley, A. W. The use of amniocentesis and fetal transfusion in erythroblastosis fetalis, Pediatrics, 35:836, 1965.

Maddock, W. G., et al. Gastrointestinal tract; observation on belching during anesthesia, operations and pyelography and rapid passage of gas, Ann. Surg., 130:512, 1949.

Podolsky, M. L., and Jester, A. W. Distribution of air in intestinal tract of infants during first twelve hours as determined by serial roentgenograms, J. Pediatr., 45:633, 1954.

Singleton, E. B. Radiologic evaluation of intestinal obstruction in the newborn, Radiol. Clin. North Am., 1:571, 1963.

Soveri, V. Der Verlauf der Luft durch den Verdauungskanal des Sauglings, Acta Paediatr. (Suppl. 3), 23:1, 1939.

Wasch, M. G., and March, A. Radiographic appearance of gastrointestinal tract during the first day of life, J. Pediatr., 32:47, 1948.

Windle, W. F. *Physiology of the Fetus* (Philadelphia: W. B. Saunders, 1940).

Atresia And Stenosis

Astley, R. Duodenal atresia with gas below the obstruction, Br. J. Radiol., 42:351, 1969.

Barnard, C. N. The genesis of intestinal atresia, Surg. Forum, 7:393, 1956.

Berdon, W. E., Baker, D. H., Santulli, T. V., Amoury, R. A., and Blanc, W. A. Microcolon in the newborn infant with intestinal obstruction: Its correlation with the level and time of onset of obstruction, Radiology, 90:878, 1968.

Bodian, M., White, L. L. R., Carter, C. O., and Louw, J. H. Congenital duodenal obstruction and mongolism, Br. Med. J., 1:77, 1952.

Brodribb, J. H. G. Intramural calcification and stenosis of the small intestine of the newborn; case reports, Br. J. Radiol., 37:63, 1964.

Dickson, J. A. S. Apple peel small bowel: an uncommon variant of duodenal and jejunal atresia, J. Pediatr. Surg., 5:595, 1970.

Fonkalsrud, E. W., deLorimier, A. A., and Hays, D. M. Congenital atresia and stenosis of the duodenum. A review compiled from the members of the surgical section of the American Academy of Pediatrics, 43:79, 1969.

Harris, P. D., Neuhauser, E. B. D., and Gerth, R. The osmotic effect of water soluble contrast media on circulating plasma volume, Am. J. Roentgenol. Radium Ther. Nucl. Med., 91:694, 1964.

Hope, J. A., and O'Hara, A. E. Use of air as a contrast medium in the diagnosis of intestinal obstruction of the newborn, Radiology, 70:349, 1958.

Kassner, E. G., Sutton, A. L., and DeGrott, T. J. Bile duct anomalies associated with duodenal atresia; paradoxical presence of small bowel gas, Am. J. Roentgenol. Radium Ther. Nucl. Med., 116:577, 1972.

Louw, J. H., and Barnard, C. N. Congenital intestinal atresia: observations on its origin, Lancet, 2:1065, 1955.

Mellins, H. Z., and Milman, D. H. Congenital duodenal obstruction: Roentgen diagnosis by insufflation of air, Am. J. Dis. Child., 72:81, 1946.

Neuhauser, E. B. D. The roentgen diagnosis of fetal meconium peritonitis, Am. J. Roentgenol. Radium Ther. Nucl. Med., 51:421, 1944.

Santulli, T. V., and Blanc, W. A. Congenital atresia of the intestine: pathogenesis and treatment, Ann. Surg., 154:939, 1961.

Steinfeld, J. R., and Harrison, R. B. Extensive intramural intestinal calcification in a newborn with intestinal atresia: case report, Radiology, 107:405, 1963.

Weitzman, J. J., and Vanderhoff, R. S. Jejunal atresia with agenesis of the dorsal mesentery with "Christmas tree" deformity of the small intestine, Am. J. Surg., 111:443, 1966.

Annular Pancreas

Atallah, N. K., and Melhem, R. E. Annular pancreas in infancy: report of three cases, Am. J. Roentgenol. Radium Ther. Nucl. Med., 90:740, 1963.

Elliott, G. B., Kliman, M. R., and Elliott, K. A. Pancreatic annulus: a sign or a cause of duodenal obstruction?, Can. J. Surg., 11:357, 1968.

Free, E. A., and Gerald, B. Duodenal obstruction in the newborn due to annular pancreas, Am. J. Roentgenol. Radium Ther. Nucl. Med., 103:321, 1968.

Hope, J. W., and Gibbons, J. F. Duodenal obstruction due to annular pancreas, Radiology, 63:473, 1954.

Anomalies of Rotation

Astley, R. *Radiology of the Alimentary Tract in Infancy* (London: Edward Arnold, 1956).

Berdon, W. E., Baker, D. H., Bull, S., and Santulli, T. V. Midgut malrotation and volvulus. Which films are most helpful?, Radiology, 96:375, 1970.

Dott, N. M. Anomalies of intestinal rotation: their embryological and surgical aspects with report of five cases, Br. J. Surg., 11:251, 1923.

Estrada, R. L. *Anomalies of Intestinal Rotation and Fixation* (Springfield, Ill.: Charles C Thomas, Publisher, 1958).

Franken, E. A., Jr. Anomalies of the anterior abdominal wall: classification and roentgenology, Am. J. Roentgenol. Radium Ther. Nucl. Med., 112:58, 1971.

Friedland, G. W., Mason, R., and Poole, G. J. Ladd's bands in older children, adolescents and adults, Radiology, 95:363, 1970.

Frimann-Dahl, J. Volvulus of the right colon, Acta Radiol. (Stockholm), 41:141, 1954.

Frye, T. R., Mah, C. L., and Schiller, M. Roentgenographic evidence of gangrenous bowel in midgut volvulus with observations in experimental volvulus, Am. J. Roentgenol. Radium Ther. Nucl. Med., 114:394, 1972.

Houston, C. S., and Wittenborg, M. H. Roentgen evaluation of anomalies of rotation and fixation of the bowel in children, Radiology, 84:1, 1965.

Lough, J. O., Estrada, R. L., and Wiglesworth, F. H. Internal hernia into Treves' field pouch. Report of 2 cases and review of the literature, J. Pediatr. Surg., 4:198, 1969.

Mall, F. P. Development of human intestine and its position in the adult, Bull. Johns Hopkins Hosp., 9:197, 1898.

McIntosh, R. M., and Donovan, E. J. Disturbances of rotation of the intestinal tract; clinical picture based on observation in 20 cases, Am. J. Dis. Child., 57:116, 1939.

Parsons, P. B. Paraduodenal hernias, Am. J. Roentgenol. Radium Ther. Nucl. Med., 69:563, 1953.

Silverman, F. N., and Caffey, J. Congenital obstructions of alimentary tract in infants and children: errors of rotation of midgut, Radiology, 53:781, 1949.

Simpson, A. J., Leonidas, J. C., Krasna, I. H., Becker, J. M., and Schneider, K. M. Roentgen diagnosis of midgut malrotation: value of upper gastrointestinal radiographic study, J. Pediatr. Surg., 7:243, 1972.

Warthen, R. O., et al. Reversed rotation of bowel, Am. J. Dis. Child., 83:487, 1952.

Meconium Ileus

Berdon, W. E., Baker, D. H., Santulli, T. V., Amoury, R. A., and Blanc, W. A. Microcolon in newborn infants with intestinal obstruction, Radiology, 90:878, 1968.

di Sant' Agnese, P. A., and Talamo, R. C. Medical progress: pathogenesis and pathophysiology of cystic fibrosis of the pancreas, N. Engl. J. Med., 277:1287, 1344, 1399, 1967.

Dolan, T. F., Jr., and Touloukian, R. J. Familial meconium ileus not associated with cystic fibrosis, J. Pediatr. Surg., 9:821, 1974.

Donnison, A. B., Schwachman, H., and Gross, R. E. A review of 164 children with meconium ileus seen at the Children's Hospital Medical Center, Boston, Pediatrics, 37:833, 1966.

Farber, S. Pancreatic function and disease in early life: pathologic changes associated with pancreatic insufficiency in early life, Arch. Pathol., 37:238, 1944.

Feldman, W., and Belmonte, M. M. The inspissated stool syndrome: an unusual mode of presentation of cystic fibrosis beyond the newborn period, Can. Med. Assoc. J., 96:158, 1967.

Frech, R. S., McAlister, W. H., Ternberg, J., and Strominger, D. Meconium ileus relieved by 40% water soluble contrast enemas, Radiology, 94:341, 1970.

Gross, R. E. *The Surgery of Infancy and Childhood* (Philadelphia: W. B. Saunders, 1953).

Grossman, H., Berdon, W. E., and Baker, D. H. Gastrointestinal findings in cystic fibrosis, Am. J. Roentgenol. Radium Ther. Nucl. Med., 97:227, 1966.

Harris, P. D., Neuhauser, E. B. D., and Gerth, R. The osmotic effect of water soluble contrast media on circulating plasma volume, Am. J. Roentgenol. Radium Ther. Nucl. Med., 91:694, 1964.

Harrison, G. Personal communication.

Holsclaw, D. S., Eckstein, H. B., and Nixon, H. H. Meconium ileus: 20 year review of 109 cases, Am. J. Dis. Child,. 109:101, 1965.

Keats, T. E., and Smith, T. H. Meconium ileus: demonstration of ileal meconium mass by barium enema examination, Radiology, 89:1073, 1967.

Landsteiner, K. Darmverschluss durch eingedicktes Meconium: Pankreatitis, Centralbl. allg. Path. Anat., 16:903, 1905.

Leonidas, J. C., Berdon, W. E., Baker, D. H., and Santulli, T. V. Meconium ileus and its complications: a reappraisal of plain film roentgen diagnostic criteria, Am. J. Roentgenol. Radium Ther. Nucl. Med., 108:598, 1970.

Neuhauser, E. B. D. Roentgen changes associated with pancreatic insufficiency in early life, Radiology, 46:319, 1946.

Noblett, H. R. Treatment of uncomplicated meconium ileus by gastrografin enema: a preliminary report, J. Pediatr. Surg., 4:190, 1969.

Wagget, J., Johnson, D. G., Borns, P., and Bishop, H. C. Nonoperative treatment of meconium ileus by gastrografin enema, J. Pediatr., 77:407, 1970.

White, H. Meconium ileus: new roentgen sign, Radiology, 66:567, 1956.

Meconium Peritonitis

Berdon, W. E., Baker, D. H., Becker, J., and DeSanctis, P. Scrotal masses in healed meconium peritonitis, N. Engl. J. Med., 277:585, 1967.

Hillcoat, B. L. Calcification of the meconium within the bowel of the newborn, Arch. Dis. Child., 37:86, 1962.

Kasmersky, C. T., and Howard, W. H. R. Significance of intraabdominal calcification in the newborn infant, Am. J. Roentgenol. Radium Ther. Nucl. Med., 68:396, 1952.

Neuhauser, E. B. D. Roentgen diagnosis of fetal meconium peritonitis, Am. J. Roentgenol. Radium Ther. Nucl. Med., 51:421, 1944.

Olnick, H. M., and Hatcher, M. B. Meconium peritonitis, J.A.M.A., 152:582, 1953.

Smith, B., and Clatworthy, H. W. Meconium peritonitis: prognostic significance, Pediatrics, 27:967, 1961.

Tucker, R. S., and Izant, R. J., Jr. Problems with meconium, Am. J. Roentgenol. Radium Ther. Nucl. Med., 112:135, 1971.

Wilson, J. J., and Engel, R. R. Anticipating meconium peritonitis from metaphyseal bands, Radiology, 92:1055, 1969.

Aganglionosis

Berdon, W. E., Koontz, P., and Baker, D. H. The diagnosis of colonic and terminal ileal aganglionosis, Am. J. Roentgenol. Radium Ther. Nucl. Med., 91:680, 1964.

Frech, R. S. Aganglionosis involving the entire colon and a variable length of the small bowel, Radiology, 90:249, 1968.

Sandegard, E. Hirschsprung disease with ganglion cell aplasia of colon and terminal ileum: report of case treated with total colectomy and ileoanostomy, Acta Chir. Scand., 106:369, 1953.

Zuelzer, W. W., and Wilson, J. L. Functional intestinal obstruction on congenital neurogenic basis in infancy, Am. J. Dis. Child., 75:40, 1948.

Duplications

Bremer, J. L. Diverticula and duplications of intestinal tract, Arch. Pathol., 38:132, 1944.

Davis, J. E., and Barnes, W. A. Intrathoracic duplications of alimentary tract communicating with small intestine, Ann. Surg., 136:287, 1952.

Favara, V. E., Franciosi, R. A., and Akers, D. R. Enteric duplications. Thirty-seven cases: a vascular theory of pathogenesis, Am. J. Dis. Child., 122:501, 1971.

Grosfeld, J. L., O'Neill, J. A., Jr., and Clatsworthy, H. W. Enteric duplications in infancy and childhood: an 18 year review, Ann. Surg., 172:83, 1970.

Gross, R. E., Holcomb, G. W., Jr., and Farber, S. Duplications of the alimentary tract, Pediatrics, 9:449, 1952.

Gross, R. E., et al. Thoracic diverticula which originates from intestine, Ann. Surg., 131:363, 1950.

Mellins, R. W. P., and Koop, C. E. Clinical manifestations of duplication of the bowel, Pediatrics, 27:397, 1961.

Neuhauser, E. B. D., et al. Roentgenographic features of neurenteric cysts, Am. J. Roentgenol. Radium Ther. Nucl. Med., 79:235, 1958.

Snodgrass, J. J. Transdiaphragmatic duplication of alimentary tract, Am. J. Roentgenol. Radium Ther. Nucl. Med., 69:42, 1953.

Meckel's Diverticulum

Cross, V. F., Wendth, A. J., Phelan, J. J., Goussous, H. G., and Moriarty, D. J. Giant Meckel's diverticulum in a premature infant, Am. J. Roentgenol. Radium Ther. Nucl. Med., 108:591, 1970.

Duszynski, D. O., Jewett, T. C., and Allen, J. E. Tc^{99m} Na pertechnetate scanning of the abdomen with particular reference to small bowel pathology, Am. J. Roentgenol. Radium Ther. Nucl. Med., 113:258, 1971.

Fortier-Beaulieu, M., Chaumont, P., Labrune, M., and Goldlust, D. M. The radiological approach to the diagnosis of Meckel's diverticulum during infancy, Progr. Pediatr. Radiol., 2:303, 1969.

Gross, R. E. The Surgery of Infancy and Childhood (Philadelphia: W. B. Saunders, 1953).

Rosenthall, L., Henry, J. N., Murphy, D. A., and Freeman, L. M. Radiopertechnetate imaging of the Meckel's diverticulum, Radiology, 105:371, 1972.

White, A. F., Oh, K. S., Weber, A. L., and James, A. E., Jr., Radiologic manifestations of Meckel's diverticulum, Am. J. Roentgenol. Radium Ther. Nucl. Med., 118:86, 1973.

Diverticulosis of the Small Bowel

Caplan, L. H., and Jacobson, H. G. Small intestinal diverticulosis, Am. J. Roentgenol. Radium Ther. Nucl. Med., 92:1048, 1964.

Miller, W. B., and Felson, B. Diverticulitis of the terminal ileum, Am. J. Roentgenol. Radium Ther. Nucl. Med., 96:361, 1966.

Parulekar, S. G. Diverticulosis of the terminal ileum and its complications, Radiology, 103:283, 1972.

Persistent Vitelline Duct

Grosfeld, J. L., Franken, E. A. Intestinal obstruction in the neonate due to vitelline duct cyst, Surg., Gynecol. Obstet., 138:527, 1974.

Shakelford, G. D., and McAlister, W. H. Pneumoperitoneography in the evaluation of congenital anomalies in the umbilical region, Radiology, 104:361, 1972.

Wilson, J. W. Diagnosis of abdominal cysts in infants and children, Radiology, 64:178, 1955.

Inguinal Hernia

Ducharme, J. C., Bertrand, R., and Chacar, R. Is it possible to diagnose inguinal hernia by x-rays? A preliminary report on herniography, J. Canad. Assoc. Radiol. 18:448, 1967.

Mustard, W. T., Ravitch, M. M., Snyder, W. H., Jr., Welch, K. J., and Benson, C. D., editors. Pediatric Surgery (Chicago: Year Book Medical Publishers, 1969).

Shackelford, G. D., and McAlister, W. H. Inguinal herniography, Am. J. Roentgenol. Radium Ther. Nucl. Med., 115:399, 1972.

Swischuk, L. E., and Stacy, T. M. Herniography: radiologic investigation of inguinal hernia, Radiology, 101:139, 1971.

White, J. J., Haller, J. A., Jr., and Dorst, J. P. Congenital inguinal hernia and inguinal herniography, Surg. Clin. North Am., 50:823, 1970.

Umbilical Hernia

Gross, R. E. The Surgery of Infancy and Childhood (Philadelphia: W. B. Saunders, 1953).

McNamara, T. O., Gooding, C. A., Kaplan, S. S. L. and Clark, R. E. Exomphalos-macroglossia-gigantism (visceromegaly) syndrome (the Beckwith-Wiedermann syndrome), Am. J. Roentgenol. Radium Ther. Nucl. Med., 114:264, 1972.

Woods, G. E. Some observations on umbilical hernia in infants, Arch. Dis. Child., 28:450, 1953.

Chapter 13

ACQUIRED LESIONS OF THE SMALL INTESTINE

DUODENAL ULCER

There are numerous reports in the literature of duodenal ulcer in infants as well as in children. The reports of this condition in young infants are especially interesting because of the discrepancy in the number of cases reported from different institutions, it being a frequent finding in a few centers but extremely uncommon in others. In our own hospital, the radiologic demonstration of a duodenal ulcer in infants and children is relatively rare. Because of the small size of the infant's duodenal bulb and because its high position often renders it inaccessible to satisfactory palpation and distention, the identification of ulceration is extremely difficult, and what often appears to be a crater is likely to be only a minute collection of barium trapped between mucosal folds. Undoubtedly duodenal ulcer in infancy is responsible for many cases of unexplained hematemesis, but usually the small size of the ulceration makes radiologic demonstration impossible. Evaluation of duodenal ulcer in older children is more accurate because the child can give voice to his subjective symptoms and the size and position of the duodenal bulb are comparable to those in the adult, making radiologic demonstration of the ulcer or deformity of the duodenal bulb easier.

A survey of many pediatric radiology departments confirms the relative rarity of peptic ulcer in the pediatric age group. The inclusion of steroid-induced ulcers increases the incidence.

Duodenal ulcer in infants and children is more common than gastric ulcer by a ratio of 3:1. The etiologic hypotheses are the same as for gastric ulcer (see Chapter 10, p. 132). In the neonatal group, the abrupt rise in gastric acidity which occurs within 24 hours after birth is probably etiologically important, especially when associated with conditions of stress. Ulceration of the duodenum in infants is acute and does not become chronic, as occasionally happens in older children.

SYMPTOMS. The symptoms of duodenal ulcer in children, as in adults, are usually subjective except when hematemesis or melena occurs. Consequently the clinical evaluation of the older child from the standpoints of diagnosis and response to treatment is considerably more reliable than in the infant. Pain is the major symptom and is usually localized to the epigastrium but may be periumbilical. The child complains of discomfort between meals and obtains relief after eating. The discomfort may be especially severe at night and on arising in the morning. The location of the pain and its relation to food occasionally does not conform to this pattern, so the possibility of duodenal ulcer should be considered in any child having abdominal pain, hematemesis, or melena. Older children with duodenal ulcer often are emotionally "high-strung," this perhaps being a contributing factor to the development of duodenal ulcer. The frequency of unexplained abdominal pain in children is appreciated by all pediatricians and, although peptic ulcer may be responsible, urinary tract problems, abdominal epilepsy, and unrecognizable causes are much more common than radiographically identifiable peptic ulcer.

RADIOLOGIC EXAMINATION. The technic of examination of the duodenum is given in Chapter 2. Fluoroscopy is an indispensable part of the examination, and often only the spot films exposed during fluoroscopy show diagnostic evidence of duodenal ulcer. The infant's duodenal bulb is more difficult to examine than the older child's because of its high posterior position, which often prevents adequate palpation. In the older child the stomach and bulb are more accessible to palpation, allowing the examiner to exert pressure on the stomach and forcefully pass barium into the duodenum. If this maneuver is timed with a peristaltic wave the duodenal bulb can be fully distended and examined in frontal and right and left oblique positions, thereby enabling each side of the bulb to be identified and recorded on spot films. Failure to distend the bulb completely should not be mistaken for deformity. Transient pylorospasm may impede fill of the bulb, especially in an apprehensive child, but after a few minutes of patient waiting this is usually overcome. Persistent pylorospasm may be the only indication of inflammatory disease of the duodenum or stomach. It is only presumptive evidence of duodenitis or gastritis, but the diagnosis may be assumed to be correct if there is favorable response to treatment. Most duodenal ulcers in children are on the posterior surface of the bulb. In the frontal view, an ulcer on the posterior or anterior surface of the duodenum may be obscured by the contrast material unless pressure is applied (Fig. 13–1A and B). Spot films made during pressure on the bulb are often helpful in demonstrating these craters and frequently show a ring-shaped filling defect representing the edema encircling the crater. Radiating mucosal folds may also be seen extending outward from the ulcer. Air swallowed at the time of ingestion of barium may be used to good advantage in obtaining double contrast studies of the duodenal bulb.

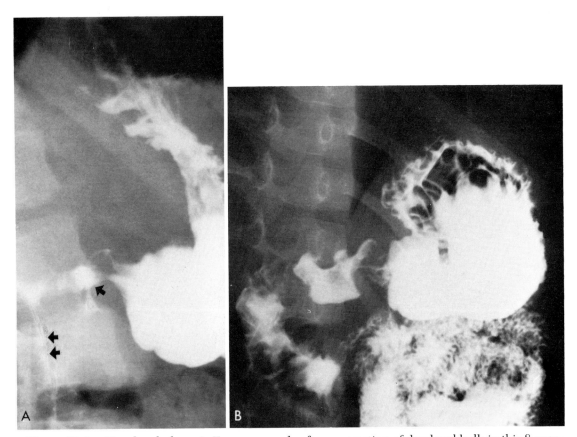

Figure 13–1. Duodenal ulcer. *A*, Exposure made after contraction of duodenal bulb in this 8-year-old child shows residual barium in a large crater *(arrow)*. Constriction of second portion of duodenum *(double arrows)* was persistent and represents associated duodenitis. *B*, Duodenal ulcer on the superior margin of the duodenal bulb in a 7-year-old boy with hematemesis.

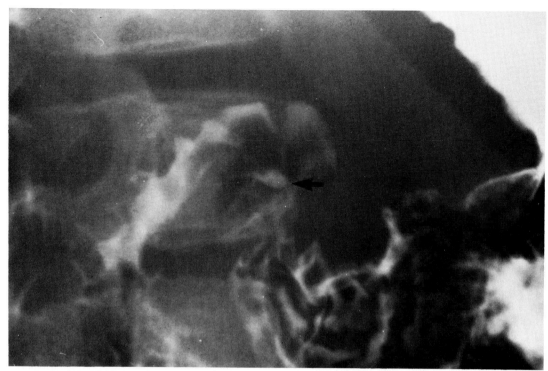

Figure 13-2. Duodenal ulcer *(arrow)* identified on the posterior wall of the duodenum utilizing ingested air to achieve double contrast effect.

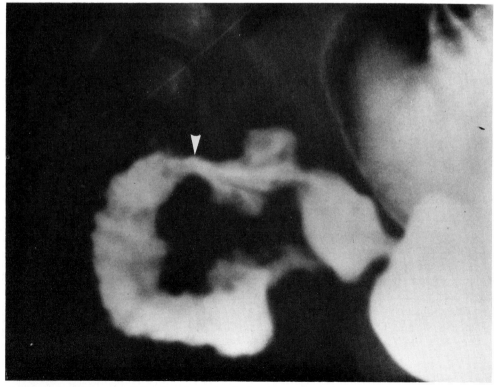

Figure 13-3. Deformity of the duodenal bulb with ulcer *(arrow)* in 1 month old infant with congenital syphilis.

This is done by exposing films of the duodenum with the patient in the supine position with the right side elevated, thereby allowing the ingested air to rise into the duodenum (Fig. 13–2).

Deformity of the bulb is less frequently encountered in the child than in the adult because the inflammatory process is less chronic in the pediatric patient. Occasionally, however, because of spasm or scarring, deformity is present, usually consisting of constriction of the midportion of the bulb and dilatation of the bulb fornix (Fig. 13–3).

Duodenitis of the second portion of the duodenum may accompany duodenal ulcer. It is identified by its narrowed appearance and coarsening of the mucosal pattern. Verification of persistence of the constriction by fluoroscopy is important to avoid misinterpreting a normal peristaltic wave as an inflammatory constriction.

Spontaneous pneumoperitoneum is extremely rare in children but may be the first evidence of duodenal ulcer. The diagnosis in such cases is made only at laparotomy but should be suspected in any child with free air in the peritoneal cavity (Fig. 13–4). If the amount of air is small, a lateral decubitus film may be more helpful than the upright film.

Follow-up examinations after medical treatment of duodenal ulcer are invaluable in determining the success of the treatment.

MALABSORPTION DISORDERS

During the past decade the term "malabsorption syndrome" has been used with increasing frequency to cover a multitude of intestinal abnormalities, all of which are clinically characterized by infants and children whose weight gain is inadequate, whose abdomen is usually protuberant, and whose stools are semisolid, pale, bulky and foul-smelling.

The majority of abnormalities produced in the malabsorption syndrome are usually diseases of the small intestine, which affect the normal metabolism or absorption of ingested food products. The basic considerations are altered anatomy of the intestinal tract, deficient secretions from the liver and pancreas, abnormalities of the intestinal mucosa, and miscellaneous causes. The following outline lists many of these abnor-

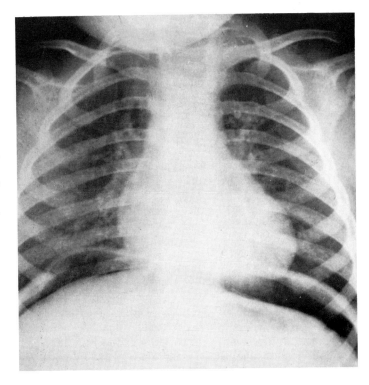

Figure 13–4. Perforated duodenal ulcer in 11 month old infant. Upright film of abdomen shows evidence of pneumoperitoneum. (Courtesy of Dr. A. O. Singleton, Jr., University of Texas.)

malities which can be suspected by radiologic examinations:

I. Anatomic Abnormalities
    1. Malrotation
    2. Duplication
    3. Small bowel stenoses or adhesions
    4. Surgically produced blind loops
    5. Small intestinal resections
II. Deficient Secretions from the Liver and Pancreas
    A. Pancreatic Exocrine Functions
        1. Cystic fibrosis
        2. Syndrome of pancreatic achylia, chronic neutropenia, and other bone marrow abnormalities
        3. General malnutrition
        4. Protein-calorie malnutrition
        5. Specific lipase deficiency
    B. Liver Disease
        1. Biliary obstruction
        2. Neonatal hepatitis and childhood cirrhosis of liver
III. Abnormalities of Intestinal Mucosa
    1. Slick-gut syndrome
    2. Celiac disease
    3. Chronic infections, including parasitic manifestations
    4. Protein-losing enteropathies
    5. Iron-deficiency anemia
    6. Intestinal lymphangiectasias
    7. Whipple's disease
    8. Acrodermatitis enteropathica
    9. Specific disaccharidase deficiencies
    10. Abetalipoproteinemia
IV. Miscellaneous Factors
    1. Emotional
    2. Zollinger-Ellison syndrome
    3. Ganglioneuromas
    4. Immune deficiency diseases
    5. Hyper- and hypoparathyroidism
    6. Renal disease
    7. Familial dysautonomia

It should be appreciated that alterations of small bowel pattern and motility may be normal variants in the infant age group. Consequently, the diagnosis of a malabsorption syndrome based on the radiologic appearance should not be made without careful clinical correlation. Radiologic evaluation becomes more significant after the first two years of life.

In the evaluation of celiac disease, inflammatory disease of bowel, parasitic infestations, lymphangiectasia, and disaccharidase deficiencies where histologic or biochemical evaluation can be made from the specimen, peroral biopsies may provide diagnostic information.

The clinical history cannot be overemphasized in the differential diagnosis of the malabsorption syndromes. Fatty stools (steatorrhea) are usually a reflection of some abnormality of the intestinal mucosa. Failure to thrive in celiac disease and in the disaccharide malabsorption conditions can usually be related to dietary changes. In celiac disease the clinical findings are more frequently seen during an earlier period of infancy. The presence of mucus in the stool is more commonly a reflection of either bacterial or parasitic infestations.

In the evaluation of suspected malabsorption it is necessary to determine if steatorrhea is present and if so, its cause. There are a number of methods of demonstrating steatorrhea, including macroscopic and microscopic examination of the stool, chemical studies of the stool for fat, absorption tests including xylose excretion, lipiodol excretion, and absorption tests utilizing ^{131}I-labeled triolein and oleic acid. After steatorrhea has been confirmed, tests to determine the cause should be performed, consisting of radiologic examination of the small intestine, bacteriologic studies, estimation of sweat sodium and chloride, determination of pancreatic exocrine functions, and peroral intestinal mucosal biopsy. The radiographic studies are particularly helpful in the anatomic abnormalities, but are less reliable in malabsorption states secondary to liver and pancreatic disease and even less specific in those conditions in which there is abnormality of the intestinal mucosa. This is particularly true in the young infant, where normal variations of the intestinal mucosal pattern frequently mimic the flocculation and segmentation of barium in the small intestine as well as the alterations of mucosal patterns seen in older children (see Figs. 11–10 and 11–11). Overfilling of the small bowel with barium may obscure abnormal patterns.

Peroral biopsy of the small intestine mucosa is helpful in celiac disease, giardiasis, the protein-losing enteropathies, and in the inflammatory lesions. Fluoroscopic localization of the Crosby capsule in the duodenal loop is necessary for accurately determining the site of biopsy (Fig. 13–5). In each of these conditions there is nonspe-

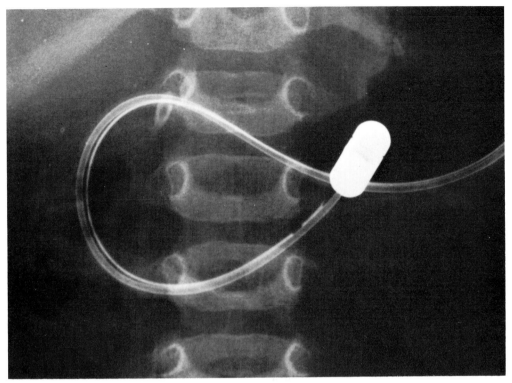

Figure 13–5. Crosby capsule positioned proximal to the ligament of Treitz.

cific flattening of the villi of the small bowel. Dilated lymphatics are characteristic of lymphangiectasia, but may also be seen in many of the other conditions. Inflammatory changes are, of course, to be expected in the inflammatory lesions.

ANATOMIC ABNORMALITIES. Radiologic studies are diagnostic in those conditions of altered anatomy. The complication of fistulae which develop in inflammatory lesions commonly produce an alteration of mucosal pattern. Careful fluoroscopic studies and radiographic interval films following the ingestion of barium (Fig. 13–6) are necessary to locate the fistula. Children with an intestinal tract fistula frequently show a lack of normal development that may be misdiagnosed as pituitary deficiency.

Blind loops secondary to end-to-end anastomoses, duplications, and congenital stenoses may also be responsible for malabsorption syndromes. In these conditions the altered bacterial flora in the dilated loop competes for vitamin B_{12}, with resulting failure of absorption of this necessary ingredient for a number of bodily needs including maturation of blood cells. Consequently macrocytic anemia is common in these conditions. The mechanism by which bacterial overgrowth in these conditions produces steatorrhea and malabsorption syndrome is not entirely clear, but is probably the result of abnormal metabolism of bile salts. The bacterial overgrowth deconjugates the bile salts and the steatorrhea is secondary to the toxic effect of the unconjugated salts on the intestinal mucosa, or secondary to a decreased amount of conjugated bile salts available for digestion of fat within the intestine. Upper gastrointestinal tract studies will usually demonstrate collection or stasis of barium within the blind loop (Fig. 13–7).

Partial small bowel obstruction secondary to either volvulus or peritoneal bands may also be responsible for the malabsorption syndrome. Whether this is the result of alteration of normal intestinal peristalsis, secondary to associated inflammatory changes of the bowel, or due to interference with normal bile salt metabolism as seen in the blind loop and duplication

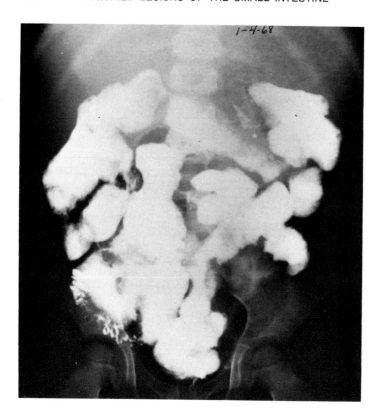

Figure 13–6. Small bowel fistulae in 8 year old child with Crohn's disease.

anomalies is not clear. Radiologic studies are of value in these conditions.

Recurrent volvulus is usually secondary to some type of intestinal malrotation. The abdominal scout film will usually show distended loops of bowel proximal to the obstruction, or scattered segmental loops within the midportion of the abdomen. Barium enema studies are helpful by demonstrating abnormal position of the cecum or abnormal mobility of the cecum. Upper gastrointestinal tract studies are usually unnecessary, but if performed will frequently show abnormal position of the ligament of Treitz. The presence of adhesions and bands may be suspected by distention of bowel proximal to the obstruction and fluoroscopic evidence of increased peristalsis. Hypoproteinemia, edema, and tetany may accompany steatorrhea. The importance of local venous obstruction in the pathogenesis is not clear.

DEFICIENT SECRETIONS FROM THE LIVER AND PANCREAS. The most common intestinal tract problem secondary to pancreatic enzyme deficiency is cystic fibrosis. Meconium ileus is the earliest clinical manifesta-

tion of this condition and has been described in the chapter on congenital intestinal obstruction. In older infants and children cystic fibrosis of the pancreas may be responsible for poor development and for a malabsorption pattern consisting of increased number of bulky, fatty stools. Infants and children with this condition usually have an enormous appetite which differentiates this particular form of malabsorption syndrome from others. Radiographic evaluation of the upper intestinal tract in infants with fibrocystic disease is unreliable because of the variability of the normal bowel pattern in this age group. However, in children with gastrointestinal symptoms of cystic fibrosis of the pancreas, the small bowel is usually dilated and the mucosal folds thickened and separated (Fig. 13–8).

Colon studies in these patients will commonly show the characteristic nodular pattern, especially in the postevacuation film, apparently the result of dilated, plugged mucous glands (Fig. 13–9A and *B*). Intussusception is not uncommon in the older patient with fibrocystic disease (Fig. 13–

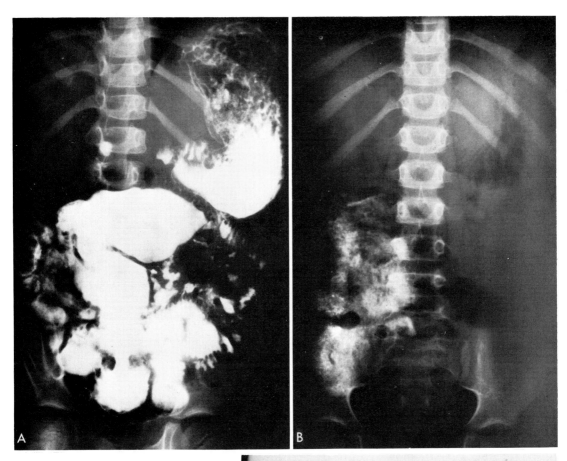

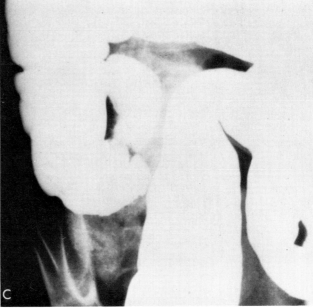

Figure 13–7. Blind loop syndrome in 4 year old child with megaloblastic anemia. *A,* Upper gastrointestinal tract shows collection of contrast media in dilated loop of bowel resembling colon. *B,* Scout film of the abdomen made 2 days later shows retention of barium within the large dilated segment of bowel. *C,* Colon examination shows no abnormality of cecum or terminal ileum but the residual contrast media within the dilated loop is seen adjacent to this. At operation a blind ileal loop was discovered incident to end-to-side anastomosis for treatment of ileal atresia at birth. (Reprinted with permission from Singleton, E. B., *Alimentary Tract Roentgenology,* 2nd ed., Margulis and Burhenne, editors. St. Louis: C. V. Mosby, 1973, p. 1491.)

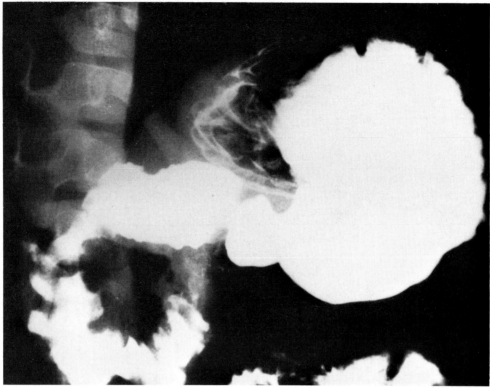

Figure 13–8. Fibrocystic disease in 8 year old child. The mucosal folds of the duodenum are coarsely thickened. Additional small bowel studies showed marked segmentation.

10). Ileocolic and colocolic intussusceptions are the most common forms. The usual expected discomfort of intussusception is often absent or markedly modified in fibrocystic patients with intussusception.

The other malabsorption syndromes associated with deficient secretion from the liver and pancreas or malnutrition as listed in the outline (p. 226) have no distinctive radiographic features other than alteration of intestinal mucosa, edema of the bowel, and segmentation of barium within the small bowel (Fig. 13–11). Severe malnutrition as best exemplified in kwashiorkor will produce a markedly altered small bowel pattern. However, this is undistinguishable from other severe malabsorption patterns (Fig. 13–12).

ABNORMALITIES OF INTESTINAL MUCOSA. The slick-gut syndrome is a term used to describe infants with chronic diarrhea and physical deterioration in whom a definitive cause is unknown. The condition is usually seen in infants under a year of age who have a history of recurrent diarrhea. The cause of the syndrome is unknown but after a variable period of hyperalimentation and no oral feedings, in which the gut is put at rest, the infant recovers. Abdominal radiographs in this condition usually show dilatation of multiple loops of small bowel as well as gas in the colon. In young infants the condition may simulate partial small bowel obstruction or total colonic Hirschsprung's disease. Studies of the gastrointestinal tract with barium are usually uninformative other than showing distended loops of bowel and absent or separated mucosal markings in the small intestine (Fig. 13–13).

Children with celiac disease (gluten-induced enteropathy) are usually asymptomatic until one year of age when the intake of wheat and rye increases and produces symptoms of irritability, loss of appetite, and abnormal bulky and fatty stools. In this condition there is not only malabsorption of fat but also slow absorption of carbohydrates, which can be determined by D-xylose absorption tests. Upper gastrointes-

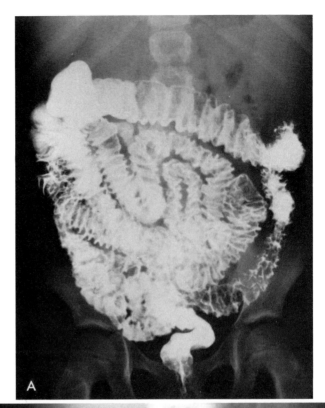

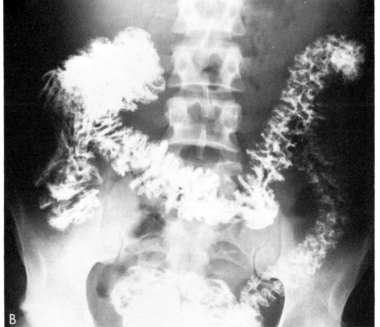

Figure 13–9. Fibrocystic disease. *A*, Barium enema in 7 year old child with fibrocystic disease, hepatospleno-megaly, and esophageal varices. The mucosal pattern of the terminal ileum is mark-edly coarsened and the mucosa of the colon shows a nodular configuration. *B*, Post-evacuation colon examina-tion of a 14 year old boy with fibrocystic disease. The mucosal pattern of the colon is nodular and coarsened.

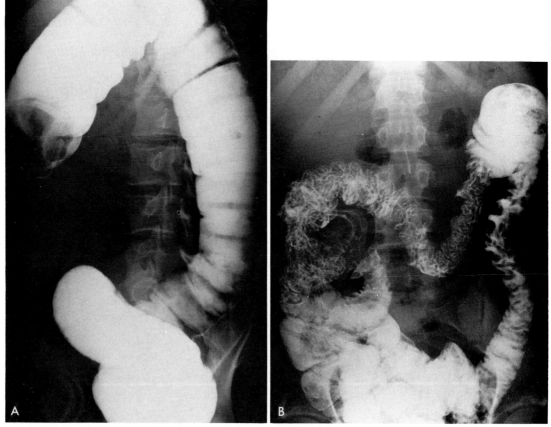

Figure 13–10. Intussusception in 17 year old boy with fibrocystic disease *A,* Preevacuation film shows the intussusception in the transverse colon. *B,* Postevacuation film shows intussusceptum has been reduced. The characteristic mucosal pattern of fibrocystic disease is obvious. The patient was relatively asymptomatic, a common feature of the older patient with fibrocystic disease who develops intussusception.

tinal tract studies show clumping or flocculation of barium throughout the small intestine and dilatation of loops with separation of mucosal folds. The radiographic features are not specifically different from many other forms of malabsorption (Fig. 13–14). Treatment consists of eliminating wheat and rye from the diet.

Chronic infections, particularly giardiasis, will produce thickening of the intestinal tract mucosa with coarsening and thickening of the mucosal folds. The radiographic features in this condition as well as in the protein-losing enteropathies and in other abnormalities of the intestinal mucosa cannot be differentiated. However, the coarse fold pattern in giardiasis is often exaggerated in the duodenum and jejunum (Fig. 13–15).

Intestinal lymphangiectasia may produce symptoms in young infants or its clinical onset may not appear until later life. Excessive loss of protein into the intestinal tract is the most significant clinical feature, usually associated with diarrhea, edema, and malabsorption symptoms. Small bowel biopsy is diagnostic. The radiographic findings consist of the edema, thickening, and separation of the mucosal folds. Segmentation and dilatation are usually minimal. In children nodular radiolucencies representing dilated lymphatics are more common than in older patients (Fig. 13–16).

Specific disaccharidase deficiency also produces a nonspecific malabsorption bowel pattern. In patients with this condition as well as in patients with milk allergy one can usually demonstrate barium dilution, bowel dilatation, and a rapid transit time of ingested barium when the specific offender is given shortly before the upper gastrointestinal tract study.

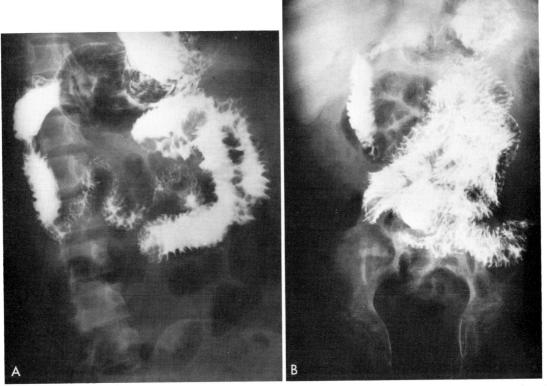

Figure 13-11. Edema of the bowel associated with cirrhosis. *A,* The mucosal pattern in this 8 year old girl is thickened and edematous with barium outlining the crevices between the edematous folds. *B,* 13 year old girl with cirrhosis secondary to bile duct atresia. Again note the prominent serrations of barium trapped between the edematous intestinal mucosa.

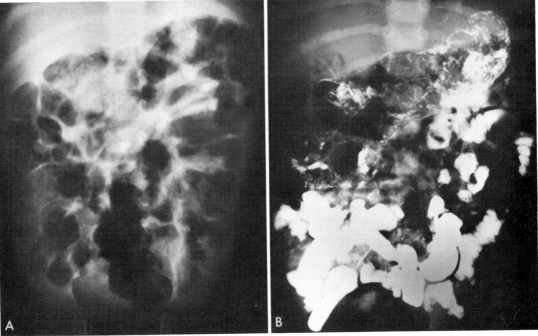

Figure 13-12. Kwashiorkor in an 18 month old infant. *A,* Scout film shows distention of small bowel and colon. *B,* Upper gastrointestinal studies show irregular segmentation of barium throughout the small bowel with alteration of mucosal pattern.

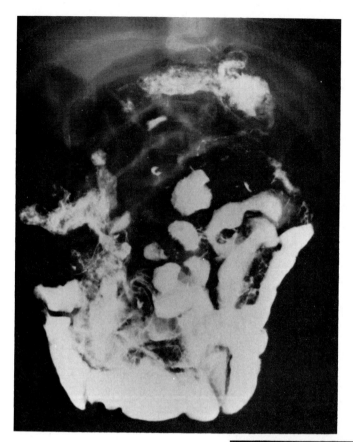

Figure 13–13. Two month old male infant with clinical findings of the "slick-gut syndrome." Upper gastrointestinal studies show barium scattered within loops of small bowel. Mucosal pattern is poorly defined. However, this radiographic pattern is not diagnostic and must be correlated with the clinical findings to be significant.

Figure 13–14. Celiac disease in 3 year old child. There is marked clumping of barium throughout the small bowel with coarsening of mucosal pattern and evidence of hypersecretion.

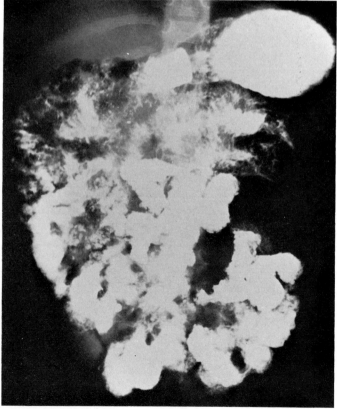

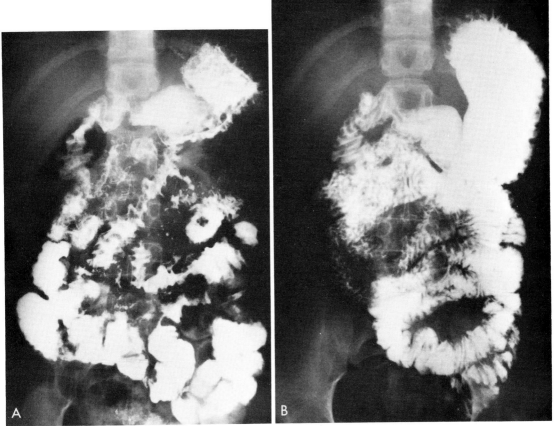

Figure 13–15. Intestinal giardiasis in an 11 year old boy. *A*, Upper gastrointestinal examination shows marked coarsening of the mucosal folds of the duodenum and jejunum with associated segmentation. *B*, Repeat examination of upper gastrointestinal tract following treatment 3½ months later. The small bowel has a normal appearance.

Abetalipoproteinemia is a rare disorder responsible for malabsorption which clinically and radiographically resembles celiac disease. The condition is due to a congenital deficiency of beta-lipoprotein, a protein responsible for membrane integrity and for the transport of fat through the mucosa of the intestinal tract. Diagnosis is made by mucosal biopsy, and with appropriate staining shows fat droplets accumulated in the form of small round bodies in the intestinal mucosa.

Miscellaneous factors listed in the outline may produce clinical and radiographic features of malabsorption syndrome but these are not specific and their identity is dependent upon excluding other conditions, and upon the identification of other abnormalities which may be responsible.

In IgA and IgM deficiencies lymphoid hyperplasia may be demonstrated not only within the terminal ileum but within other areas of the small bowel as well. Associated segmentation of the bowel is usually present and giardiasis is a common complication.

In the Zollinger-Ellison syndrome there is peptic ulceration, which is frequently postbulbar, and gastric hypersecretion due to nonbeta cell islet adenoma. Because of the hypersecretions the duodenum is dilated and may resemble the colon (colonization) (Fig. 13–17). Steatorrhea and diarrhea are common clinical findings.

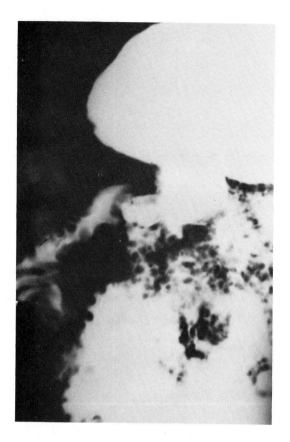

Figure 13–16. Intestinal lymphangiectasia in 2 year old child. The mucosal folds of the proximal small bowel are thickened, and nodular filling defects representing dilated lymphatics are present.

Figure 13–17. Zollinger-Ellison syndrome in a 12 year old boy. A large gastric ulcer is seen on the lesser curvature of the stomach. The duodenum is dilated (colonization) with separation of the mucosal folds.

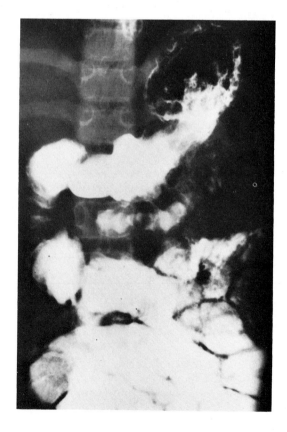

TRANSITORY INTUSSUSCEPTION

During examination of the upper gastrointestinal tract of children, one or several segments of small bowel having the radiographic characteristics of intussusception may be seen. The jejunum is most often involved and shows a coiled-spring configuration of barium trapped between the opposing feathery plicae of the intussusceptum and intussuscipiens, with a thin line of barium in the compressed central lumen (Figs. 13–18 and 13–19). The finding is transitory and rarely seen on more than one film of a single examination. Whether or not it is significant is debatable. When discovered in a child who is being examined for abdominal pain it provides a logical explanation for the discomfort; on the other hand, it is seen occasionally in children without abdominal discomfort, so its signficance is questionable.

SUPERIOR MESENTERIC ARTERY SYNDROME

Although compression of the third portion of the duodenum between the aorta and superior mesenteric artery is more commonly found in the young adult, it may occur in children in an acute form and be responsible for abdominal pain and vomiting. These children, as their adult counterparts, are usually thin, hypersthenic fe-

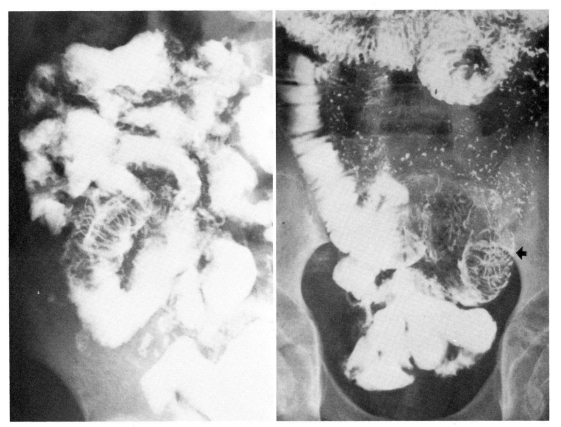

Fig. 13–18   Fig. 13–19

Figure 13–18. (*left*) Transitory small bowel intussusception in child aged 3½ years with vague abdominal pain. Two hour delayed film made during gastrointestinal tract examination shows coiled-spring silhouette with central column of contrast material in ileum characteristic of intussusception. Additional exposures showed no abnormalities.

Figure 13–19. (*right*) Transitory small bowel intussusception (*arrow*) in child aged 9 years with mild recurrent abdominal pain. Radiologic findings are similar to those in Figure 13–18.

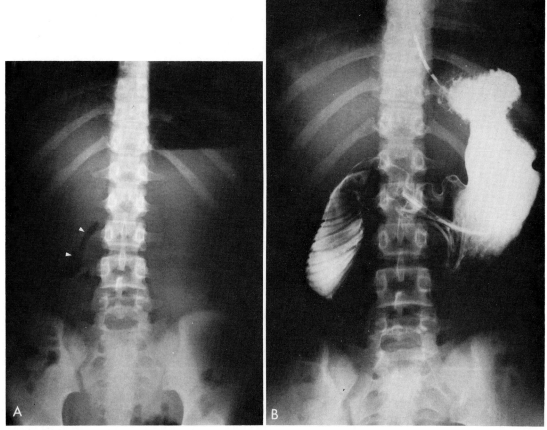

Figure 13–20. Superior mesenteric artery syndrome in 7 year old child. *A,* Scout film of the abdomen shows retention of fluid in the stomach. Persistent collection of gas was identified in the duodenal loop *(arrow). B,* Upper gastrointestinal study shows obstruction of the duodenum in the region of the superior mesenteric artery.

males (commonly) and frequently have a history of sudden weight loss which may have been self-imposed or due to illness or to being placed in a hyperextension cast. Loss of retroperitoneal fat about the superior mesenteric artery and duodenum is one explanation offered. X-ray examination shows dilatation and hyperactivity of the second portion of the duodenum with partial obstruction of the distal duodenum (Fig. 13–20). The findings may be identical to duodenal trauma. Lateral abdominal aortography may be helpful in showing interposition of the duodenum beneath the acute angle formed by the superior mesenteric artery.

INFLAMMATORY LESIONS

Regional Enteritis

Regional enteritis (Crohn's disease, terminal ileitis, regional ileitis) is a chronic inflammatory process of unknown etiology affecting any portion of the gastrointestinal tract but most often involving the terminal ileum and extending frequently into the cecum. Selective involvement of the colon (granulomatous colitis) is discussed in Chapter 17. The condition is more common in young adults, but children of any age may be affected, especially teen-agers. Although the condition is unusual in infants, it is more common than once thought. The process is chronic, with periodic remissions and exacerbations. Regional ileitis may have an acute onset with fever, leukocytosis, and right lower quadrant pain. These cases are usually mistaken for appendicitis, the correct diagnosis being made at laparotomy. The entire thickness of the bowel wall is involved, resulting in edema and thickening of the wall, ulceration and destruction of the mucosa and, in later stages, fibrosis and narrowing of the lumen. There may be involvement either of a single segment of short or greater length or of multiple segments separated by normal bowel.

SYMPTOMS. Diarrhea and cramping abdominal pain are the predominant symptoms at all ages. There may be fever, anorexia, and loss of weight, depending on the severity of the process. Unexplained growth failure is not an unusual feature. The abdomen over the involved areas is tender, and occasionally thickened seg-ments of bowel may be palpated through the abdominal wall.

ROENTGENOLOGIC EVALUATION. In young children the appearance of the small intestine may be similar to that seen in severe malabsorption disorders. The bowel is irritable, and hypermotility is frequently present. This may be the only finding in the very early stages. With persistence of the process the mucosal plicae become thickened, coarsened, and more widely spaced due to edema (Figs. 13-21 and 13-22). Even then the evidence of enteritis is only suggestive, and a definite diagnosis is rarely possible. In older children, localized disease is more easily identified (Fig. 13-23). Although any area of the small bowel may be affected, the terminal ileum is most commonly involved (Fig. 13-24). The bowel is irritable, the mucosal pattern poorly defined or ulcerated, and often spastic with temporary hold-up of barium at the affected site. In the more chronic cases strictures are present with dilatation of the

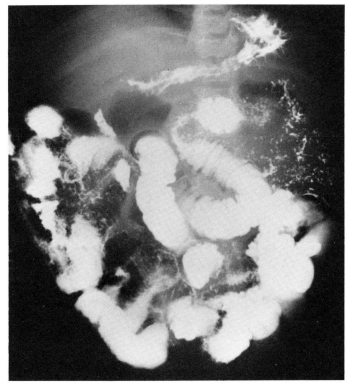

Figure 13-21. Probable Crohn's disease in 8 month old infant with vomiting and diarrhea. Upper gastrointestinal tract studies resemble pattern seen in malabsorption syndrome.

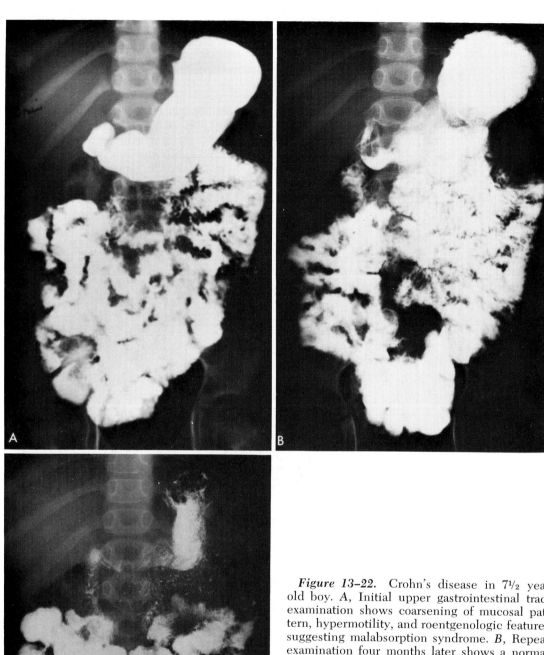

Figure 13–22. Crohn's disease in 7½ year old boy. *A,* Initial upper gastrointestinal tract examination shows coarsening of mucosal pattern, hypermotility, and roentgenologic features suggesting malabsorption syndrome. *B,* Repeat examination four months later shows a normal bowel pattern which correlated with the patient's clinical recovery. *C,* Examination one year later shows alteration of mucosal pattern in the ileum with polypoid filling defects and early cicatricial changes. Spreading of several loops of bowel secondary to edema is also noted.

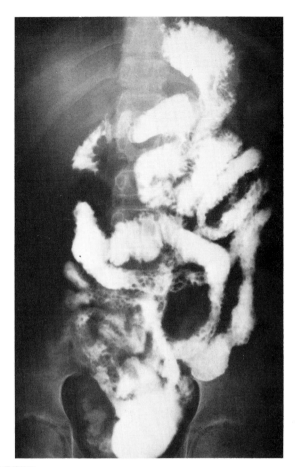

Figure 13-23. Longstanding Crohn's disease in 8 year old boy. The mucosa of the lower jejunum and ileum is abnormal and replaced by multiple granulomatous polyps. (Reprinted with permission from Singleton, E. B., in *Alimentary Tract Roentgenology*, 2nd ed., Margulis and Burhenne, editors. St. Louis: C. V. Mosby, 1973, p. 1498.)

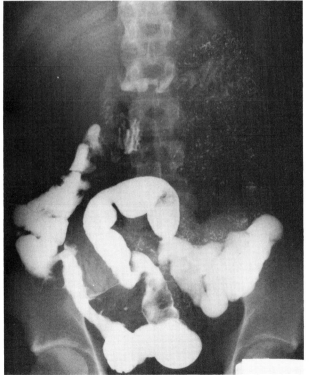

Figure 13-24. Crohn's disease in 15 year old boy. The mucosal pattern of the ileum is destroyed and multiple small sinuses extend into the surrounding soft tissues.

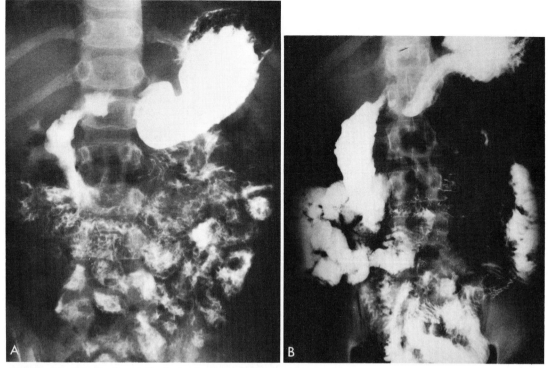

Figure 13–25. Isolated Crohn's disease of the duodenum. *A*, 4 year old girl with Crohn's disease of the duodenum. *B*, 11 year old boy who developed isolated Crohn's disease of the duodenum seven years after having clinical evidence of Crohn's disease manifested only by perianal ulceration.

proximal bowel. Isolated Crohn's disease of the duodenum is rare but an awareness of this condition is important (Fig. 13–25A and B). At this stage the roentgen appearance is diagnostic when correlated with the clinical findings, but unfortunately the disease is then in an advanced stage. Fistulae, sinus tracts, and localized abscesses are common complications.

Follow-up radiologic examinations are useful in determining the regression or advance of the disease. However, it should be remembered that symptomatic amelioration precedes the radiographic evidence of improvement; therefore the clinical evaluation is a more accurate index of the activity of the disease.

Tuberculous Enteritis

Tuberculous infections of the intestinal tract may be the result of direct invasion of the bowel after infected sputum is swallowed or of hematogenous implantation. Invariably, pulmonary tuberculosis, usually advanced, is present. Pasteurization and tuberculin testing of dairy cows has eliminated primary tuberculosis of the intestine.

It is unusual, even in large sanatoriums, to find radiographic examples of tuberculous enteritis. This is the result of the relatively fewer cases of advanced pulmonary tuberculosis today as compared with former years.

Tuberculous enteritis usually involves the terminal ileum and cecum but may be present in either alone (Fig. 13–26). Symptoms, when present, are similar to other types of enteritis, with diarrhea, cramping, abdominal pain, and fever being predominant.

ROENTGENOLOGIC APPEARANCE. The radiologic appearance is indistinguishable from regional enteritis. The involved ileum is hyperirritable and constricted, with dilatation of the bowel proximal to the stenosis (Fig. 13–26). The wall of the ileum is irregular and mucosal markings are indistinct or absent. The presence of pulmonary tuberculosis is helpful in differentiation from regional enteritis and also tuberculous enteritis more often involves the cecum. Bacteriologic identification of the pathogenic mycobacterium is necessary, however, for a definite diagnosis.

Acute Bacterial and Viral Enteritis

Infants and young children with acute enteritis or gastroenteritis of bacterial or viral origin occasionally present radiographic evidence of marked ileus. As pointed out in Chapter 12, air-fluid levels are frequently seen in radiographs of the abdomen of the normal infant in upright position. However, in the presence of acute enteritis, the air-fluid levels may be abnormally prominent and are accompanied by gaseous distention of the stomach, small bowel, and colon. In the child past infancy these findings may be especially confusing, and the appearance is frequently identical to that of low colonic obstruction.

The radiographic appearance in these cases is the exact opposite of the deficient gas pattern described by Margulis, et al., occasionally seen in severely dehydrated infants with diarrhea. Also the difference is apparent clinically, some children showing abdominal distention and others a scaphoid abdomen due to the collapsed intestinal loops. It seems unlikely that the degree of dehydration or electrolyte imbalance is solely responsible for this difference, and probably factors which are as yet unknown are responsible for these variations in gas pattern.

The scout film of the abdomen shows gas in the stomach, small bowel, and usually all portions of the colon. Upright or decubitus films show multiple air-fluid levels in all segments of the bowel (Fig. 13–27A and B). Differentiation from an obstructive lesion is based on the presence of gas in all segments of the bowel, including lower portions of the colon and rectum (frequently best demonstrated in a prone abdominal radiograph), and the clinical evidence of profuse diarrhea.

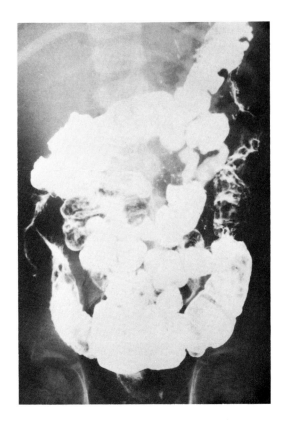

Figure 13–26. Tuberculous enteritis in 4 year old child with pulmonary changes of miliary tuberculosis. Upper gastrointestinal tract studies show deformity of the cecum and terminal ileum with associated dilatation of the proximal ileum and ulceration in the region of the ileocecal valve.

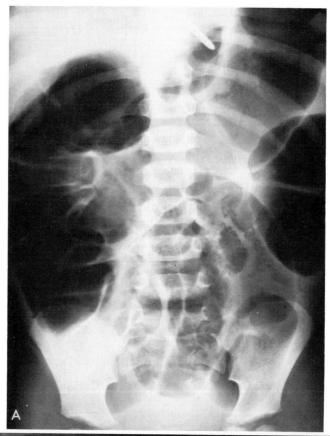

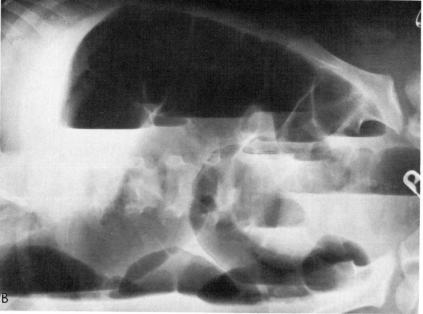

Figure 13-27. Severe gastroenteritis in a 5 year old child. Patient had acute onset of fever, vomiting, and diarrhea which abated in 24 hours. *A*, Abdominal scout film showing gaseous distention of colon and small intestine simulating low mechanical obstruction. *B*, Lateral decubitus film showing multiple air-fluid levels in colon and small intestine.

NECROTIZING ENTEROCOLITIS (ISCHEMIC BOWEL DISEASE)

In the first edition published in 1959 this condition was described under the heading of "noninfectious enterocolitis." Subsequent articles have popularized the term "necrotizing enterocolitis," and it is now a commonly recognized condition in large pediatric intensive care units.

Ischemic gastroenterocolitis in the young infant is usually found in the premature and low birth weight infant who for a variety of reasons may be subjected to conditions of stress. These include premature rupture of membranes, umbilical cord problems, infected amniotic fluid, central nervous system damage, sepsis, respiratory distress, and a variety of other conditions which may affect the neonate during the physiologic transition to extrauterine environment. The typical symptom complex includes anorexia, labile temperature, abdominal distention, gastric retention, vomiting, and bloody diarrhea. Two to four per cent of all deaths of premature infants are due to necrotizing enterocolitis. There is a questionably slight increased incidence in the male, but no racial differences have been found.

The underlying pathogenesis is probably based upon a reaction to intestinal ischemia due to either recognized or unrecognized perinatal distress for reasons already described. This hypothesis has evolved primarily due to work by Scholander, who studied regulation of arterial blood distribution in the seal during diving, by Aakhus and Johansen, who studied ducks during submersion asphyxia, and by Touloukian, who performed similar studies in piglets undergoing various stages of asphyxia. Briefly, these investigators determined that cessation of respirations invoked a reflex mechanism producing diminished arterial blood flow to the extremities, the mesentery, and the kidneys with resulting increase in coronary artery and cerebral blood flow. In the normal birth process, studies have shown that there is a similar mechanism which increases cerebral blood flow and coronary artery blood flow at the expense of arterial blood flow elsewhere. Consequently a logical conclusion is that if circumstances exist which result in persistence of the stress or hypoxic condition then ischemic disease of the bowel may result. Associated observations by Gruenwald and others of esophageal ulcerations related to anoxia supported these concepts. Other theories of pathogenesis, including swallowing of infected amniotic fluid, lysozyme deficiency in artificial milk, and Swartzman-type reaction, are less convincing than the "dive reflex" theory.

RADIOGRAPHIC FINDINGS. The earliest radiographic finding in our experience is a decrease in the normal amount of gas within the intestinal tract although others have observed an increase in the amount of gas in the small bowel. The most significant finding is a change in the normal gas pattern associated with the clinical findings (Figs. 13–28 and 13–29).

Pneumatosis cystoides intestinalis is a manifestation of the condition and is characterized by the presence of bubbles or

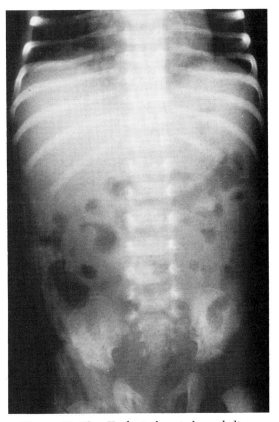

Figure 13–28. Early ischemic bowel disease in 10 day old infant with clinical findings of necrotizing enterocolitis. Film of the abdomen shows deficiency of the normal gas pattern.

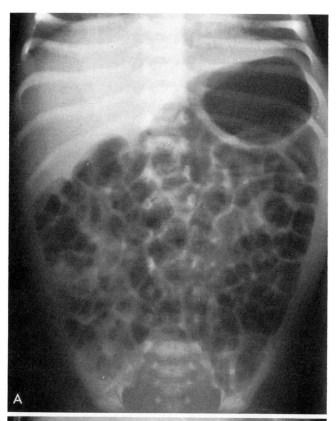

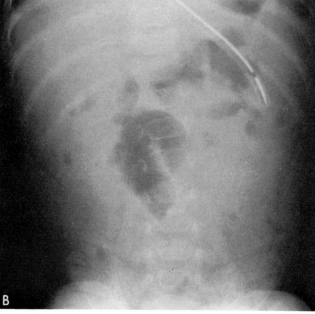

Figure 13-29. Ischemic bowel disease in 2 week old infant. *A,* Prior to onset of symptoms of ischemic bowel disease scout film of the abdomen showed excessive but normal accumulation of gas within stomach, small bowel, and colon. *B,* Two days later following onset of clinical findings of necrotizing enterocolitis, there is a decrease in the gas pattern.

linear streaks of gas within the bowel wall, more common in the small bowel than in the colon (Fig. 13–30). The gas that is in the bowel wall is identified as persistent radiolucent lines or fine bubbles conforming to and restricted to the bowel wall (Fig. 13–31). The colonic segments which are seen "on end" show a double radiolucent ring, the inner ring representing the intestinal gas lying between fecal material and mucosa, and the outer ring being gas in the submucosa. Only a single ring may be identified in the small intestine because of lack of solid intraluminal contents (Fig. 13–32A and B). Gaseous distention of bowel of varying degree is usually present. The combination of gas surrounding solid feces in the colon may present a radiographic appearance similar to pneumatosis. However, in the former condition the double ring is not present, and at some point in the linear air column the fecal material is seen to be in contact with the bowel wall.

Although there previously were many theories regarding the etiology of the intramural gas, the most plausible cause is that because of bowel ischemia, there is necrosis of mucosa with dissection of gas from the intestinal lumen into the submucosal layer. This may be followed by the additional complication of pneumoperitoneum (Figs. 13–33 and 13–34A and B) and gas within the portal circulation (Fig. 13–35), both of which represent ominous prognostic findings. Surgical intervention is necessary if the patient fails to respond to conservative treatment or if pneumoperitoneum or peritonitis develop. Coagulopathy may be an additional serious complication.

Conservative treatment, particularly the use of hyperalimentation rather than oral feedings, antibiotics, and careful radiographic follow-up studies, has resulted in more survivals than formerly seen. It is estimated that over 80 per cent will recover from necrotizing enteritis (per se) with conservative management. Consequently an

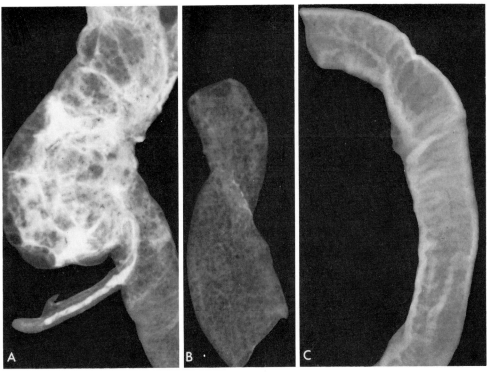

Figure 13–30. Pneumatosis intestinalis. Radiographs of autopsy specimens. A, Multiple blebs identified in wall of cecum. Barium residue is present in cecum and appendix. B, Radiograph of ileum shows the multiple blebs in contrast with segment of normal ileum shown in C.

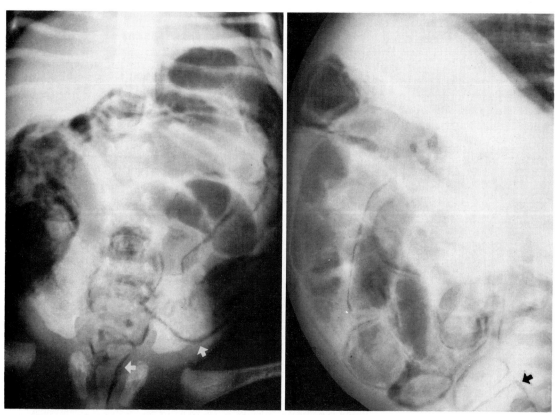

Figure 13–31. Pneumatosis cystoides intestinalis in 1 week old infant. Abdominal scout films show rectum and colon sharply outlined by collection of gas in bowel wall. (Courtesy of Dr. A. O. Stiennon, Madison, Wis.; *Pneumatosis Intestinalis in Newborn*, reprinted with permission from A. J. Dis. Child, *81*:651, 1951.)

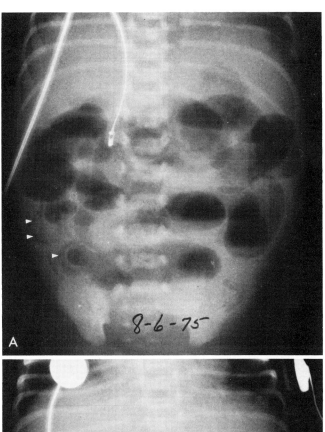

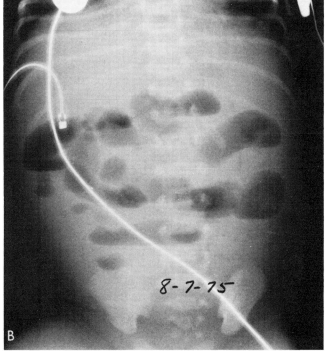

Figure 13–32. Necrotizing enterocolitis in 1 week old infant following respiratory distress syndrome. *A,* Abdominal scout film shows increase in the amount of gas and air-fluid levels in the small bowel. Pneumatosis intestinalis is identified as ring shadows in the right lower quadrant *(arrows). B,* Repeat examination 24 hours later shows free fluid in the peritoneal cavity suggesting peritonitis.

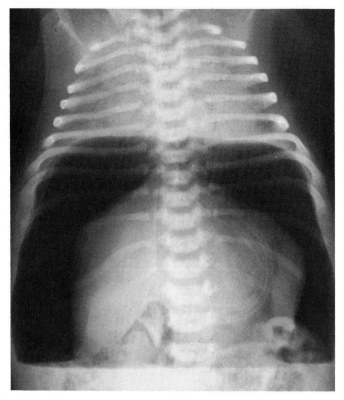

Figure 13–33. Massive pneumoperitoneum complicating necrotizing enterocolitis in a 6 day old infant.

increasing number of acquired bowel obstructions are being seen in infants surviving ischemic bowel disease. This is undoubtedly the result of the life-saving measures now utilized in the treatment. Ileal stenoses comprise the majority of the obstructions (Figs. 13–36, 13–37, and 13–38), but colon strictures may also occur (Fig. 13–39).

The spectrum of ischemic bowel disease varies, depending upon the time of the ischemic insult. Tandler's theory of atresia due to failure of recanalization has now been largely replaced by the more recent work of Louw. By interfering with the mesenteric blood supply of fetal puppies and allowing these puppies to complete their gestation, it was shown that bowel atresia as well as a number of other anomalies could develop due to interference of arterial blood supply. This work was subsequently confirmed by Santulli. Consequently the spectrum of ischemic bowel disease may be projected retrogradely into

intrauterine life to explain most of the cases of bowel atresia, particularly where there is meconium-containing bile and amniotic cells distal to the point of obstruction. The development of an ischemic insult in the immediate prenatal or perinatal period may result in the birth of an infant with necrotic segment of bowel and perforation. Radiographically this does not show the progression of the changes seen in the slightly older infant with necrotizing enterocolitis but shows pneumoperitoneum as the initial radiographic finding. The common sites of perforation are the terminal ileum, stomach, and colon areas which normally have a decreased mucosal profusion of blood during stress conditions. Many of the cases of "incomplete development of the gastric musculature" are probably the result of ischemic disease of the stomach. Another part of the spectrum of ischemic bowel disease in intrauterine life is meconium peritonitis, except those cases associated with fibrocystic disease. The

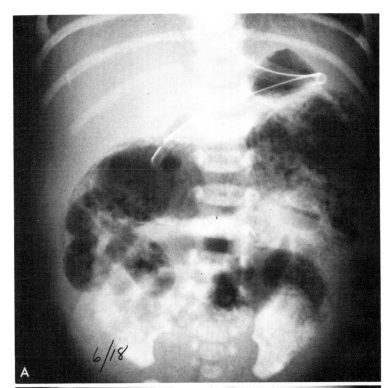
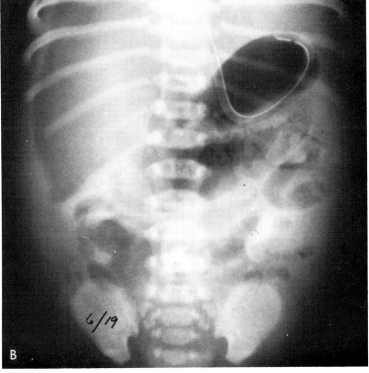

Figure 13–34. Necrotizing enterocolitis in 8 day old infant. *A,* Pneumatosis intestinalis is identified in the colon. *B,* Repeat examination 24 hours later shows free air in the peritoneal cavity as evidenced by the radiolucency in the right upper quadrant.

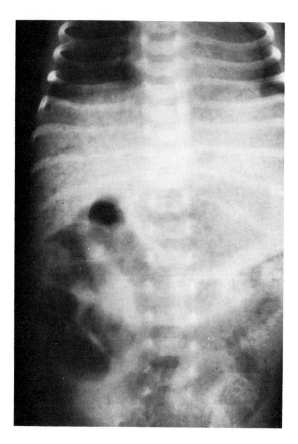

Figure 13–35. Gas within the portal venous circulation complicating pneumatosis intestinalis in a 2 week old infant recovering from respiratory distress syndrome.

presence of calcified meconium in the peritoneal cavity indicates that perforation of the bowel has occurred, probably secondary to ischemic bowel disease.

Pneumoperitoneum in the critically ill infant does not always indicate perforation of the intestinal tract. Infants with respiratory distress, especially those receiving mechanically assisted ventilation, may develop pneumomediastinum with dissection of air into the retroperitoneum and rupture into the peritoneal cavity. Although the presence of air-fluid levels in the peritoneal cavity indicates perforation of the bowel, the absence of fluid is not proof that the peritoneal air developed as a result of respiratory air block. The use of water-soluble contrast material to determine if bowel perforation is present may be helpful, but because of the usual critical condition of the patient, immediate surgical investigation is probably preferable if the infant has not been on ventilatory assistance.

Iatrogenic ischemic conditions may be secondary to umbilical vein catheterization with compromise of blood flow into the portal circulation and with obstruction of the superior mesenteric vein, or may be due to umbilical artery catheterization with improper positioning of the catheter so that it obstructs the superior mesenteric artery (Fig. 13–40).

Compromise of the blood supply to the intestinal tract may follow surgical correction of coarctation of the thoracic aorta in young children. Presumably the sudden increased profusion of blood through the mesenteric vessels produces an arteritis with resulting temporary ischemic changes of the bowel. Clinically there is abdominal distention and vomiting. Radiographically there is an increase in the intestinal gas with distention of small bowel and colon.

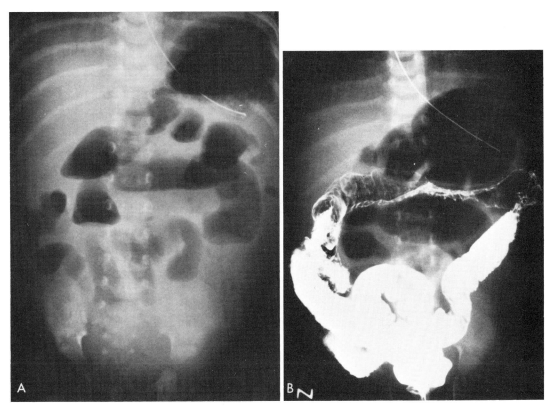

Figure 13-36. Ileal obstruction complicating ischemic bowel disease. *A*, Abdominal scout film shows an obstructive pattern occurring approximately 3 weeks following recovery from necrotizing enterocolitis. *B*, Barium enema study shows the colon to be uninvolved, with obstruction in the terminal ileum. At operation ileal stenosis was found.

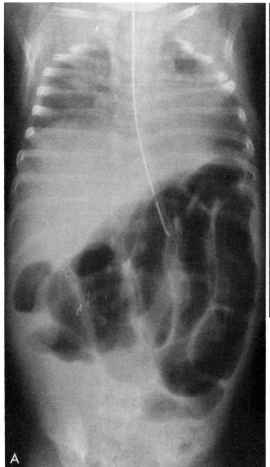

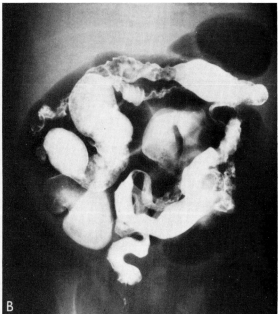

Figure 13–37. Ileal and colon strictures complicating necrotizing enterocolitis. *A*, Scout film of the abdomen shows evidence of small bowel obstruction. *B*, Barium enema shows multiple strictures involving the colon and ileum.

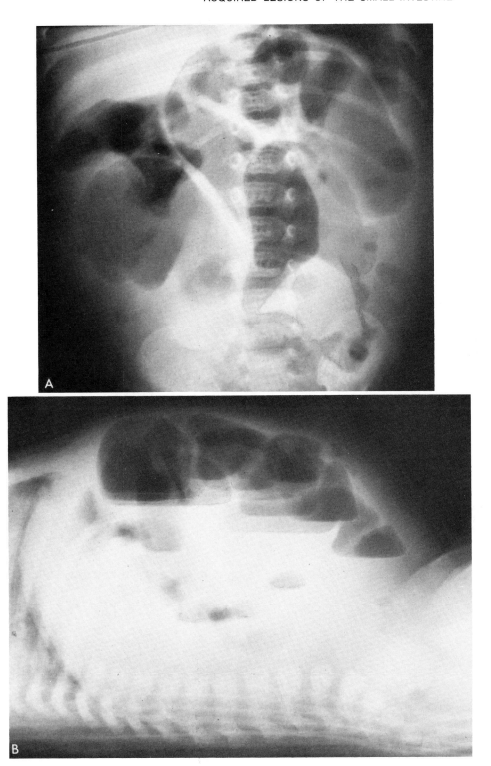

Figure 13–38. Postischemic stenosis of terminal ileum in 2 month old infant. *A*, Abdominal scout film showing distended loop of small bowel with a few scattered areas of gas in colon, indicating partial ileal obstruction. *B*, Lateral supine film showing multiple air-fluid levels. Exploration showed marked stenosis of terminal ileum.

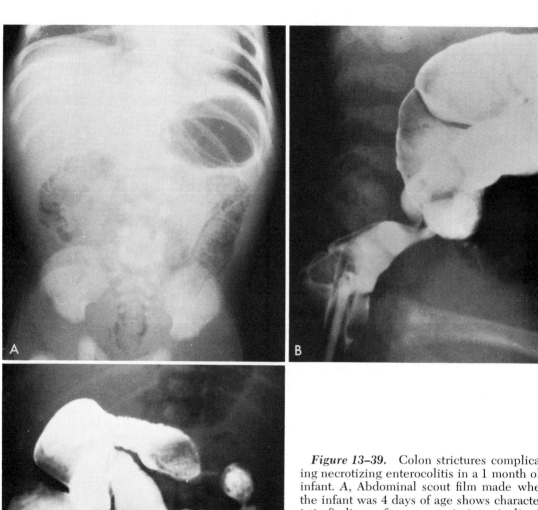

Figure 13–39. Colon strictures complicating necrotizing enterocolitis in a 1 month old infant. *A*, Abdominal scout film made when the infant was 4 days of age shows characteristic findings of penumatosis intestinalis. *B*, Barium enema shows stricture at the rectosigmoid junction as well as *C*, two strictures at the splenic flexure.

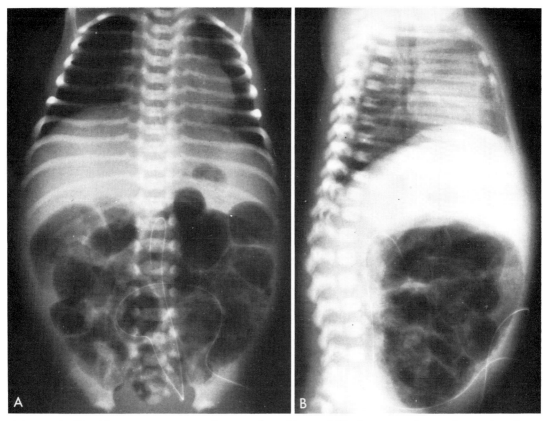

Figure 13–40. Necrotizing enterocolitis produced by umbilical artery catheter obstructing the superior mesenteric artery. *A*, Frontal projection shows the loop in the catheter which has been positioned in the abdominal aorta. *B*, Lateral view shows tip of the catheter directed anteriorly in what was later identified as being in the superior mesenteric artery.

INTUSSUSCEPTION

Intussusception is the invagination or telescoping of a segment of bowel into the adjacent distal segment. The invaginated portion is known as the intussusceptum, and the recipient segment as the intussuscipiens. The nomenclature of the various types of intussusception depends on the relationship of the intussusceptum to the intussuscipiens. For example, ileoileal refers to intussusception involving only the ileum; ileocolic refers to invagination of the ileum (the intussusceptum), into the colon, (the intussuscipiens). Other combinations include ileoileocolic, colocolic, and appendicealcolic. Regardless of the type, unless the intussusception is reduced the result is usually intestinal obstruction, occlusion of the blood supply to the involved bowel, peritonitis and death.

Intussusception occurs most often in Caucasian male infants from 9 months to 2 years of age. Males are affected more commonly than females in a ratio of approximately 3:1.

A definite lesion responsible for the intussusception is present in about 5% of cases, the frequency of a responsible lesion increasing in children past infancy. One exception to this generalization is the rare type of intussusception reported in the newborn which is associated with specific lesions (duplications, polyps, hamartomas) in a high percentage of cases. The most common causative lesion is Meckel's diverticulum and the next most common is polyp. Other direct causes may be hypertrophied Peyer's patch, lymphoma, aberrant pancreas in the ileum, enlarged mesenteric lymph nodes, ileal duplication, and hematoma of the ileum secondary to trauma or Schönlein-Henoch purpura. In the absence of definite lesions such as these, the etiology is unknown. Redundancy of the ileal mucosa has been considered as a cause, as well as allergy, acute enteritis, and change from a liquid to a solid diet. Intussusception in older children with fibrocystic disease of the pancreas has been described in the section on malabsorption disorders (pp. 228 and 230).

Locations of intussusceptions in order of frequency are: ileocolic, 75%; ileoileocolic, 15%; the remaining 10% is distributed among mixed intussusceptions, colocolic, and intussusceptions localized to the small intestine (jejunoileal or ileoileal). Appendicealcolic intussusceptions are so unusual as to be insignificant in the recording of percentages.

SYMPTOMS. Intussusception usually occurs in the healthy, well-nourished, and thriving infant. The proportionately small group of infants who have had enteritis or upper respiratory infection before the attack has led to the opinion that diarrhea or mesenteric adenitis may occasionally initiate the intussusception. The onset is sudden, the first symptom being abdominal pain which causes the infant to cry and draw up his legs. The pain frequently abates for 15 to 30 minutes, then returns with increased and persistent severity accompanied by vomiting. In young infants vomiting is frequently the initial symptom noticed by the parents because of the difficulty in differentiating in this age group the crying due to pain from that due to other causes. In the older more articulate infant and in children pain is invariably the first predominant symptom. One or more normal bowel movements often occur with the first attack of pain and are followed by passage of a bloody stool or bloody mucus (currant-jelly stool). The abdomen is usually scaphoid at the onset, but as the condition persists, abdominal distention appears, the degree depending on the completeness of obstruction. After the first few hours, if the intussusception is not reduced, pallor, sweating, dehydration, and prostration appear. Without treatment, death occurs in a few days.

Examination of the abdomen frequently discloses an abdominal mass which is often of tubular shape and located in the lateral or superior boundaries of the abdomen,

depending on the extent of migration of the intussusception. In extreme cases, the intussusception may be palpated in the rectum.

In all cases of acute intussusception, the prognosis depends on the duration. The longer the condition is present, the more depleted the child and the more likely there is to be devitalization and gangrene of the bowel.

Intussusception limited to the small intestine, in either jejunum or ileum, causes symptoms of high intestinal obstruction. Vomiting is more severe than in the ileocolic type, and bright blood in the stool is less likely.

Chronic forms of intussusception may occur. In such cases bowel obstruction is not complete, and the blood supply to the involved intestine is not compromised. In our experience the chronic type of intussusception has been limited to children with fibrocystic disease.

REDUCTION: SURGERY VS. BARIUM ENEMA. In previous years there was considerable diversity of opinion as to whether the initial approach to reduction of an intussusception should be by laparotomy and manual reduction or by hydrostatic pressure exerted by an enema.

Treatment by hydrostatic pressure dates back to the days of Hippocrates, who advocated the use of enemas in all forms of ileus. The instillation of effervescent powders in the rectum, insufflation of hydrogen sulfide in the colon, and the retrograde passage of bougies are examples of ancient ways of reducing an intussusception. In 1876 Hirschsprung reported his experience with the treatment of intussusception by enema, and in 1905 a detailed account of his results gave the first statistical analysis of the value of this method of treatment.

The first successful surgical correction of an intussusception in an infant was described in 1871 by Hutchinson. The mortality rates after surgery during the following years were considerably higher than the 35% mortality reported by Hirschsprung using hydrostatic pressure. Lehmann, reporting in 1913, is credited with being the first to describe the radiographic diagnosis of an intussusception, and in 1927 Pallin and Olsson in Sweden, Retan in the United States, and Pouliquen in France first reported the reduction of intussusception by barium enema under fluoroscopy. This approach was popularized by Ravitch.

Although a comparison of the mortality rates for the operative and nonoperative forms of treatment over a long period favors the latter, the improvement of anesthesia, operative technics, and postoperative care has gradually equalized the mortality rates until today the prognosis, regardless of the method of reduction, depends mainly on the duration of the illness and the resulting condition of the patient. The problem now resolves itself into whether to make an initial attempt to reduce the intussusception by hydrostatic pressure and, if this fails, to send the child to surgery, or to proceed immediately with operative reduction. The proponents of operative reduction claim that: (1) hydrostatic pressure may reduce or rupture devitalized bowel, which can only be recognized by direct inspection; (2) the intussusception may be caused by a polyp or lymphoma, which can only be determined by laparotomy; (3) the barium enema depletes the child's remaining physical reserve and thereby enhances the surgical risk if reduction by hydrostatic pressure fails, and (4) the child is exposed to too much radiation if hydrostatic reduction is attempted. The objections to these claims are: (1) there is little likelihood of reducing or perforating gangrenous bowel by enema as long as the reservoir is no more than 3 or 3½ feet above the tabletop; (2) in children under 2 years who have 70 to 90% of the intussusceptions, the incidence of tumor is only 2.5% and, also, the lesions which may cause intussusceptions are rarely dangerous in themselves; (3) manual reduction of intussusception is far more traumatic and more likely to rupture the bowel than hydrostatic pressure, and there is no convincing evidence that unsuccessful attempts at nonoperative reduction create a greater surgical risk as long as supportive measures are being provided; (4) morbidity resulting from surgical complications is obviated if hydrostatic pressure can successfully reduce the intussusception; (5) the length of hospital stay is shorter when the nonoperative procedure is used. The objection regarding radiation exposure is probably the most valid argument against reduction under fluoroscopy. However, the amount of exposure by the experienced radiologist who keeps the size of the field to a minimum and whose observations during the reduction are limited to split-second glances is scarcely more than encountered in a routine colon examination.

The success of either method depends largely on the duration of the condition. The mortality in early uncomplicated cases treated by surgeons experienced in pediatrics is very low. The improvement in mortality figures during recent years is undoubtedly the result of earlier recognition and better surgical care than in former years. The success of reduction by barium enema is largely dependent on the length of time the intussusception has been present. Irreducibility is due to edematous enlargement of the intussusceptum which prohibits its passage back through the proximal part of the intussuscipiens. The time necessary for the bowel to become irreducible is unknown. Experiments by Ravitch on the reduction of induced intussusception in dogs showed that all were reducible at 38 hours, but at 48 hours most were irreducible by hydrostatic pressure. The excellent results of both operative and nonoperative reduction in the first 24 hours suggest that devitalization and irreducibility of bowel are unusual during this period. There are, of course, exceptions, as when early interference of the blood supply leads to rapid onset of necrosis. This is especially likely in ileoileal intussusceptions, probably because of the small size of the recipient segment as compared to the size of the colon in ileocolic intussusceptions. This, together with the obstructive action of the ileocecal valve, explains the ineffectiveness of hydrostatic pressure in reducing this type of intussusception.

Every infant or child suspected of having an intussusception should have a barium enema to confirm the diagnosis unless there is evidence of advanced intestinal obstruction and peritonitis. Decision to attempt hydrostatic reduction depends on the age of the patient, the presence or absence of radiographic signs of advanced intestinal obstruction, and clinical evidence of peritonitis. If the child is over 2 years of age, reduction by enema is usually not attempted. We feel that after this age a definite lesion may be responsible for the intussusception, and although such a lesion is usually benign an occasional lymphosarcoma may be missed without surgical intervention. Our success in reducing an intussusception by enema in the presence of advanced radiographic signs of obstruction (marked distention of small bowel, multiple air-fluid levels) has been poor and usually due either to ileoileal intussusception or to extensive edema or gangrene of the intussusceptum. Attempts at hydrostatic reduction are also contraindicated if there are signs of peritonitis (high fever, leukocytosis, and acute abdominal tenderness). We have not seen peritonitis associated with intussusception without radiographic evidence of advanced obstruction. If evidence of bowel obstruction as determined by the initial abdominal scout film is minimal or lacking, hydrostatic reduction is to be expected in the majority of cases. The greater the degree of obstruction seen on the initial film, the poorer the probability of hydrostatic reduction. However, even in these cases the intussusception was partially reduced, often to the region of the ileocecal valve, thereby facilitating surgical reduction.

Although the duration of the process is considered by some to be the determining factor in the choice of method of reduction, we have not found this to be necessarily true. If long duration has led to a greater degree of obstruction, there will be considerable difficulty in accomplishing the reduction by enema; but if not accompanied by obstruction, there apparently is no relation between the duration and the ease of reduction by hydrostatic pressure.

In none of our cases has there been evidence that a barium enema was harmful. In cases showing definite clinical evidence of recurrence, surgery is undertaken without barium enema because of the high incidence of a definite causative lesion in the recurrent case. If there is questionable recurrence, a diagnostic barium enema is given, and if intussusception is found no attempt at reduction by the enema is made.

We have not considered the operative and nonoperative approaches to the treatment of intussusception as being competitive. Each is useful and often complementary to the other, depending on the circumstances of the particular case.

RADIOLOGIC EXAMINATION. Abdominal scout films made with the patient in both supine and upright positions should be obtained in every suspected case of intussusception. Frequently a vague area of density corresponding to the location of the palpable mass is observed. This is usually in the right lower quadrant or right flank but may be in the epigastrium or left side of the abdomen, depending on the distal extension of the intussusceptum (Fig. 13–41). The normal outline of the colon proximal to the mass cannot be identified. The degree of distention of the small bowel depends upon the amount of obstruction. In many cases the quantity and distribution of gas in the small intestine are within normal limits. Usually there is mild distention of the ileum, especially in the early stages. Later, as the intussusception persists, the degree of obstruction and associated dilatation of the small intestine are increased. In ileoileal intussusception the radiographic appearance is identical to other forms of low small bowel obstruction. However, Rigler has reported a gas shadow having the configuration of a bicycle seat in the right upper quadrant in a child with ileoileal intussusception. This configuration is the result of gas within the apex of the intussusception (Fig. 13–42). Hydrostatic reduction is facilitated if the child is sedated. We prefer to give this intravenously, prior to fluoroscopy, at the time intravenous fluids are begun. In this way the patient is less resistant to the procedure, retains the enema more readily, and reduction, if possible, is carried out more quickly.

Fluoroscopy is begun after insertion of an unlubricated No. 16 Foley or Bardex catheter. Although inflatable catheters are unnecessary and even contraindicated for colon examination of pediatric patients, we have found that the one exception is its use in the hydrostatic reduction of intussusception. The large size is required to permit a sufficiently forceful flow to maintain the necessary hydrostatic pressure. It is occasionally difficult to insert this type of catheter past the anal sphincter without lubrication; but by simply wetting it, passage is facilitated. A lubricant enables the infant to expel the inflated bag, and the ease with which this is accomplished by a straining infant is always astonishing. After the catheter is passed into the rectum, the sides

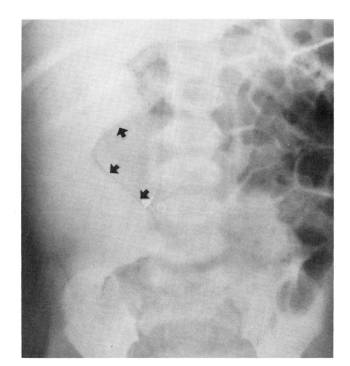

Figure 13-41. Intussusception in 10 month old infant with history of abdominal pain. Abdominal scout film shows soft tissue mass occupying the right flank *(arrows)*, representing ileocolic intussusception.

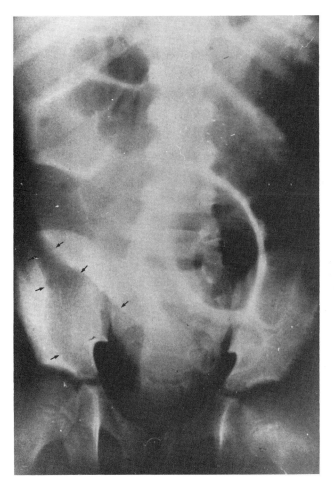

Figure 13-42. Ileoileal intussusception. There are multiple distal loops of small bowel. The dilated loop in the right lower quadrant has been compared to the configuration of a bicycle seat *(arrows)*, the narrow segment being the front part of the seat.

of the buttocks are pressed together by adhesive tape and the Foley bag is inflated under fluoroscopic control. The barium container should be 3 feet above the tabletop. The hydrostatic pressure exerted by the barium column at this height is not enough to damage the colon, yet sufficient over a sustained period to accomplish reduction in the reducible cases. With the infant supine and an attendant at the head of the fluoroscopy table holding the infant's shoulders, and the fluoroscopist's right hand or the hands of another on the infant's thighs, the enema is begun.

As a rule the colon fills rapidly until the head of the intussusception is encountered, when there is an abrupt obstruction to the retrograde flow of the barium. The configuration of the lead point of the barium column is that of a concave meniscus, the concavity produced by the head of the intussusceptum. As continued hydrostatic pressure is applied, there is extension of the margins of the meniscus with engulfing of the intussusceptum, which persists as a filling defect in the head of the barium column. As the intussusception is reduced, the filling defect is displaced proximally along the path of the colon until it reaches the region of the ileocecal valve. At this point, barium is often visualized extending around the mass and filling the cecum and appendix (Fig. 13–43). Attempts to reduce the intussusception by palpation through the abdominal wall while the enema is administered are of little value and may be harmful by increasing the intraluminal pressure to the point of bowel damage. However, gentle palpation in the direction of the ileocecal valve is permissible after the intussusception is nearly completely reduced. The cecum and proximal portion of the ascending colon often appear to be angulated medially, probably owing to traction by the mesentery of the ileal intussusceptum. Reduction is complete when barium can be identified in the terminal ileum (Fig. 13–44B). This may at times be difficult because of the overlapping of the distended rectosigmoid, but by careful po-

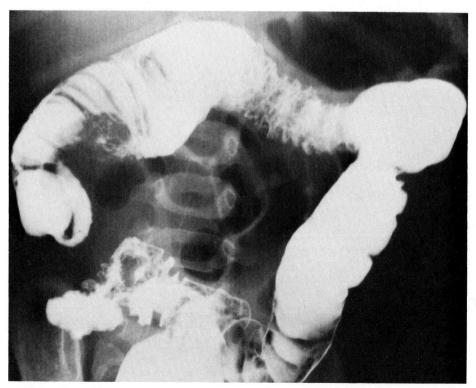

Figure 13–43. Ileocolic intussusception in 10 month old infant. Contrast material has flowed into cecum and appendix, leaving filling defect in area of ielocecal valve. Continued hydrostatic pressure reduced the intussusception.

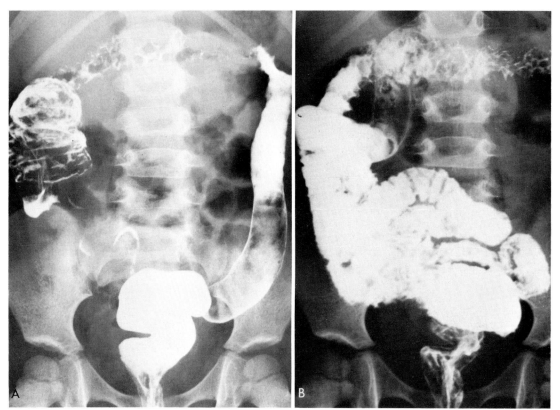

Figure 13-44. Ileocolic intussusception in child, aged 2½ years. *A,* Coiled-spring appearance of the intussusception visualized in ascending colon. *B,* With continued hydrostatic pressure, intussusception is reduced as is evident from extensive fill of ileum.

sitioning and spot films the entrance of barium into the ileum can be visualized. It is necessary to fill an adequate portion of the terminal ileum in order to exclude an ileoileal intussusception.

The reduction of an ileocolic intussusception as described here may be accomplished speedily, but more often a period of patient waiting is necessary. The radiologist should be aware of this and should not be talked out of a fair attempt at reduction by the waiting surgeon if immediate reduction does not occur. This is often the case, especially if the surgeon is a senior staff member and the fluoroscopist a resident. Fluoroscopy should be kept at a minimum, with brief interval glimpses of the head of the barium column and with the field narrowed to include only this area.

The first site of resistance to the reduction is usually in the hepatic flexure. If a few minutes of sustained hydrostatic pressure fail to displace the intussusceptum,

the infant is allowed to expel the barium and the process repeated. Films made after evacuation show the pathognomonic coiled-spring sign, which is due to barium trapped between the opposing mucosa of the intussusceptum and intussuscipiens (Fig. 13-44A). A central linear column of contrast material is frequently seen in the compressed lumen of the intussusceptum (Fig. 13-45). The second attempt will usually reduce the intussusceptum to the proximal portion of the ascending colon or ileocecal valve. Again, if the process of reduction stops, the infant is allowed to expel the enema and once more the procedure is repeated. If the third attempt does not succeed in brisk filling of the terminal ileum, the intussusception is considered irreducible and the patient taken to surgery. Even in such cases, the major portion of the reduction has been accomplished and final reduction by surgery facilitated.

The completeness of the reduction is de-

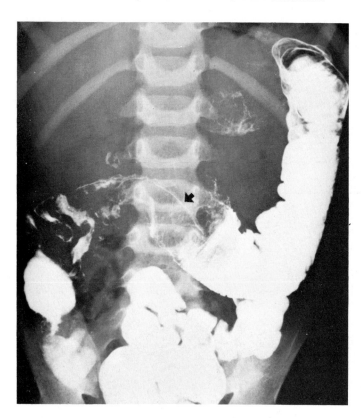

Figure 13–45. Ileocolic intussusception in child aged 2 years. Intussusception is identified as a filling defect in transverse colon. Central linear density *(arrow)* represents barium in compressed lumen of the intussusceptum.

termined by adequate filling of the ileum, relief of the clinical symptoms, and return of normal bowel movements. The recovery in the stool of charcoal introduced into the stomach has been used by Ravitch as a proof of complete reduction. We have not felt this was necessary if the radiologic and clinical signs of reduction were present.

Several types of intussusception deserve special mention. Reduction of the colonic component of an ileoileocolic intussusception may be accomplished, but the ileal component persists. This is evident from inability to fill more than a few inches of the terminal ileum and occasionally from a filling defect within the ileum (Figs. 13–46A and B, and 13–47). No attempt is made to reduce an ileoileal intussusception by hydrostatic pressure because of the frequency of devitalized bowel in this condition.

Colocolonic intussusception may be suspected from the abrupt disappearance of the intussusception during fluoroscopy without the gradual displacement of the intussusceptum into the region of the ileocecal valve.

In cecocolic intussusception there is fill of the ileum before the cecum is distended. This may be impossible to differentiate from an inverted appendiceal stump, but the history of previous appendectomy is a differentiating point.

Appendiceal cecocolic intussusception is extremely rare and may present unusual radiographic and clinical findings (Fig. 13–48).

Intussusception occurring in the upper portions of the small intestine, especially in the postoperative patient, cannot be identified or reduced by barium enema. The clinical and radiographic signs are those of high small bowel obstruction. Positive identification is made after the oral ingestion of barium and identification of the coiled-spring configuration of the point of obstruction.

Transitory small bowel intussusceptions are functional disturbances and are described on page 237.

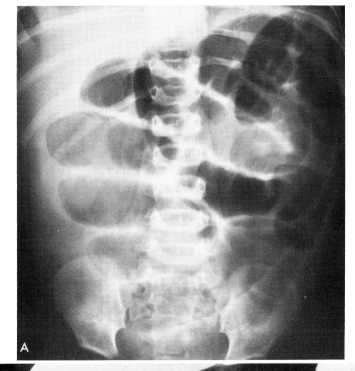

Figure 13–46. Ileoileo-colic intussusception in 5 month old infant. *A*, Abdominal scout film showing distention of small intestine without evidence of gas in the colon. Note absence of gas in extreme right side of abdomen. *B*, Barium enema studies succeeded in reducing colonic portion of the intussusception but persistent filling defect due to ileal intussusception was encountered when barium entered ileum (*arrow*).

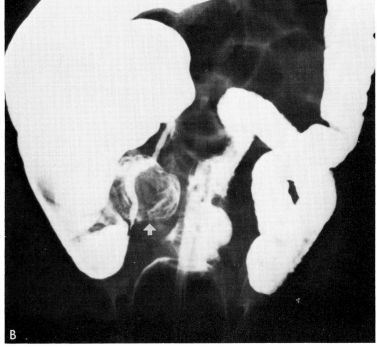

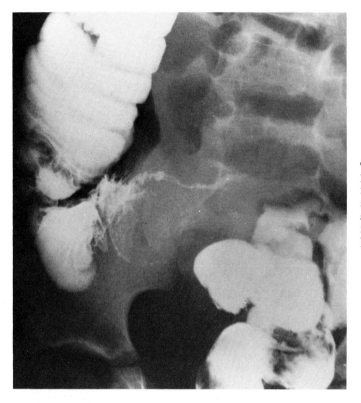

Figure 13-47. Ileoileal intussusception in a 5 year old boy with purpura. Spot film demonstrates filling defect within the terminal ileum secondary to the ileoileal component around which barium is seen to flow. Surgical exploration demonstrated a hematoma of the terminal ileum.

INTESTINAL PARASITES

Ascaris lumbricoides (roundworm or eelworm) is the most common intestinal parasite which has been identified radiographically in children. Other parasitic diseases of the small bowel may produce malabsorption patterns and have been described in a previous section.

In 1922 Fritz, using a barium contrast meal, first recognized the roentgen appearance of intestinal ascarides, and Lenarduzzi, 1938, was probably the first to describe the direct visualization of ascaris on roentgenograms of the abdomen without barium.

The life cycle of ascaris begins after human ingestion of ova from polluted soil. The ova hatch in the small intestine and the young larvae migrate through the intestinal wall into the mesenteric lymphatic or venules and then are carried in the bloodstream to the lungs. Here they enter the alveoli, and after a period of development pass up the bronchial tree into the hypopharynx and are swallowed. They reach maturity in the small intestine, usually the jejunum. Each day the females lay 100,000 to 200,000 ova, which pass out with the feces. Diagnosis is usually based on identification of the ova in the stool. However, if there are only a few female ascarides, discovery of the ova may be extremely difficult. It is in these cases, i.e., when the female worms are absent or scarce, that roentgenologic investigation is especially valuable.

The male worm is 10 to 20 cm long and the female somewhat longer, measuring 17 to 30 cm. Both are several millimeters wide. Their large size is responsible for their easier identification in the small jejunum or ileum of the child than in the larger bowel of the adult.

SYMPTOMS. The usual symptoms of ascaris infection are vague abdominal discomfort and colicky pain in the epigastrium and midabdomen. Vomiting is common, and with an overwhelming infestation, adult worms may be vomited as well as passed with the stools. Anemia, anorexia, weight loss, low-grade fever, and poor nu-

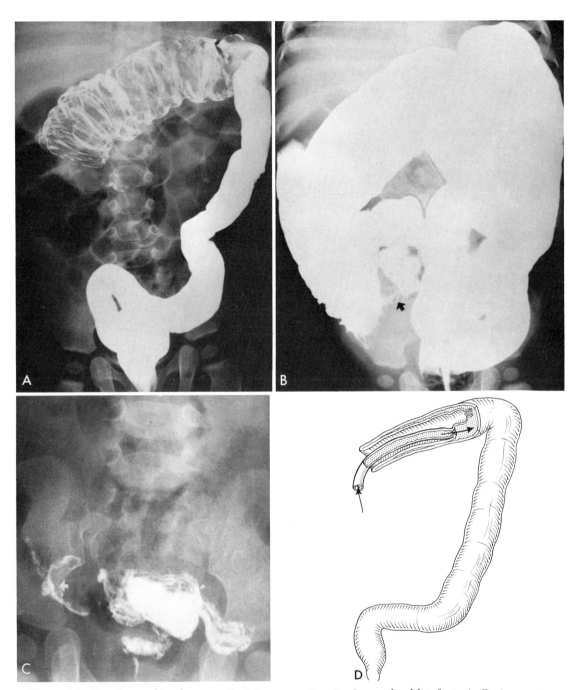

Figure 13–48. Appendiceal cecocolic intussusception in 8 month old infant. *A,* Barium enema study showing intussusception with head of intussusceptum at splenic flexure. *B,* Sustained hydrostatic pressure succeeded in filling terminal ileum *(arrow),* but cecal tip is not fully distended. *C,* Radiograph of the abdomen exposed 24 hours after colon examination, showing concave linear collection of barium in cecum *(arrow)* outlining appendiceal cecocolic intussusception (proved at operation). *D,* Diagram of the original intussusception. Ileum virtually opens into fecal stream of distal colon, explaining why the intussusception was present for six weeks without causing constipation or intestinal obstruction.

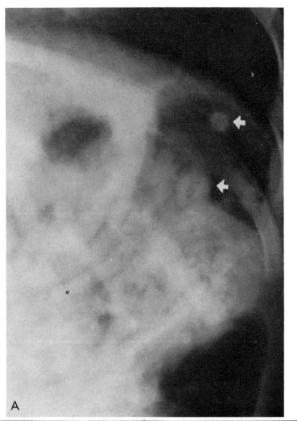

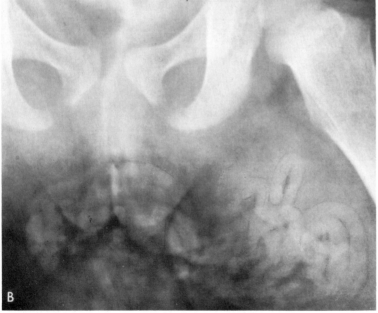

Figure 13–49. Ascaris lumbricoides in infant. *A*, Abdominal scout film, showing outlines of ascarides *(arrows)* in splenic flexure. *B*, Film of abdomen made the next day during gastrointestinal tract examination, disclosing many ascarides lying free in the diaper. (Courtesy of Dr. J. F. Holt, University of Michigan.)

trition are invariably present, the degree depending upon the severity of the infestation. If enough worms are present, obstruction of the terminal ileum may occur, resulting in abdominal distention, vomiting, dehydration, etc. This is especially likely after treatment with a vermifuge or purgative, the mass of worms passing through the small intestine and becoming lodged in the narrower terminal ileum. Symptoms caused by worms blocking the appendiceal lumen, perforating the intestinal wall, obstructing the common bile duct, or invading the liver and pleural cavity have been reported. The passage of a large number of larvae into the pulmonary alveoli will cause an atypical form of pneumonitis. The collection of enough worms in a segment of bowel will form a mass which may be palpable through the abdominal wall. Ochsner, et al. reported a case of intussusception produced by ascaris.

RADIOLOGIC EVALUATION. When a great number of worms are concentrated in one portion of the small intestine, the abdominal scout film may be diagnostic. The identification of such worm masses is made possible by the gas content of the bowel which outlines the parasites as multiple tubular filling defects. An enormous accumulation of the worms in one or several loops of bowel produces a whorled effect (Fig. 13–49A and B). Whenever ascarides can be identified directly, as in such instances, they are invariably present in the stool. The radiologic identification of ascarides is more likely during examination of the small intestine with barium. A worm is visible within the barium column as a radiolucent tubular filling defect several centimeters long and several millimeters wide (Fig. 13–50A and B). After the barium meal has passed into the terminal ileum or colon, the worms may be identified by the parallel lines of barium coating the outside of each worm or, more often, as a single stringlike density of barium in the enteric canal of the worm (Fig. 13–51). At such

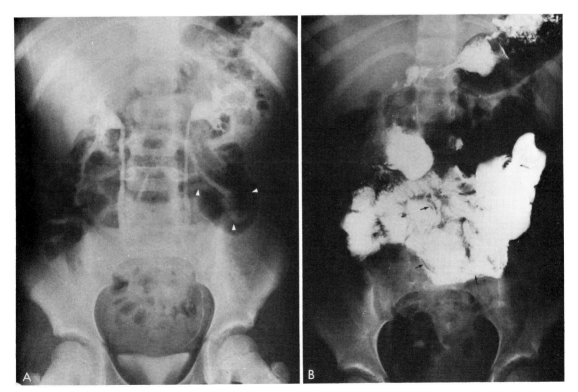

Figure 13–50. Ascaris lumbricoides in 7 year old girl being evaluated for abdominal pain. *A,* Intravenous pyelogram shows linear structure within a loop of jejunum *(arrows). B,* Upper gastrointestinal examination shows barium within the proximal small bowel as well as within the intestinal lumen of the ascaris (arrow).

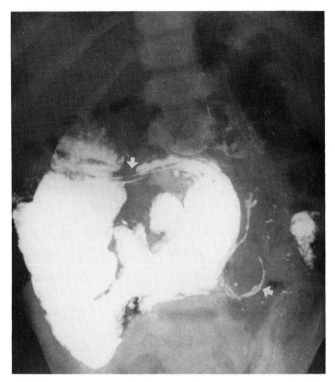

Figure 13–51. *Ascaris lumbricoides* in child aged 4. Ascarides appear as linear areas of contrast material *(arrows)*, due apparently to their ingestion of barium.

times, movement of the parasite may be seen on fluoroscopy. According to Archer, if the patient has eaten shortly before the examination, barium is not ingested by the worm, presumably because its enteric canal is already filled.

Although identification of ova or adult worms in the stool usually establishes the diagnosis of intestinal ascariasis, making roentgen examination unnecessary, radiologic study is of value when ova cannot be found in the stool because of absence or scarcity of female ascarides. Since the parasite may be identified either by the negative image it casts in the barium column or by the positive image after the barium meal has passed, examination at intervals is necessary. At two hours the barium has, as a rule, passed into the terminal ileum and permits identification of ascarides in the upper segments of the intestine.

Another parasitic infection which may be suspected radiographically is whipworm infestation *(Trichuris trichiura)*. These par-asites flourish mainly in warmer climates about the world and often in areas of poor sanitation. The infection is obtained by oral ingestion of the eggs which temporarily become attached to the duodenum until the larvae hatch. They then migrate to the cecum or appendix when they reattach and become mature worms, varying in length from 3 to 5 cm. Clinical features depend upon the severity of the infestation. In mild cases symptoms such as malaise, anorexia, or weight loss may be present, while the more severe cases present with bloody diarrhea or even rectal prolapse. The diagnosis is established by recovery of trichuris eggs from the stool.

Radiographically the organisms are best demonstrated by the use of the double contrast barium enema. The worms are well defined, thin, linear radiolucencies which are of varying shape, generally rounded or serpentine. There may be difficulty in identifying the lesions in mild infestations for they are found mostly in the cecum or appendix, but in severe cases the terminal ileum may be involved as well as the entire colon and rectum (Fig. 13–52).

NEOPLASMS

Benign

There are a number of benign small bowel neoplasms, many of them associated with recognizable syndromes. In our experience the most common small bowel neoplasm is the hamartomatous polyp associated with the Peutz-Jeghers syndrome. Adenomatous polyps may occur in the small bowel in Gardner's syndrome, in ju-

venile polyposis, and in the Cronkite-Canada syndrome. Isolated adenomas of the small bowel may also occur. With the exception of Peutz-Jeghers syndrome, most of the syndromes having polyposis involve the colon predominantly and will be discussed in Chapter 17. Benign adenomatous polyp usually occurs as a single isolated lesion or as a few lesions in a single segment of the intestine, but also may be extensive, involving larger areas. Polyposis of the small intestine or generalized throughout the intestinal tract associated with pigmentation of the oral mucosa and lips is known as the Peutz-Jeghers syndrome. The pigmentation is helpful in differentiating this

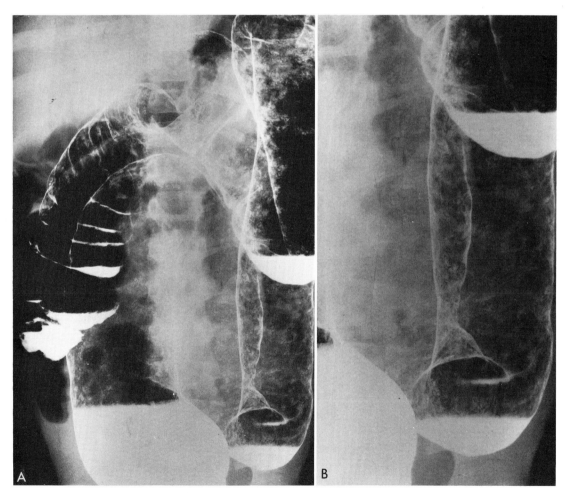

Figure 13–52. Three year old child with whipworm infection. *A,* Double-contrast colon study shows innumerable thin tortuous and well defined lucent defects throughout the entire large bowel. *B,* Close-up view of the descending colon showing the worms to better advantage. (Courtesy of Drs. R. M. Fisher and B. J. Cremin, University of Cape Town and Red Cross War Memorial Children's Hospital, Cape Town, South Africa.)

condition from other forms of polyposis (Fig. 13–53). The association of malignancy with Peutz-Jeghers syndrome is controversial at this time, but some investigators believe there is an undefined small malignant potential not found in the general populace.

SYMPTOMS. Small intestinal polyps are silent lesions until obstruction occurs as a result of intussusception or until bleeding is sufficient to appear in the stool. The symptoms usually do not occur until middle or late childhood, presumably because a considerable time is required for the lesion to reach significant size. Recurrent bouts of abdominal pain due to transitory intussusception often precede an attack severe enough to instigate clinical or surgical investigation.

Recognition of the characteristic pigmentation in cases of Peutz-Jeghers syndrome is sufficient reason, before symptoms appear, to investigate the gastrointestinal tract by radiologic methods, and direct examination of the intestinal tract is indicated if bleeding occurs, with or without x-ray evidence of polyps.

Other neoplasms of the small intestine

such as hemangioma, fibroma, leiomyoma, and lipoma produce symptoms by intestinal obstruction due either to an intussusception or to direct occlusion of the bowel lumen.

RADIOLOGIC EVALUATION. X-ray demonstration of a solitary small bowel polyp is very difficult and often impossible because of its small size and the difficulty in adequately examining all portions of the small intestine. The exception is the duodenal polyp, which is more easily identified as a filling defect because of the relatively fixed position of the duodenum and ease of fluoroscopic examination.

After the ingestion of barium its passage through the stomach and small intestine is carefully followed by frequent interval fluoroscopic observation and radiographs. The polyp is seen as a small radiolucent defect measuring several millimeters to more than a centimeter in diameter within the bowel lumen (Fig. 13–54). The polyp may be attached to the wall by a broad flat base or may be pedunculated, floating on a stalk several centimeters long. It is just as important for the radiologist to examine all segments of the small bowel fluoroscopically and with pressure films as it is for the surgeon to examine the entire small bowel at the time of laparotomy. Only in this way may an intestinal polyp be located. In attempts to locate small bowel polyps the interval films between the fluoroscopic examinations should be made with the patient prone. This position induces pressure on the small bowel and will demonstrate a polyp more readily than if pressure is not applied, the polyp then being obscured by the contrast material (Fig. 13–55).

The discovery of a single polyp, either by radiographic means or by surgery, implies that others may appear or are already present but undetectable. Thus, follow-up examinations are required. There is no set time for the repeat examination of the stomach, small bowel, and colon. Once a year is advisable, or more often if symptoms occur.

If intussusception is present, the characteristic coiled-spring appearance may be seen without a definite intraluminal mass. This is particularly true of an intramural or sessile lesion (Fig. 13–56). Angiography may be useful in locating hemangiomas as well as other vascular lesions (Fig. 13–57) and in the Peutz-Jeghers syndrome.

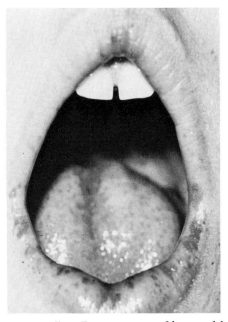

Figure 13–53. Pigmentation of lips and buccal mucosa in child with Peutz-Jeghers syndrome.

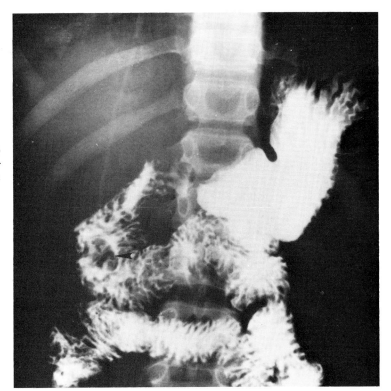

Figure 13–54. Polyp (*arrow*) in the duodenal loop in 10 year old child with Peutz-Jeghers syndrome.

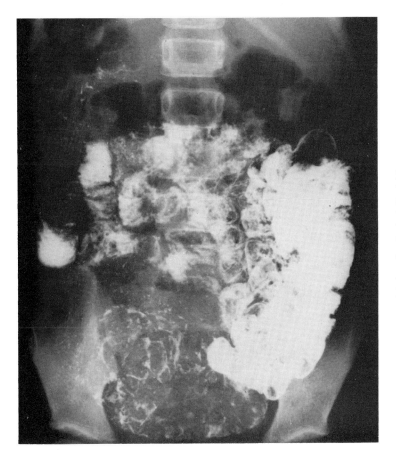

Figure 13–55. Multiple polyps scattered throughout the small intestine with massive collection of the tumors in the terminal ileum. (Reprinted with permission from Singleton, E. B., *Alimentary Tract Roentgenology,* 2nd ed., Margulis and Burhenne, editors. St. Louis: C. V. Mosby, 1973, p. 1500.)

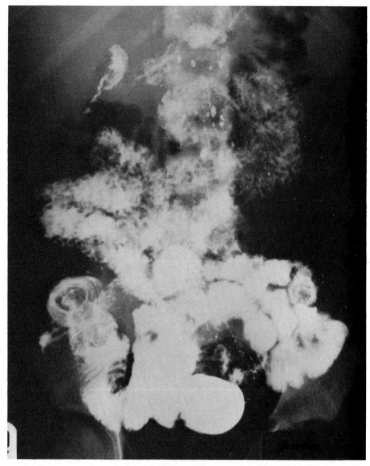

Figure 13–56. Multiple small bowel hemangiomas in 14 year old boy. Intussusception is identified in the terminal ileum, and at exploration was found to be the result of a sessile hemangioma.

Malignant

Except for true adenomatous polyps, most intestinal tumors encountered in early life are sarcomatous, and lymphosarcoma is the most frequent type of this group. The tumor arises in the lymphoid tissue of the bowel, the usual site being the terminal ileum. Other forms of lymphoma, including Hodgkin's disease and reticulum cell sarcoma, may arise in the small intestine of children but are less common than lymphosarcoma.

Whatever the type, the predominant symptom is usually abdominal pain, often secondary to intussusception. If the lesion becomes ulcerated, blood may be identified in the stools. Associated signs consisting of weight loss, anorexia, and fever may be present. Leukemia often occurs in terminal cases.

RADIOLOGIC EVALUATION. In the presence of intussusception, the radiographic findings are identical to those described earlier for that condition. In the absence of intussusception, partial obstruction may be present with slight dilatation of bowel proximal to the ileal lesion. The bowel at the site of the lesion is irregular and the normal mucosal pattern is destroyed or disrupted. The involved segments may be slightly dilated or constricted (Fig. 13–58A, B, and C). Accurate estimation of the extent of the lesion is seldom possible and can be made only at the time of surgery. However, multiple sites of involvement may occasionally be identified radiographically (Fig. 13–59).

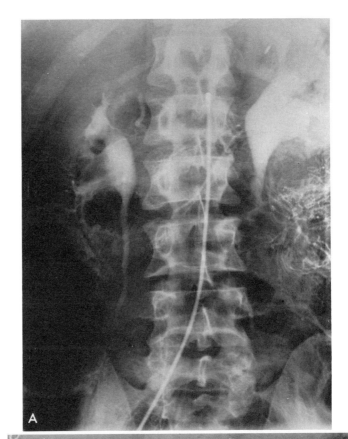

Figure 13–57. Multiple telangiectases of the bowel in patient with Osler-Weber-Rendu syndrome. *A,* Delayed film of a superior mesenteric arteriogram shows collection of anomalous vessels in the proximal small bowel. *B,* Subtraction film enhances the angiodysplastic lesions *(large arrows)* and also shows the filling of the draining vein *(small arrows).*

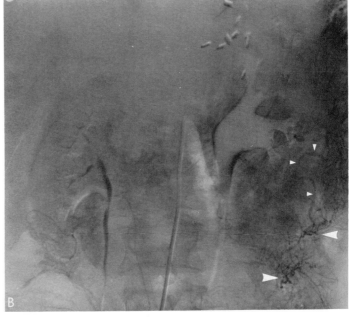

The fact that a lymphosarcoma of the ileum may form an intussusception is a major argument advanced by those opposed to barium enema reductions. However, a malignant lesion producing intus- susception in the infant is so rare as to be outweighed by the advantages of hydro- static reduction given earlier in this chapter. Intussusception in a child past 2 years has a greater possibility of being sec-

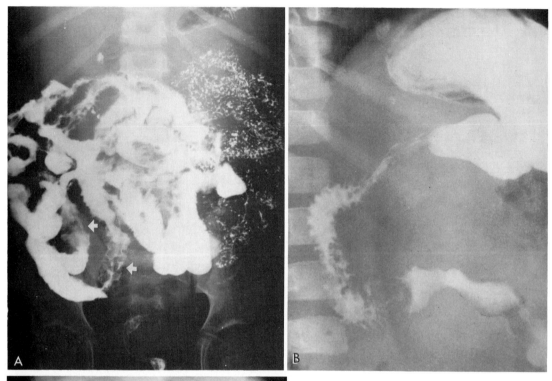

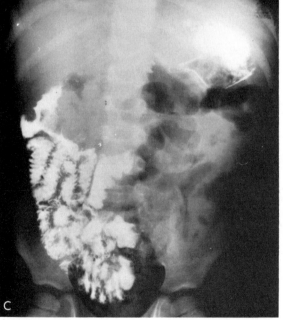

Figure 13-58. *A*, Lymphosarcoma of ileum in child, aged 6. Irregularity and disruption of the mucosal pattern *(arrows)* in ileum were a persistent finding on several examinations. Pathologic diagnosis: lymphosarcoma. *B*, Lymphosarcoma invading jejunum and duodenum in a 2 year old child. Note abrupt loss of mucosal pattern in distal duodenum. *C*, Reticulum cell sarcoma of the duodenum in a 4 year old boy. There is loss of normal mucosal pattern. Location of the jejunum on right indicates associated nonrotation of the bowel. (*C* reprinted with permission from Singleton, E. B., *Alimentary Tract Roentgenology*, 2nd ed., Margulis and Burhenne, editors. St. Louis: C. V. Mosby, 1973, p. 1500.)

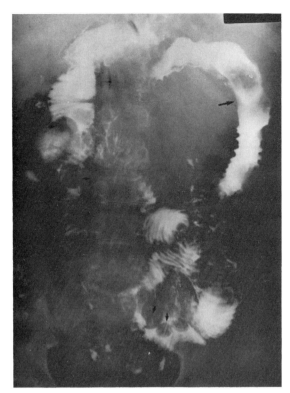

Figure 13–59. Lymphosarcoma of the bowel involving several locations. There is loss of normal mucosal pattern in proximal jejunal loop *(arrow)*, and multiple nodular intramural filling defects are seen in other portions of the small intestine *(small arrows).*

ondary to a lymphoma, and operative reduction should be undertaken in order to ascertain the cause.

FOREIGN BODIES

Any foreign body which goes through the pylorus usually passes through the remainder of the alimentary tract without difficulty. Occasionally elongated objects, particularly sharp-pointed ones, have difficulty in making the turn at the angle formed by the junction of the second and third portions of the duodenum and especially at the angulation produced by the ligament of Treitz at the duodenojejunal junction. It may be difficult in some instances to decide whether the object is in the stomach or the proximal small bowel. Lateral roentgenograms of the abdomen readily determine this. If the object lies in the posterior portion of the abdomen and is below the level of the gastric fundus, it is in the duodenum. By giving the patient a small amount of contrast material, this can be confirmed (Fig. 13–60). Rarely, an object which has passed into the jejunum becomes lodged in the distal portions of the small intestine or at the ileocecal valve (Fig. 13–61). A sharp-pointed object remaining in the bowel is a potential threat of perforation, and many instances of serious sequelae of perforation, such as peritonitis, psoas abscess, and even renal infections, are recorded in the medical literature.

Therefore if an object having the physical properties that might lead to perforation becomes lodged in the small intestine its removal is necessary. The length of time one may safely wait before removing such an object is purely empiric. Many objects of various shapes and sizes have been reported as remaining in the intestinal tract for several weeks before they were spontaneously evacuated. If there is clinical evidence of perforation, such as abdominal pain, rigidity, and pneumoperitoneum, laparotomy is performed immediately. In the absence of clinical symptoms our policy has been to allow 48 hours for an elongated object, once in the duodenum, to pass the ligament of Treitz. If after this time the object has not changed its position, surgical removal is usually necessary. At one time magnetic removal was common, but now is rare because of the nonmagnetic properties of most objects. The hold-up of small ingested foreign objects in the duodenum sugegsts congenital duodenal anomalies such as annular pancreas or disorders of stenosis.

Fortunately, most swallowed objects are opaque and readily localized on radiographs of the abdomen. The locating of radiolucent objects may be aided by ingested contrast material, and this should be attempted if the foreign body is known to be of sufficient size or shape to cause obstruction or perforation. Frequent fluoroscopic examinations are necessary to examine each portion of the small bowel, and with patience it may be possible to identify the object as a filling defect within the barium column. Films made after the contrast material has passed through the intestinal tract may show the radiolucent object coated with barium.

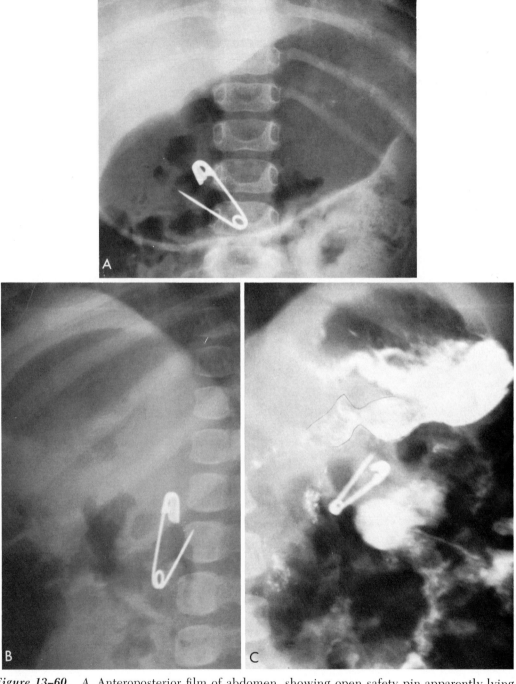

Figure 13–60. A, Anteroposterior film of abdomen, showing open safety pin apparently lying in stomach. B, Lateral view, showing posterior location of pin below level of gastric fundus, indicating its location in duodenum. C, After ingestion of small amount of barium, pin is definitely localized to duodenum.

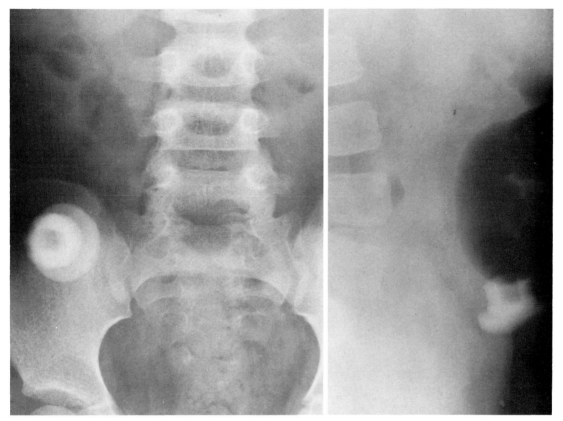

Figure 13-61. Foreign object lodged in terminal ileum. Anteroposterior and lateral radiographs of abdomen showing rubber penicillin bottle cap in ielocecal region. It remained there for six days before spontaneous passage into colon.

EXTERNAL TRAUMA TO THE ABDOMEN

External trauma to the abdomen may alter the intestinal gas pattern. The usual radiographic appearance is that of mild to severe paralytic ileus, gas being present in the stomach, small bowel, and colon. In the milder forms, differentiation by radiographic means alone from the moderate accumulation of gas in the intestinal tract of debilitated individuals is impossible.

Localized injury to the solid viscera, the pancreas, spleen, kidneys, or liver may result in localized ileus of the bowel adjacent to the damaged organ. Radiographically this appears as one or two loops of small intestine slightly distended with gas, limited to the area occupied by the affected organ. An occurrence such as this is impossible in the infant and young child because of the normal quantity of gas in the small intestine of this age group.

Pneumoperitoneum will be observed if the injury was severe enough to rupture the bowel. Upright or lateral decubitus radiographs of the abdomen are usually necessary to detect free air in the peritoneal cavity (Fig. 13-62).

Intestinal obstruction may develop as a result of hematoma in the bowel wall. This is particularly true in duodenal trauma where the third portion of the duodenum is compressed between the adjacent vertebrae and the external force (Figs. 13-63 and 13-64). In such cases there is progressive distention of bowel proximal to the obstruction accompanied by clinical signs of obstruction several hours after the injury. Similar changes occur in intramural hemorrhage due to other causes such as Schön-lein-Henoch purpura.

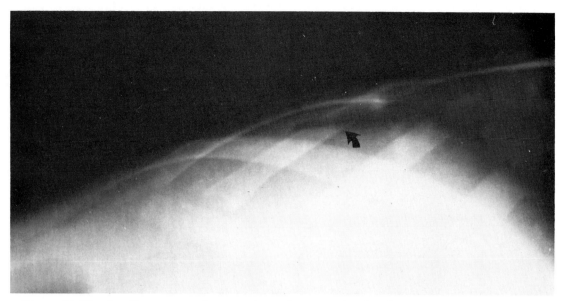

Figure 13-62. Small pneumoperitoneum (*arrow*) seen in the decubitus view in an 8 year old boy who received trauma to the abdomen. At exploration a perforation was found in the jejunum.

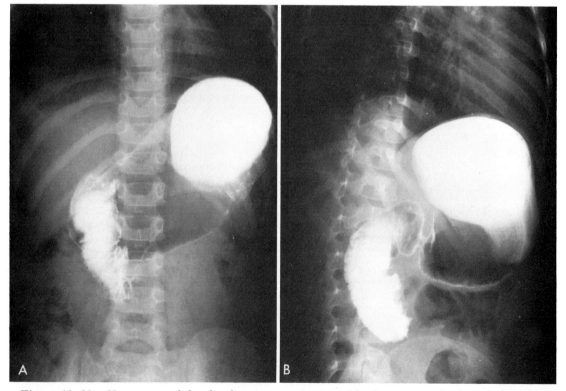

Figure 13-63. Hematoma of the duodenum in a young child who sustained a bicycle handlebar injury to the abdomen. *A*, Upper gastrointestinal examination shows obstruction to the flow of barium through the duodenum. *B*, Oblique view shows the obstruction to better advantage. The child recovered without operative intervention.

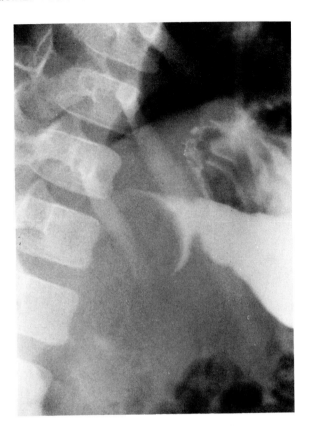

Figure 13–64. Trauma to the upper abdomen in 4 year old child who fell from the back of a truck. Spot film of the duodenum made at fluoroscopy shows filling defect obstructing the duodenal bulb. At exploration a large hematoma was found in the third portion of the duodenum which extended proximally to the duodenal bulb.

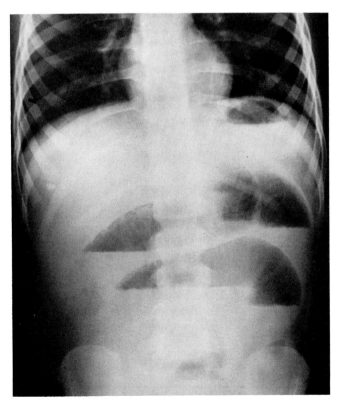

Figure 13–65. Intestinal obstruction secondary to trauma. Child, aged 4, received direct blow to abdomen 10 days before this examination. Abdominal scout film shows distention of jejunum and air-fluid levels. At operation, inflammatory adhesions secondary to hemorrhage in the mesentery were found completely obstructing the jejunum.

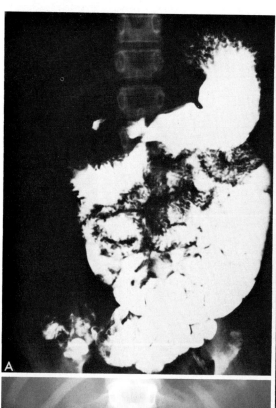
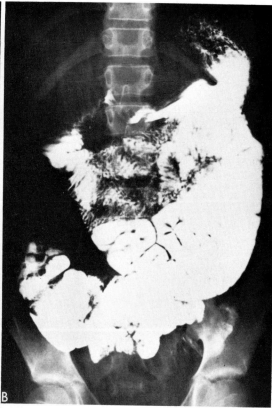
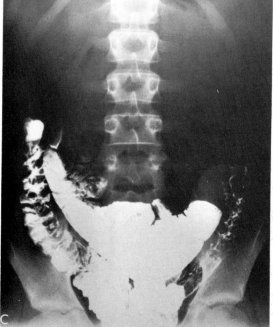

Figure 13–66. Paraduodenal hernia in 11 year old girl with recurrent abdominal pain. *A,* Upper GI studies show no abnormality of mucosal pattern. There is slight dilatation of the duodenal loop. *B,* Delayed film shows evidence of encapsulation of the small bowel. *C,* Barium enema post-evacuation film shows depression of the distal transverse colon and separation between the colon and stomach. At operation no free small bowel was found in the peritoneal cavity, having herniated through the defect in the paraduodenal fossa. (Courtesy of Dr. Garry LeQuesne, Children's Hospital, Cincinnati, Ohio.)

Obstruction may have its onset several days after the injury, and in such cases is due to adhesion formation adjacent to the injured bowel (Fig. 13–65).

INTERNAL HERNIA

The most common internal hernia in children is the retrocecal or transmesenteric (Treves' field pouch) hernia. An unusual form of acquired small bowel obstruction usually seen in older children and young adults is the result of herniation of small bowel through a defect in the paraduodenal fossa of Landzert (paraduodenal hernia). This fossa is lateral to the fourth portion of the duodenum and bounded anteriorly by the peritoneal fold containing the inferior mesenteric vein.

Clinically there is usually a history of recurrent crampy intermittent abdominal pain with or without a history of vomiting or diarrhea. Because this condition occurs in an age group which is usually very active, a history of trauma may be elicited. However, the chronicity of the complaint and the history of similar attacks over a span of several months or years is important in the differential considerations.

The radiographic findings are usually very subtle, and the radiographic diagnosis can be made only if the radiologist is aware of this condition. Abdominal scout films may show distention of small bowel but may be within normal limits. Upper GI studies show encasement of the small intestine, the loops of which appear encapsulated during the entire small bowel study. Barium enema may show a depressed transverse colon with separation of the stomach and colon by the encased small bowel (Fig. 13–66).

REFERENCES

Duodenal Ulcer

Apley, J. The Child with Abdominal Pains (Springfield, Ill.: Charles C Thomas, 1959).
Girdany, B. R. Peptic ulcer in children, Pediatrics, 12:56, 1953.
Miller, R. A. Observations on gastric acidity during the first month of life, Arch. Dis. Child., 16:22, 1941.
Oeconomopoulos, C. T. Perforated duodenal ulcer in an infant, J. Pediatr., 53:324, 1958.
Robb, J. D. A., Thomas, P. S., Orszulok, J., and Odling-Smee, G. W. Duodenal ulcer in children, Arch. Dis. Child., 47:688, 1972.
Rosenlund, M. L., and Koop, C. E. Duodenal ulcer in childhood, Pediatrics, 45:283, 1970.
Singleton, E. B. Incidence of peptic ulcer as determined by radiologic examination in the pediatric age group, J. Pediatr., 65:858, 1964.

Malabsorption Disorders

Ament, M. E. Malabsorption syndromes in infancy and childhood, J. Pediatr., 81:685, 867, 1972.
Anderson, C. M. Intestinal malabsorption in children, Arch. Dis. Child., 41:571, 1966.
Astley, R., and French, J. M. Small intestine pattern in normal children and in coeliac disease, Br. J. Radiol., 24:321, 1951.
Bartram, C. I., and Small, E. The intestinal radiologic changes in older people with pancreatic cystic fibrosis, Br. J. Radiol., 44:195, 1971.
Bayes, B. J., and Hamilton, J. R. Blind loop syndrome in children: Malabsorption secondary to intestinal stasis, Arch. Dis. Child., 44:76, 1969.
Berdon, W. E., Baker, D. H., Bull, S., and Santulli, T. V. Midgut malrotation and volvulus. Which films are most helpful? Radiology, 96:375, 1970.
Berk, R. N., and Lee, F. A. The late gastrointestinal manifestations of cystic fibrosis of the pancreas, Radiology, 106:377, 1973.
Challacombe, D. N., Richardson, J. M., Edkins, S., and Hay, I. F. Ileal blind loop in childhood, Am. J. Dis. Child., 128:719, 1974.
Davidson, M. Disaccharide intolerance, Pediatr. Clin. North Am., 14:93, 1967.
Djurhuus, M. J., Lykkegaard, E., and Pock-steen, O. C. Gastrointestinal radiologic findings in cystic fibrosis, Pediatr. Radiol., 1:113, 1973.
Donaldson, R. M. Normal bacterial population of the intestine and their relation to intestinal function, N. Engl. J. Med., 270:938, 994, and 1050, 1964.
Golden, R. Abnormalities of small intestine in nutritional disturbances: Some observations on their physiologic basis, Radiology, 36:286, 1941.
Gotto, A. M., Phil, D., Levy, R. I., John, K., and Fredrickson, D. S. On the protein defect in abetalipoproteinemia, N. Engl. J. Med., 284:813, 1971.
Grossman, H., Berdon, W. E., and Baker, D. H. Gastrointestinal findings in cystic fibrosis, Am. J. Roentgenol. Radium Ther. Nucl. Med., 97:227, 1966.
Haworth, E. M., Hodson, C. J. Pringle, E. M., and Young, W. F. The value of radiological investigation of the alimentary tract in children with coeliac syndrome, Clin. Radiol., 19:65, 1968.
Hermans, P. E., Huizenga, K. A., Hoffman, H. N., Brown, A. L., and Markowitz, H. Dysgammaglobulinemia associated with nodular lymphoid hyperplasia of the small intestine, Am. J. Med., 40:78, 1966.
Hodges, F. J., et al. Roentgenologic study of small intestine. II. Dysfunction associated with neurologic diseases, Radiology, 49:659, 1947.
Hodgson, J. R., Hoffman, H. N., and Huizenga, K. A. Roentgenologic features of lymphoid hyperplasia of the small intestine associated with dysgammaglobulinemia, Radiology, 88:883, 1967.
Holsclaw, D. S., Rocmans, C., and Shwachman, H. In-

tussusception in patients with cystic fibrosis, *Pediatrics, 48*:51, 1971.

Ingelfinger, F. J., and Moss, R. E. Motility of the small intestine in sprue, *J. Clin. Invest., 22*:345, 1943.

Isbell, R. G., Carlson, H. C., and Hoffman, H. N. Roentgenologic-pathologic correlation in malabsorption syndromes, *Am. J. Roentgenol. Radium Ther. Nucl. Med., 107*:158, 1969.

Kowalski, R. Roentgenologic studies of the alimentary tract in kwashiorkor, *Am. J. Roentgenol. Radium Ther. Nucl. Med., 100*:100, 1967.

Lemy, M., Frezal, J., Polonovski, J., Druez, G., and Rey, J. Congenital absence of beta-lipoproteins, *Pediatrics, 31*:277, 1963.

Lifshitz, F., Coello-Ramirez, P., and Gutierrez, M. L. C. Monosaccharide intolerance and hypoglycemia in infants with diarrhea. II. Metabolic studies in 23 infants, *J. Pediatr., 77*:604, 1970.

Marshak, R. H., and Lindner, A. E. Malabsorption syndrome, *Semin. Roentgenol. 1*:138, 1966.

Marshak, R. H., Ruoff, M., and Lindner, A. E. Roentgen manifestations of giardiasis, *Am. J. Roentgenol. Radium Ther. Nucl. Med., 104*:557, 1968.

Marshak, R. H., Khilnani, N., Eliasoph, J., and Wolf, B. S. Intestinal edema, *Am. J. Roentgenol. Radium Ther. Nucl. Med. 101*:379, 1967.

Nelson, S. W., and Christoforidis, A. J. Roentgenologic features of the Zollinger-Ellison syndrome — Ulcerogenic tumors of the pancreas, *Semin. Roentgenol., 3*:254, 1968.

Neuhauser, E. B. D. Roentgen changes associated with pancreatic insufficiency in early life, *Radiology, 46*:319, 1946.

Nichols, B. L., and Klish, W. J. "Slick-gut syndrome," personal communication.

Panish, J. F. Experimental blind loop steatorrhea, *Gastroenterology, 45*:394, 1963.

Preger, L., and Amberg, J. R. Sweet diarrhea: Roentgen diagnosis of disaccharidase deficiency, *Am. J. Roentgenol. Radium Ther. Nucl. Med. 101*:287, 1967.

Shimkin, P. M., Waldmann, T. A., and Krugman, R. L. Intestinal lymphangiectasia, *Am. J. Roentgenol. Radium Ther. Nucl. Med., 110*:827, 1970.

Shwachman, H. Gastrointestinal manifestations of cystic fibrosis, *Pediatr. Clin. North Am., 22*:787, 1975.

Silverman, F. N. Regional enteritis in children, *Aust. Paediatr. J., 2*:207, 1966.

Singleton, E. B. Radiologic evaluation of intestinal obstruction in the newborn, *Radiol. Clin. North Am., 1*:571, 1963.

Taussig, L. M., Saldino, R. N., and di Sant'Agnese, P. A. Radiographic abnormalities of the duodenum and small bowel in cystic fibrosis of the pancreas (mucoviscidosis), *Radiology, 106*:369, 1973.

Waldmann, T. A. Progress in gastroenterology: Protein-losing enteropathy, *Gastroenterology, 50*:422, 1966.

White, H., and Rowley, W. F. Cystic fibrosis of the pancreas: Clinical and roentgenographic manifestations, *Radiol. Clin. North Am., 1*:539, 1963.

Transitory Intussusception

Caffey, J. *Pediatric X-Ray Diagnosis*, p. 635 (6th ed.; Chicago: Year Book Medical Publishers, 1972).

Superior Mesenteric Artery Syndrome

Altman, D. H., and Puranik, S. R. Superior mesenteric artery syndrome in children, *Am. J. Roentgenol. Radium Ther. Nucl. Med., 118*:104, 1973.

Berk, R. N., and Coulson, D. B. The body cast syndrome, *Radiology, 94*:303, 1970.

Burrington, J. D., and Wayne, E. R. Obstruction of the duodenum by the superior mesenteric artery—does it exist in children? *J. Pediatr. Surg., 9*:733, 1974.

Hearn, J. D. Duodenal ileus with special reference to superior mesenteric artery compression, *Radiology, 86*:305, 1966.

Mindell, H. J., and Holm, J. L. Acute superior mesenteric artery syndrome, *Radiology, 94*:299, 1970.

Ogduokiri, C. G., Law, E. J., and MacMillan, B. G. Superior mesenteric artery syndrome in burned children, *Am. J. Surg., 124*:75, 1972.

Wallace, R. G., and Howard, W. B. Acute superior mesenteric artery syndrome in the severely burned patient, *Radiology, 94*:307, 1970.

Wayne, E. R., and Burrington, J. D., Duodenal obstruction by superior mesenteric artery in children, *Surgery, 72*:762, 1972.

Inflammatory Lesions

Ament, M. E., and Ochs, H. D. Gastrointestinal manifestations of chronic granulomatous disease, *N. Engl. J. Med., 288*:382, 1973.

Brombart, M., and Massion, J. The radiologic differences between ileocecal tuberculosis and Crohn's disease. I. Diagnosis of ileocecal tuberculosis, *Am. J. Dig. Dis., 6*:589, 1961.

Chrispin, A. R., and Tempany, E. Crohn's disease of the jejunum in children, *Arch. Dis. Child., 42*:631, 1967.

Crohn, B. B., Ginzberg, L., and Oppenheimer, G. D. Regional ileitis: A pathologic and clinical entity, *J.A.M.A., 99*:1323, 1932.

Ehrenpreis, P. H., Gierup, J., and Lagercrantz, R. Chronic regional enterocolitis in children and adolescents, *Acta Paediatr. Scand., 60*:209, 1971.

Frimann-Dahl, J. *Roentgen Examinations in Acute Abdominal Disease*, pp. 160–162 (3rd ed.; Springfield, Ill.: Charles C Thomas, 1974).

Law, D. H. Regional enteritis, *Gastroenterology, 56*:1086, 1969.

Legge, D. A., Carlson, H. C., and Hoffman, H. N., II. A roentgenologic sign of regional enteritis of the duodenum, *Radiology, 100*:37, 1971.

Legge, D. A., Carlson, H. C., and Judd, E. S. Roentgenologic features of regional enteritis of the upper gastrointestinal tract, *Am. J. Roentgenol. Radium Ther. Nucl. Med., 110*:355, 1970.

Margulis, A. R., et al. Deficiency in intestinal gas in infants with diarrhea, *Radiology, 66*:93, 1956.

Marshak, R. H., and Lindner, A. E. *Radiology of the Small Intestine*, pp. 179–245, (2nd ed.; Philadelphia: W. B. Saunders Co., 1976).

Miller, R. C., and Larsen, E. Regional enteritis in early infancy, *Am. J. Dis. Child., 122*:301, 1971.

Moseley, J. E., Marshak, R. H., and Wolf, B. S. Regional enteritis in children, *Am. J. Roentgenol. Radium Ther. Nucl. Med., 84*:532, 1960.

Rubin, S., Lambie, R. W., and Chapman, J. Regional

ileitis in childhood, *Am. J. Dis. Child., 114*:106, 1967.

Silverman, F. N. Regional enteritis in children, *Aust. Paediatr. J.,* 2:207, 1966.

Welch, K. J. Regional enteritis, *In* Benson, C. D., Mustard, W. T., Ravitch, M. M., et al., editors, *Pediatric Surgery,* p. 880 (2nd ed.; Chicago: Year Book Medical Publishers, 1969).

Necrotizing Enterocolitis

Aakhus, T., and Johansen, K. Angiocardiography of the duck during submersion asphyxia, *Acta Physiol. Scand.,* 62:10, 1964.

Bell, R. S., Graham, C. B., and Stevenson, J. K. Roentgenologic and clinical manifestations of neonatal necrotizing enterocolitis, *Am. J. Roentgenol. Radium Ther. Nucl. Med., 112*:123, 1971.

Berdon, W. E., Grossman, H., Baker, D. H., Mizrahi, A., Barlow, O., and Blanc, W. A. Necrotizing enterocolitis in the premature infant, *Radiology,* 83:879, 1964.

Castor, W. R. Spontaneous perforation of the bowel in the newborn following exchange transfusion, *Can. Med. Assoc. J.,* 99:934, 1968.

Fetterman, G. H. Neonatal necrotizing enterocolitis—Old pitfall or new problem? *Pediatrics,* 48:345, 1971.

Friedman, A. B., Abellera, R. M., Lidsky, I., and Lubert, M. Perforation of the colon after exchange transfusion in the newborn, *N. Engl. J. Med.,* 282:796, 1970.

Goldstein, W. B., Cusmano, J. V., Gallagher, J. J., and Hemley, S. Portal vein gas: A case report with survival, *Am. J. Roentgenol. Radium Ther. Nucl. Med.,* 97:220, 1966.

Gruenwald, P. The pathology of perinatal distress, *Arch. Pathol.,* 60:170, 1955.

Hopkins, G. B., Gould, V. E., Stevenson, J. K., and Oliver, T. K., Jr. Necrotizing enterocolitis in premature infants, *Am. J. Dis. Child.,* 120:229, 1970.

Irving, L., Scholander, P. F., and Grinnell, S. W. The regulation of arterial blood pressure in the seal during diving, *Am. J. Physiol.,* 135:557, 1942.

Johansen, K. Regional distribution of the circulating blood during submersion asphyxia in the duct, *Acta Physiol. Scand.,* 62:1, 1964.

Joshi, V. V., Winston, Y. E., and Kay, S. Neonatal necrotizing enterocolitis. Histologic evidence of healing, *Am. J. Dis. Child.,* 126:113, 1973.

Krasner, I. H., Becker, J. M., Schneider, K. M., et al. Colonic stenosis following necrotizing enterocolitis of the newborn, *J. Pediatr. Surg.,* 5:200, 1970.

Leonidas, J., Berdon, W. E., Baker, D. H., and Amoury, R. Perforations of the GI Tract and pneumoperitoneum in newborns treated with continuous lung distending pressures, *Pediatr. Radiol.,* 2:241, 1974.

Lloyd, D. A., and Cywes, S. Intestinal stenosis and enterocyst formation as late complications of neonatal necrotizing enterocolitis, *J. Pediatr. Surg.,* 8:479, 1973.

Lloyd, J. R. The etiology of gastrointestinal perforations in the newborn, *J. Pediatr. Surg.,* 4:77, 1969.

Louw, J. H. Congenital intestinal atresia and stenosis in the newborn. Observations on its pathogenesis and treatment, *Ann. R. Coll. Surg. Engl.,* 25:209, 1959.

Louw, J. H., and Barnard, C. E. Congenital intestinal atresia: Observations on its origin, *Lancet,* 2:1065, 1955.

Macklin, M. T., and Macklin, C. C. Malignant interstitial emphysema of the lungs and mediastinum as an important occult complication in many respiratory diseases and other conditions: An interpretation of the clinical literature in light of laboratory experiment, *Medicine,* 23:281, 1944.

Mizrahi, A., Barlow, O., Berdon, W. E., Blanc, W. A., and Silverman, W. A. Necrotizing enterocolitis in premature infants, *J. Pediatr.,* 66:697, 1965.

Pochaczevsky, R., and Kassner, E. G. Necrotizing enterocolitis of infancy, *Am. J. Roentgenol. Radium Ther. Nucl. Med.,* 113:283, 1971.

Rabinowitz, J. G., Wolf, B. S., Feller, M. R., and Krasna, I. Colonic changes following necrotizing enterocolitis in the newborn, *Am. J. Roentgenol. Radium Ther. Nucl. Med.,* 103:359, 1968.

Santulli, T. V., and Blanc, W. A. Congenital atresia of the intestine: Pathogenesis and treatment, *Ann. Surg., 154*:939, 1961.

Santulli, T. V., Schullinger, J. N., Heird, W. C., Gongaware, R. D., Wigger, J., Barlow, B., Blanc, W. A., and Berdon, W. E. Acute necrotizing enterocolitis in infancy: A review of 64 cases, *Pediatrics,* 55:376, 1975.

Scholander, P. F. The master switch of life. *Sci. Am.,* 208:92, 1963.

Seaman, W. B., Fleming, R. J., and Baker, D. H. Pneumatosis intestinalis of the small bowel, *Semin. Roentgenol.,* 1:234, 1966.

Singleton, E. B., Rosenberg, H. M., and Samper, L. Roentgenologic considerations of the perinatal distress syndrome, *Radiology,* 76:200, 1961.

Stevenson, J. K., Oliver, T. K., Jr., Graham, C. B., Bell, R. S., and Gould, V. E. Aggressive treatment of neonatal necrotizing enterocolitis: 38 patients with 25 survivors, *J. Pediatr. Surg.,* 6:28, 1971.

Touloukian, R. J., Posch, J. N., and Spencer, R. The pathogenesis of ischemic gastroenterocolitis of the neonate: Selective gut mucosal ischemia in asphyxiated neonatal pigs, *J. Pediatr. Surg.,* 7:194, 1972.

Waldhausen, J. A., Herendeen, T., and King, H. Necrotizing colitis of the newborn: Common cause of perforation of the colon, *Surgery,* 54:365, 1963.

Intussusception

Benson, C. D., Lloyd, J. R., and Fischer, H. Intussusception in infants and children: An analysis of 300 cases, *Arch. Surg.,* 86:745, 1963.

Dennison, W. M., and Shaker, M. Intussusception in infancy and childhood, *Br. J. Surg.,* 57:679, 1970.

Ein, S. H., and Stephens, C. A. Intussusception: 354 cases in ten years, *J. Pediatr. Surg.,* 6:16, 1971.

Franken, E. A., Jr., and King, H. Postoperative intussusception in children, *Am. J. Roentgenol. Radium Ther. Nucl. Med.,* 116:584, 1972.

Frye, T. R., and Howard, W. H. R. The handling of ileocolic intussusception in a pediatric medical center (editorial), *Radiology,* 96:187, 1970.

Girdany, B. R., Bass, L. W., and Grier, G. W. Reduction of ileocecal intussusception by hydrostatic pressure, *Radiology,* 60:518, 1953.

Girdany, B. R., Bass, L. W., and Sieber, W. K. Roentgenologic aspects of hydrostatic reduction of ileocolic intussusception, *Am. J. Roentgenol. Radium Ther. Nucl. Med.* 82:455, 1959.

Gross, R. E. *The Surgery of Infancy and Childhood* (Philadelphia: W. B. Saunders Co., 1953).

Hays, D. M. Intussusception as a postoperative complication in pediatric surgery, *Surg. Gynecol. Obstet.*, 112:583, 1961.

Hellmer, H. Intussusception in children: Diagnosis and therapy with barium enema, *Acta Radiol.*, Suppl. 65, 1948.

Hipsley, P. L. Intussusception and its treatment by hydrostatic pressure, based on analysis of 100 consecutive cases so treated, *Med. J. Aust.*, 2:201, 1926.

Hirschsprung, H. Tilfaelde af subakut Tarminvagination, *Hospitalstidende*, 3:321, 1876.

Hutchinson, J. A successful case of abdominal section for intussusception, Proc. R. M. Chir. Soc., 57:31, 1874.

Lehmann, C. Ein Fall von Invaginatio ileocecalis im Röntgenbilde, *Fortschr. Geb. Roentgenstr.*, 21:561, 1913.

LeVine, M., Schwartz, S., Katz, I., Burko, H., and Rabinowitz, J. Plain film findings in intussusception, *Br. J. Radiol.*, 37:678, 1964.

Nordentoft, J. M. Value of barium enema in diagnosis and treatment of intussusception in children, *Acta Radiol.*, Suppl. 51, 1943.

Olsson, Y., and Pallin, G. Über das Bild der akuten Darminvagination bei Röntgenuntersuchung und über Desinvagination mit Hilfe von Kontrastlavements, *Acta Chir. Scand.*, 61:371, 1927.

Pouliquen, et al. Un cas d'invagination intestinale chez le nourrisson "tentative de réduction sous écran," *Bull. Mem. Soc. Radiol. Med. France*, 14:191, 1926.

Ravitch, M. M. Non-operative treatment of intussusception: Hydrostatic pressure reduction by barium enema, *Surg. Clin. North Am.*, 36:1495, 1956.

Ravitch, M. M. *Intussusception in Infants and Children* (Springfield, Ill.: Charles C Thomas, 1959).

Ravitch, M. M. Intussusception, In Mustard, W. T., Ravitch, M. M., et al., editors, *Pediatric Surgery*, vol. 2, pp. 914–931 (2nd ed.; Chicago: Year Book Medical Publishers, 1969).

Retan, G. M. Non-operative treatment of intussusception, *Am. J. Dis. Child.*, 33:765, 1927.

Rigler, L., and Godfrey, H. E. The roentgen diagnosis of ileo-ileal intussusception, *Am. J. Roentgenol. Radium Ther. Nucl. Med.*, 79:837, 1958.

Singleton, E. B. Hydrostatic reduction of intussusception, *Pediatr. Clin. North Am.*, 10:175, 1963.

Talwalker, B. C. Intussusception in the newborn, *Arch. Dis. Child.*, 37:203, 1962.

Wayne, E. R., Campbell, J. B., Burrington, J. D., and Davis, W. S. Management of 344 children with intussusception, *Radiology*, 107:597, 1973.

Yoo, R. P., and Touloukian, R. J. Intussusception in the newborn: A unique clinical entity, *J. Pediatr. Surg.*, 9:495, 1974.

Intestinal Parasites

Archer, V. W., and Peterson, C. H. Roentgen diagnosis of ascariasis, *J.A.M.A.*, 95:1819, 1930.

Barrett-Connor, E., Connor, J. D., and Beck, J. W. Common parasitic infections of the intestinal tract, *Pediatr. Clin. North Am.*, 14:235, 1967.

Bean, W. J. Recognition of ascariasis by routine chest or abdominal roentgenograms, *Am. J. Roentgenol. Radium Ther. Nucl. Med.*, 94:379, 1965.

Fisher, R. M., and Cremin, B. J. Rectal bleeding due to *Trichuris trichiura*, *Br. J. Radiol.*, 43:214, 1970.

Fritz, O. Askariden des Magendarmtraktes im Röntgenbild, *Fortschr. Geb. Roentgenstr.*, 29:591, 1922.

Isaacs, I. Roentgenographic demonstration of intestinal ascariasis in children without using barium, *Am. J. Roentgenol. Radium Ther. Nucl. Med.*, 76:558, 1956.

Krause, G. R., and Crilly, J. A. Roentgenologic changes in small intestine in presence of hookworm, *Am. J. Roentgenol. Radium Ther. Nucl. Med.*, 49:719, 1943.

Lenarduzzi, G. L'indagine radiologica nelle occlusione intestinali da oscaridi, *Arch. Ital. Chir.*, 51:645, 1938.

Makidono, J. Observations of ascaris during fluroscopy, *Am. J. Trop. Med. Hyg.*, 5:699, 1956.

Ochsner, A., et al. Complications of ascariasis requiring surgical treatment, *Am. J. Dis. Child.*, 77:389, 1949.

Reeder, M. M., and Hamilton, L. C. Tropical diseases of the colon, *Semin. Roentgenol.*, 3:62, 1968.

Reeder, M. M., and Hamilton, L. C. Radiologic diagnosis of tropical diseases of the intestinal tract, *Radiol. Clin. North Am.*, 7:57, 1969.

Reeder, M. M., Astacio, J. E., and Theros, E. G. Massive trichuris infection of the colon, *Radiology*, 90:382, 1968.

Vaughan, V. C., and McKay, R. J., editors, *Nelson Textbook of Pediatrics* (10th ed.; Philadelphia: W. B. Saunders Co., 1975).

Neoplasms

Balikian, J. P., Nassar, N. T., Shamma'a, M. H., and Shahid, M. J. Primary lymphomas of the small intestine including the duodenum, *Am. J. Roentgenol. Radium Ther. Nucl. Med.*, 107:131, 1969.

Bussey, H. J. R. Gastrointestinal polyposis, *Gut*, 11:970, 1970.

Cupps, E., Hodgson, J. R., Dockerty, M. B., and Adson, M. A. Primary lymphoma of the small intestine: Problems of roentgenologic diagnosis, *Radiology*, 92:1355, 1969.

Dargeon, H. W. Lymphosarcoma in childhood, *Am. J. Roentgenol. Radium Ther. Nucl. Med.*, 85:729, 1961.

Dodds, W. J., Schulte, W. J., Hensley, G. T., Hogan, W. J. Peutz-Jeghers syndrome and gastrointestinal malignancy, *Am. J. Roentgenol. Radium Ther. Nucl. Med.*, 115:374, 1972.

Dozois, R. R., Judd, E. S., Dahlin, D. C., and Bartholomew, L. G. Peutz-Jeghers syndrome: Is there predisposition to development of intestinal malignancy? *Arch. Surg.*, 98:509, 1969.

Fenlon, J. W., and Shackelford, G. D. Peutz-Jeghers syndrome: Case report with angiographic evaluation, *Radiology*, 103:595, 1972.

Godard, J. E., Dodds, W. J., Phillips, J. C., and Scanlon, G. T. Peutz-Jeghers syndrome: Clinical and roentgenographic features, *Am. J. Roentgenol. Radium Ther. Nucl. Med.*, 113:316, 1971.

Good, C. A. Tumors of the small intestine, *Am. J. Roentgenol. Radium Ther. Nucl. Med.*, 89:685, 1963.

Good, C. A. Benign tumors of the stomach and duodenal bulb, *J. Can. Assoc. Radiol.*, *16*:92, 1965.

Jeghers, H., et al. Generalized intestinal polyposis and melanin spots of oral mucosa, lips and digits. Syndrome of diagnostic significance, *N. Engl. J. Med.*, *241*:993, 1949.

Koehler, P. R., Kyaw, M. M., and Fenlon, J. W. Diffuse gastrointestinal polyposis with ectodermal changes: Cronkhite-Canada syndrome, *Radiology*, *103*:589, 1972.

Pickett, L. K., and Briggs, H. C. Cancer of the gastrointestinal tract in childhood, *Pediatr. Clin. North Am.*, *14*:223, 1967.

Reid, J. D. Intestinal carcinoma in the Peutz-Jeghers syndrome, *J.A.M.A.*, *229*:833, 1974.

Sherman, R. S., and Wolfson, S. L. Roentgen diagnosis of lymphosarcoma and reticulum cell sarcoma in infancy and childhood, *Am. J. Roentgenol. Radium Ther. Nucl. Med.*, *86*:693, 1961.

Shey, W. L., White, H., Conway, J. J., and Kidd, J. M. Lymphosarcoma in children: A roentgenologic and clinical evaluation of 60 children, *Am. J. Roentgenol. Radium Ther. Nucl. Med.*, *117*:59, 1973.

Foreign Bodies

Alexander, W. J., Kadish, J. A., and Dunbar, J. S. Ingested foreign bodies in children, *Progr. Pediatr. Radiol.*, *2*:256, 1969.

Brizzolara, A. J. Magnet extraction of bobby pins from gastro-intestinal tract, *Arch. Otolaryngol.*, *61*:237, 1955.

Laff, H. I., and Allen, R. P. Management of foreign objects in alimentary tract, *J. Pediatr.*, *48*:563, 1956.

External Trauma to the Abdomen

Collins, D. L., and Miller, K. E. Intussusception in hemophilia, *J. Pediatr. Surg.*, *3*:599, 1968.

Dickinson, S. J., Shaw, A., and Santulli, T. V. Rupture of the gastrointestinal tract in children by blunt trauma, *Surg. Gynecol. Obstet.*, *130*:655, 1970.

Erkalis, A. J. Abdominal injury related to trauma of birth, *Pediatrics*, *39*:421, 1967.

Felson, B., and Levin, E. J. Intramural hematoma of the duodenum: A diagnostic roentgen sign, *Radiology*, *63*:823, 1954.

Gornall, P., Ahmed, S., Jolleys, A., and Cohen, S. J. Intra-abdominal injuries in battered baby syndrome, *Arch. Dis. Child.*, *47*:211, 1972.

Hood, J. M., and Smyth, B. T. Nonpenetrating intra-abdominal injuries in children, *J. Pediatr. Surg.*, *9*:69, 1974.

Lough, J. O., Estrada, R. L., and Wiglesworth, F. W. Internal hernia into Treves' field pouch. Report of two cases and review of literature, *J. Pediatr. Surg.*, *4*:198, 1969.

Mahour, G. H., Wolley, M. M., Gans, S. L., and Payne, V. C., Jr. Duodenal hematoma in infancy and childhood, *J. Pediatr. Surg.*, *6*:153, 1971.

Meyers, M. A. Arteriographic diagnosis of intestinal (left paraduodenal) hernia, *Radiology*, *92*:1035, 1969.

Meyers, M. A. Paraduodenal hernias: Radiologic and arteriographic diagnosis, *Radiology*, *95*:29, 1970.

Parsons, P. B. Paraduodenal hernias, *Am. J. Roentgenol. Radium Ther. Nucl. Med.*, *69*:563, 1953.

Silber, D. L. Henoch-Schoenlein syndrome, *Pediatr. Clin. North Am.*, *19*:1061, 1972.

Stone, H. H. Pancreatic and duodenal trauma in children, *J. Pediatr. Surg.*, *7*:670, 1972.

Welch, K. J. Abdominal and thoracic injuries, pp. 708–731, *In* Mustard, W. T., Ravitch, M. M., et al., editors. *Pediatric Surgery* (2nd ed.; Chicago: Year Book Medical Publishers, 1969).

Chapter 14

TECHNIC OF COLON EXAMINATION

As in the examination of the upper gastrointestinal tract, both fluoroscopy and radiography are necessary for an accurate radiologic examination of the large intestine. Although the fluoroscopic portion is often time-consuming and more difficult than in the adult subject, its omission during the administration of barium enema denies the examiner the most informative part of the examination. The success of the procedure is partially dependent on the preparation of the colon. If the colon is empty, the enema is accomplished speedily and without discomfort to the child, whereas a colon that contains feces delays the examination, causes discomfort, and seriously interferes with the radiographic interpretation. On the other hand, a clean colon is not always necessary in the pediatric patient, nor are attempts to eradicate all fecal material advisable or practical, particularly in small infants. The oral administration of an unpalatable laxative to a child is frequently difficult and its administration to an infant often hazardous. Also, an effective cathartic is contraindicated in the seriously ill, dehydrated patient and in any child who has intestinal obstruction or active inflammatory disease of the colon.

The method employed by us in the usual case, and found effective, follows. A patient over 10 years old and of normal size and development is given 1½ oz of senna syrup (or some other comparable cathartic) the evening before the examination. We have found it advisable to give the cathartic at about 3:00 or 4:00 P.M. in order for its action to be accomplished by the child's bedtime. A light, low-residue supper may be eaten. The morning of the examination cleansing enemas are given and the child may eat a light breakfast before coming to the x-ray department. Enemas are of value not only in cleansing the colon but, if the child is told that this is similar to the x-ray examination he is to receive, may frequently allay his anxiety at the time of fluoroscopy.

The preparation of children between 5 and 10 years old is identical to that just described except that 1 oz of senna syrup is given. Considerable patience is frequently needed to entice a member of this age group to swallow the cathartic, but can be accomplished by properly "doctoring" it with a sweet carbonated beverage or with orange juice.

In children under 5 years, the cathartic is omitted, the preparation consisting only of two or three cleansing enemas in the evening and morning before the examination. Without use of a cathartic, a variable amount of fecal material may be encountered at the time of fluoroscopy, depending on the enthusiasm with which the preparatory enema was administered. Consequently we often utilize the first barium filling as a cleansing enema, allowing it to be evacuated and then refilling the colon.

These methods of preparation apply in the ordinary patient having a colon examination, especially if for the investigation of rectal bleeding. If feasible, a low-residue diet for one or two days prior to the examination is helpful in cleansing of the colon. In the investigation of abdominal pain as the only symptom, barium enema is usually unnecessary; a 24-hour delayed film following upper gastrointestinal tract examination will usually suffice. Barium enema studies in these patients are rarely informative and only puts the child through an uncomfortable procedure, with additional expense to the parents.

A 24-hour delayed radiograph will demonstrate the position of the cecum, which is necessary in determining the possibility of recurrent volvulus as a cause for the abdominal discomfort, and the colon is sufficiently filled with barium to exclude intussusception and other etiologic possibilities. Also, the appendix is frequently visualized, thereby excluding it as a responsible cause.

In the investigation of intestinal obstruction and Hirschsprung's disease, a cathartic is not given. We also withhold the cleansing enemas in such cases. The procedure used in cases of intussusception is described in Chapter 13.

The use of inflatable balloon catheters is not only unnecessary, but when used in the young infant may damage the rectal mucosa and cause rectal fissures. We have seen one case from another hospital where an overdistended balloon catheter was responsible for rupture of the rectum (Fig. 14–1A, and B). Also, inflatable catheters distend the rectum and prohibit adequate evaluation of this structure, which is important in the evaluation of aganglionosis. The only exception to the use of an inflated bag catheter is in the hydrostatic reduction of intussusception.

In the usual colon examination we prefer to use either an infant or adult plastic enema tip which is fixed in place by firmly taping the infant's buttocks together (Fig. 14–2). An uninflated Foley catheter is preferable for the newborn and small infant. If this is done properly, and if the infant's thighs are kept together during the examination, there is rarely any difficulty in studying the colon adequately. Before insertion of the enema tip, it is frequently advantageous to shorten its length in order to prevent undue pressure on the rectum and kinking or obstruction at the junction of the tubing and the plastic tip. In all situations it is advantageous to place a bath towel or some absorbent material beneath the patient's buttocks. The barium is allowed to flow in under hydrostatic pressure from a height of 3 feet above the tabletop.

If the patient is over 4 years old, bowel-trained and cooperative, no attempt is made to secure the enema tip. Then, with the patient supine and with the gloved right hand of the fluoroscopist or the hands of an attendant holding the child's thighs together, the flow is begun and the entrance of barium into the rectum observed

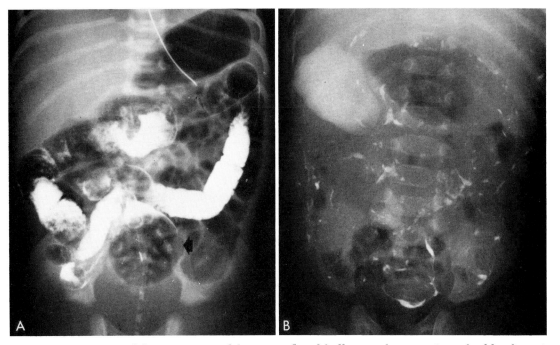

Figure 14–1. Tear of the rectosigmoid by overinflated balloon catheter in 1 week old infant. *A,* Barium enema examination shows the hyperinflated balloon catheter in a high position *(arrow). B,* Radiograph of the abdomen made several weeks later following colostomy for treatment of the rectosigmoid perforation shows residual barium scattered throughout the peritoneal cavity.

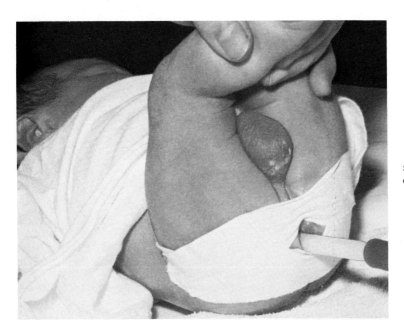

Figure 14-2. Method of securing enema tip before colon examination.

under the fluoroscope. After the rectum is filled, the flow is stopped and the patient turned to a right anterior oblique position in relation to the fluoroscopic screen. The enema is continued, and after the rectosigmoid segment is filled a spot film is obtained showing this area in profile. The patient is turned back to the supine position and the flow continued while the fluoroscopist follows the ascent of barium in the descending colon. Fill of the splenic flexure is observed by rotating the patient to the right; the hepatic flexure is seen more completely by turning the patient in the opposite direction. Routine "spotting" of the splenic and hepatic flexures are usually unnecessary and should not be encouraged because of the additional radiation incurred. However, these areas should be carefully inspected fluoroscopically with the patient turned into the appropriate oblique position. Spot films are obtained of any abnormality encountered along the path of fill. Slight delay in the progress of barium is normally encountered at the flexures, particularly the hepatic flexure, and the fill of the ascending colon is normally slower than that of the descending and transverse portions. Evaluation of the cecal position and of the degree of fixation of this structure is important in the evaluation of malrotation problems. It is frequently difficult to observe the terminal ileum in young children because of the competency of the ileal-cecal valve in this age group. Consequently, evaluation of the terminal ileum is more properly and conveniently performed by upper gastrointestinal studies. Fill of the cecum is assured if barium can be identified in the appendix or terminal ileum. Identification of the ileum may require several seconds of steady pressure, which may be aided by palpation. Fluoroscopy and enema are then discontinued and anteroposterior films of the abdomen are obtained.

The enema tip is removed and the child allowed to evacuate the mixture. If the child is bowel-trained the enema tip is withdrawn and he is taken to the toilet. In the untrained patient the tip is left in the rectum and the enema reservoir placed below the level of the tabletop, allowing the major portion of the barium to be siphoned back into the container. Then, with a large bath towel under the infant's buttocks, the tube is withdrawn. By inserting and withdrawing the tip of the tube in and out of the anus several times, the infant is stimulated to evacuate most of the barium.

After evacuation, anteroposterior films of the abdomen or other views considered necessary are obtained. Air-contrast studies are much less commonly performed in the pediatric patient than in the adult but may be helpful in attempting to locate a polyp or other intraluminal defect (lymphoid hyperplasia, whipworms, etc.) if the post-evacuation film is unsatisfactory in demonstrating the mucosal pattern. Quality diagnostic air-contrast studies can only be obtained by preliminary cleaning of the colon with a cathartic and enemas as described above. A low-residue diet for three days prior to examination is desirable. When this has been accomplished, we have obtained excellent studies using a thick barium suspension which is commercially available as a 95% weight/volume preparation.* The enema is allowed to reach the mid-ascending colon following which as much as will drain is removed with the enema tip in place. Air is then introduced under fluoroscopic control until all segments of the colon have been filled and distended. Spot films of any suspicious findings are then made. Reflux into the ileum is to be avoided. Following this, overhead radiographs in the AP, PA, upright and decubitus positions are obtained.

In the evaluation of congenital intestinal obstruction, abdominal scout films should precede any contrast media studies of the alimentary tract. In distal small bowel obstruction, loops of small bowel may be displaced from their normal location and assume a peripheral position simulating the colon. Barium enema examination will determine if the obstruction is in the colon; if not, it may be assumed the dilated small bowel is secondary to an obstructive lesion proximal to the colon. An abnormally small colon (microcolon) indicates that the obstruction is probably due to ileal atresia or meconium ileus. Abnormal position or motility of the cecum will suggest that the obstruction is the result of volvulus or peritoneal bands or a combination of these causes. The radiographic findings of different types of colon obstruction are given in Chapter 16. Water-soluble contrast medium has been used recently in the evaluation of neonatal distal bowel obstructions, principally meconium ileus and meconium plug syndrome. Diluted Gastrografin or sterile 25 to 30% Hypaque may be used. These agents have been helpful in breaking up thick deposits of meconium, but they are hypertonic, and care must be taken that secondary hemoconcentration

does not occur. Oral contrast media in small bowel obstructions is rarely indicated and is contraindicated in colon obstructions.

The most common symptom requiring colon examination in the pediatric patient is that of chronic constipation. The clinical considerations are usually those of functional constipation or Hirschsprung's disease. Clinical differentiation is usually possible by history alone. The child with functional or habitual constipation usually develops difficulties at toilet training age. The stools, although infrequent, are usually voluminous, and there is commonly a history of soiling of undergarments. Conversely the child or infant with Hirschsprung's disease has a history of constipation dating to birth and although bowel movements are infrequent, they are usually small and there is an absence of undergarment soiling.

The fluoroscopic evaluation of chronic constipation should be limited to the rectosigmoid in an effort to determine if the rectum and sigmoid colon are both dilated, as is seen in functional constipation, or if there is a transition between normal rectum and dilatation of the more proximal sigmoid as seen in aganglionosis of the rectum.

There is no excuse for filling the entire colon with contrast media—this only complicates the presenting problem. If the examination is done with careful fluoroscopy of the colon, limited to the rectosigmoid area, it is not necessary to use saline as the barium solvent. On the other hand, if the entire colon is filled, water intoxication may be a complication.

In infants with imperforate anus or rectal atresia accurate evaluation of the distance between the distal rectal pouch and the perineum is frequently impossible. However, if the infant is kept in an inverted position for several minutes and lateral radiographs of the pelvis and abdomen are made of the infant in this position, the degree of inaccuracy is reduced. Meconium is frequently impacted in the distal rectum, giving the erroneous impression of a greater distance between the gas in the rectum and the perineum than is found at surgery. It is important to search for air in the urinary bladder because a comparatively great number have rectovesical fistulae. Excretory pyelograms which are performed

---

*Liquid Polibar, E-Z-EM Co., Inc., Westbury, N.Y.

in infants with rectovesical fistula may show contrast media in the colon on delayed films.

Percutaneous injection of a small amount of sterile water-soluble iodide contrast material for more accurate evaluation of imperforate anus is described in Chapter 16.

REFERENCES

Berdon, W. E., Baker, D. H., Santulli, T. V., and Amoury, R. The radiologic evaluation of imperforate anus: An approach correlated with the current surgical concept, *Radiology, 90*:466, 1968.

Eklof, O., and Ringertz, H. The value of barium in establishing nature and level of intestinal obstruction, *Pediatr. Radiol., 3*:6, 1975.

Fonkalsrud, E. W., and Clatworthy, H. W., Jr. Accidental perforation of the colon and rectum in newborn infants, *N. Engl. J. Med., 272*:1097, 1965.

Frech, R. S., McAlister, W. H., Ternberg, J., and Strominger, D. Meconium ileus relieved by 40% water soluble contrast enema, *Radiology, 94*:341, 1970.

Hope, J., O'Hara, E., Tristan, T. A., and Lyon, J. A., Jr. Pediatric radiography, *Med. Radiogr. Photogr., 33*: 25, 1957.

Kurlander, G. J. Roentgenology of imperforate anus, *Am. J. Roentgenol. Radium Ther. Nucl. Med, 100*: 190, 1967.

Margulis, A. R., and Golberg, H. I. The current state of radiologic technique in the examination of the colon: A survey, *Radiol. Clin. North Am., 7*:27, 1969.

Noblett, H. R. Treatment of uncomplicated meconium ileus by Gastrografin enema: A preliminary report, *J. Pediatr. Surg., 4*:190, 1969.

Rowe, M. I., Furst, A. J., Altman, D. H., and Poole, C. A. The neonatal response to Gastrografin enema, *Pediatrics, 48*:29, 1971.

Santulli, T. V. Perforation of the rectum or colon in infancy due to enema, *Pediatrics, 23*:972, 1959.

Singleton, E. B. Radiologic evaluation of intestinal obstruction in the newborn, *Radiol. Clin. North Am., 1*:571, 1963.

Wagget, J., Johnson, D. G., Borns, P., and Bishop, H. C. The nonoperative treatment of meconium ileus by Gastrografin enema, *J. Pediatr., 77*:407, 1970.

Welin, S., The technical approach in the study of the large bowel with particular emphasis on the examination for polyps, *Progr. Pediatr. Radiol., 2*: 52, 1969.

Chapter 15

THE NORMAL COLON

The colon can be identified on radiographs of the abdomen by its air and fecal content (Fig. 15–1). The air either surrounds the fecal matter or is interspersed with it, but in either case the silhouette of the radiolucent and opaque densities in the path of the colon is characteristic. As a rule, the more intimate mixture of air and feces in the right half of the colon produces a mottled fecal pattern. A similar pattern is often noted in the rectum and sigmoid. In the more distal portions of the colon and in the rectum, however, the fecal particles have usually combined into solid individual masses (scybala) that are outlined by the surrounding colonic gas. This is particularly noticeable on radiographs of the constipated child. Before solid feedings are started, the fecal content of the entire colon is likely to have a mottled appearance, but after solids are begun and the number of liquid feedings is decreased the variations in the fecal pattern become more evident.

Although the radiographic evaluation of the colon is possible following the oral administration of barium, barium enema is necessary for an accurate study, especially in the evaluation of constipation or suspected inflammatory or neoplastic disease.

If the examination of the gastrointestinal tract is being made for evaluation of unexplained abdominal pain, delayed films (usually 12 to 24 hours) following an upper gastrointestinal examination usually suffice to outline the colon. By 48 hours, most of the barium has been evacuated, although small residues may remain in the cecum, sigmoid or rectum. The appendix may contain barium residue for several weeks (Fig. 15–2).

Radiographs obtained with the colon filled with barium and again after evacuation are the most conclusive means of evaluating the alterations in colonic anatomy resulting from different diseases. The diameter of the infant's and young child's colon demonstrated by barium enema appears relatively larger in comparison with the size of the abdomen than in the older child or adult (Fig. 15–3). This enlargement in both length and diameter may be enhanced by an increase in the hydrostatic pressure of the enema and should not be mistaken for megacolon. After evacuation, each of the colonic segments is appreciably shorter (Fig. 15–4). The cecum may be drawn up out of the right lower quadrant into the region of the iliac crest. The caliber of the colon decreases from right to left, reaching its smallest diameter in the distal sigmoid, with the rectum forming a terminal dilatation.

The haustral markings are localized sacs or dilatations between the semilunar folds. These folds are ridges on the mucosal surface of the colon produced by an infolding of the colonic wall as a result of the taenia coli being shorter than the other components of the colonic structures. Each fold is composed of all layers of the colonic wall except the taenia coli, which represents the outer muscular coat and the serosa. The mucosa between the folds is smooth and devoid of the valvulae characteristic of the small intestine. Haustral markings are found normally in all portions of the colon and are most prominent in the transverse portion. Their absence from this segment of the colon is usually indicative of chronic inflammatory disease, but failure to identify them in other portions is not necessarily significant. It should be remembered that overdistention of the colon with barium may efface many of the semilunar folds. The overall appearance of the colon in infancy is similar to that found in the older hypersthenic individual. The splenic and hepatic flexures are at a lower level in the abdomen and the configuration is more square than the rectangular shape seen in most older individuals (Fig. 15–3). The mucosal pattern of the colon is seen to best

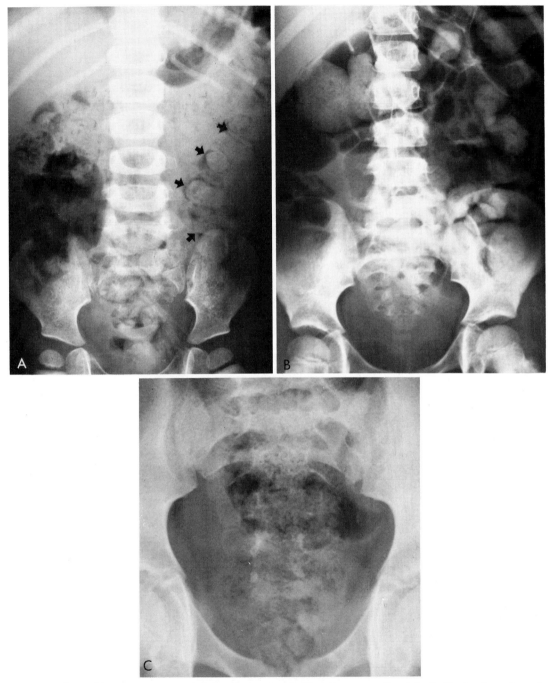

Figure 15–1. Variations in normal fecal pattern. *A,* Usual pattern. In right half of colon, the mixture of gas and semisolid feces produces mottled appearance. In left half, larger individual fecal masses *(arrows)* are present, outlined by surrounding colonic gas. *B,* Multiple large fecal masses (scybala) in transverse and descending portions of colon of child with history of constipation. *C,* Frequently the mottled fecal pattern usually seen in right portion of colon is seen in more distal portions and rectum. This is probably a reflection of consistency of the stool.

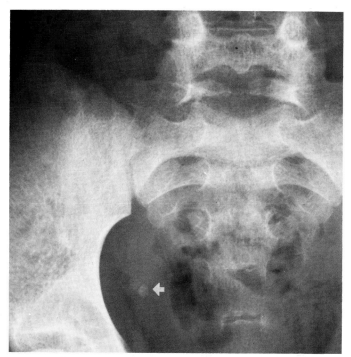

Figure 15–2. Barium residue in appendix *(arrow)* six weeks after upper gastrointestinal examination. Care should be taken not to mistake this for a ureteral calculus or appendiceal fecalith.

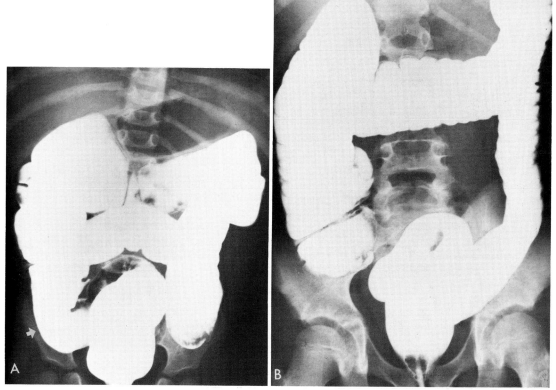

Figure 15–3. Relative sizes of colon and abdomen. *A,* In infants the barium-filled colon fills nearly the entire abdomen. Sigmoid is very redundant, extending far to right *(arrow)* and often overlying cecum. Configuration is more square than rectangular, as found in older children and adults. *B,* Colon of child, aged 8, is relatively smaller in relation to abdomen than in infants. Sigmoid is not as redundant and splenic flexure is higher.

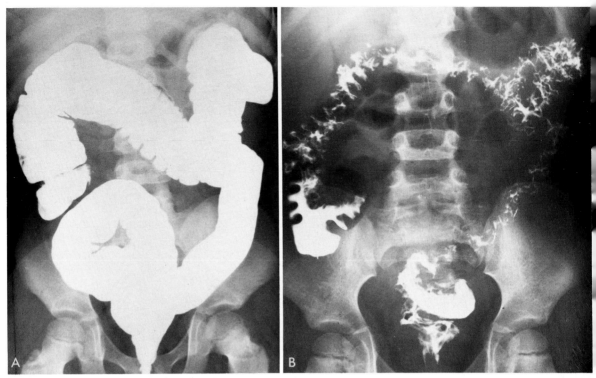

Figure 15–4. Changes in size of colon in relation to evacuation. *A*, Preevacuation. *B*, Postevacuation.

advantage after evacuation of the contrast material. It usually has a crinkled pattern, depending upon the completeness of colonic contraction (Fig. 15–4). Occasionally the mucosal pattern of the descending colon appears as longitudinal folds (Fig. 15–5).

The *cecum* is normally situated in the right lower quadrant, although it is frequently somewhat higher in infants and young children, and assumes a lower position as a result of the longitudinal growth of the abdomen (Fig. 15–6*A*, *B*, and *C*). Occasionally the cecum is in a retroverted position, i.e., angulated dorsally and cephalad or simply angulated medially with its tip approaching the midline. In such cases, as well as when the cecum is abnormally high or freely movable, there is incomplete fixation of its peritoneal attachments. The significance of this associated with intestinal obstruction is discussed in Chapter 12. The cecum is occasionally cone-shaped during infancy, similar to the fetal configuration (Fig. 15–7*A* and *B*), and variations of this configuration may persist into adulthood (Fig. 15–8). Its change to a more rounded form with elevation of the base of

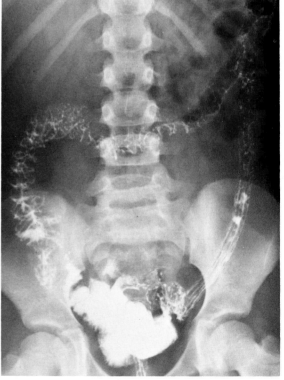

Figure 15–5. Longitudinal mucosal folds in descending colon in child, aged 7.

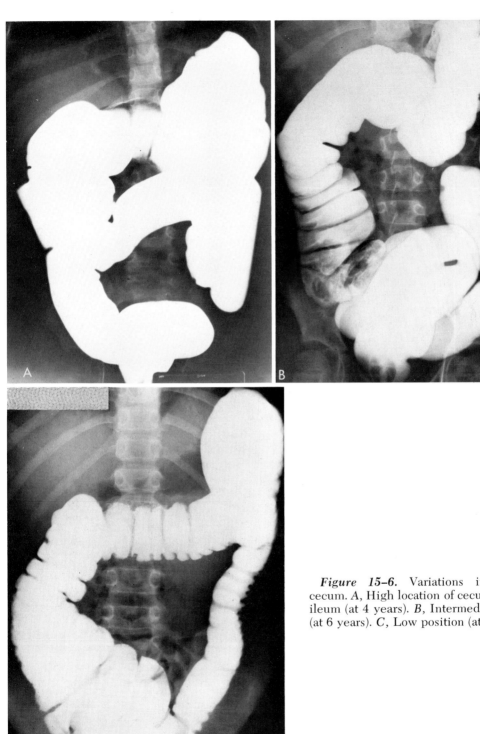

Figure 15-6. Variations in level of cecum. *A*, High location of cecum at crest of ileum (at 4 years). *B*, Intermediate position (at 6 years). *C*, Low position (at 12 years).

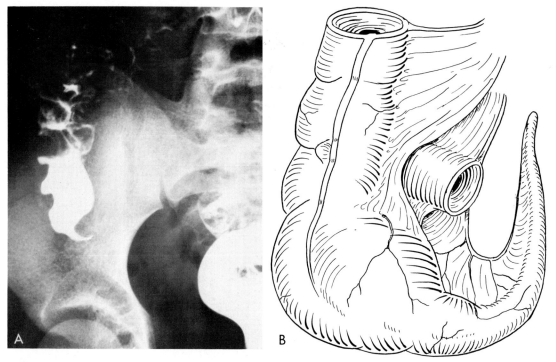

Figure 15–7. Fetal type cecum and appendix. *A,* Cone-shaped appendix at tip of cecum in child aged 7. *B,* Drawing of persistent cone-shaped cecum and fetal type of appendix.

the appendix is perhaps due to the shortening effect of the taenia coli, the other components of the wall of the cecum having a more rapid rate of growth.

Barium will enter the normal *appendix* in approximately 30% of infants and in one half to two thirds of older children. The appendix is extremely variable in length and in the infant frequently appears to be unusually long compared to that in the older child and adult (Fig. 15–9). In the retroverted cecum the appendix may extend cephalad, a variation one should remember when considering the site of pain in cases of appendicitis (Fig. 15–10). Failure to fill the appendix during either upper or lower intestinal tract examination is not indicative of appendiceal abnormality. On the other hand, if barium enters this structure, it indicates patency of the lumen and signifies that in all probability inflammatory disease of the appendix is not present. This should not, however, be considered a diagnostic test for appendicitis. The dangers of attempting to fill the appendix by barium enema in a suspected case of appendicitis far outweigh the value of information

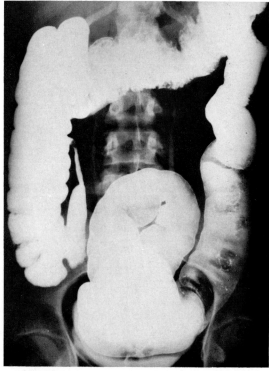

Figure 15–8. Colonization of the appendix in a 15 year old girl—a normal variant.

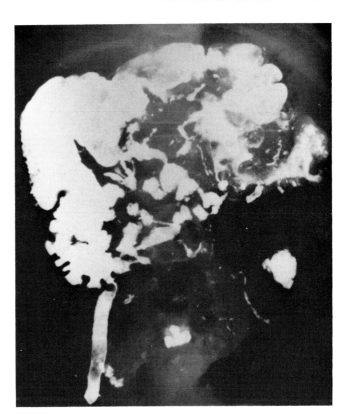

Figure 15–9. Unusually long appendix in a 6 month old infant.

which may be gained by such a procedure. In addition, the time taken in an attempt to visualize the appendix after the ingestion of contrast material may allow an acutely inflamed appendix to rupture.

The *ileocecal valve* is located on the medial wall of the colon, although occasionally it enters the colon more posteriorly. It projects into the lumen for a short distance (1 to 2 cm in older children) and may be identified on pressure films of this area. If visualized in profile, the lumen of the valve is seen to be wedge-shaped and considerably narrower than the contiguous ileum. The superior and inferior lips of the valve are identified as narrow filling defects above and below the narrowed barium wedge. The upper lip is usually longer than the lower, and both fuse at their lateral margins and continue across the dorsal wall of the colon as a single fold, the frenulum (Fig. 15–11). When the ileocecal valve is implanted on the posterior wall of the colon its identification in profile view is usually impossible because of the overlapping of the redundant sigmoid when the patient is turned to an oblique position. In such cases pressure over the barium-filled

cecum will often show the posteriorly situated valve as a round filling defect, and as such should not be mistaken for abnormality. The ileocecal valve is more easily demonstrated in children than in infants.

The *hepatic flexure* is in a lower position in the infant than in the older child because of displacement by the relatively larger liver. As the infant matures into childhood the vertical dimension of the abdomen increases, the liver becomes proportionately smaller, and the hepatic flexure comes to occupy a relatively higher position than it did during the first year of life. At the hepatic flexure the colon turns anteriorly and becomes the *transverse colon.* This structure extends across the abdomen, sagging a variable degree in its midportion before turning posteriorly in the left upper quadrant to form the *splenic flexure.* The haustral markings are more prominent in the transverse segment of the colon than in any other portion. The splenic flexure is normally at a higher level than the hepatic flexure, and in the taller and more slender child this height is enhanced. The *descending portion* of the colon has a narrower diameter than the

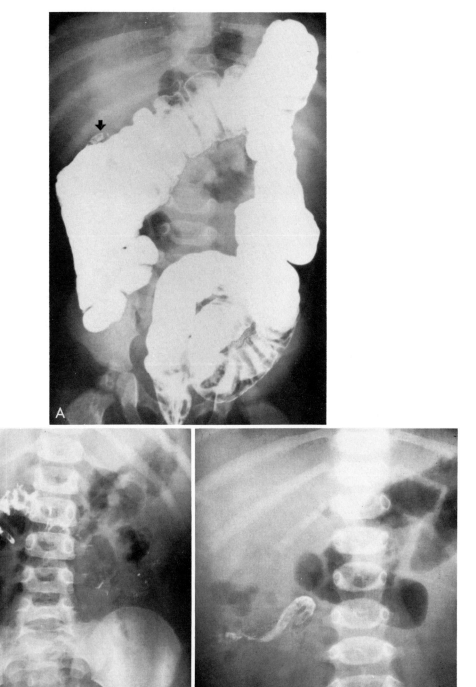

Figure 15–10. Retrocecal appendix. *A,* Appendix lying above hepatic flexure *(arrow)* of infant of one year. *B,* Appendix extending upward, parallel to ascending colon, in child aged 4. *C,* Residual barium in high-positioned appendix 48 hours after upper gastrointestinal examination.

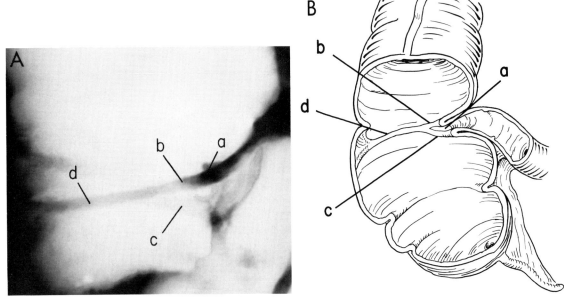

Figure 15–11. Ileocecal valve. A: *a,* orifice of ileum; *b,* superior lip of valve; *c,* inferior lip of valve; *d,* frenulum. B, Anatomy of ileocecal valve.

transverse portion and the haustral markings are less prominent. It descends down the left flank and at the level of the pelvic brim becomes the *sigmoid* colon. In infants this segment is normally very redundant, extending well to the right of midline (Fig. 15–3). Similar redundancy is occasionally seen in older children and in adults and may at times be of severe degree, forming a high loop. In such cases there is always the potentiality of volvulus formation. A slight narrowing is usually identified at the rectosigmoid junction, and this should not be mistaken for aganglionosis. The *rectum* lies parallel and closely overlies the sacrum. Its distensibility is readily appreciated at the time a barium enema is given, when it may double its volume as the hydrostatic pressure increases. The width of the rectum in relation to the width of the osseous pelvis is greater in infants and young children than in older age groups.

Aside from the many anatomic variants of the colon, there are also variations in the physiologic activity. As a rule, the movements of the large intestine are slow and sluggish as compared with those of the stomach and small intestine. Owing to the inertia of peristaltic contractions in the colon, fluoroscopic study of its functional activity is difficult because of the time limit imposed. Occasionally a contraction appears, usually in the transverse colon, in front of which the haustrations disappear and a segment of barium is propelled distally. With relaxation the haustrations reappear. At other times the barium may appear to be moved caudally en masse without significant colonic contractions, or contractions of portions of the colon accompanied by abdominal discomfort may be encountered during the retrograde fill with barium. This occurs most often in the descending and sigmoid segments. It may occasionally be a manifestation of colitis but more often has a functional basis.

REFERENCES

Caffey, J. *Pediatric X-Ray Diagnosis* (6th ed.; Chicago: Year Book Medical Publishers, 1972).

Dreyfuss. J. R., and Janower, M. L. *Radiologic Examination of the Colon* (Baltimore: Williams & Wilkins, 1969).

Henderson, S. G. Colon in the healthy newborn infant, *Radiology,* 39:201, 1942.

Margulis, A. R. Examination of the colon, *In* Margulis, A. R. and Burhenne, H. J., editors, *Alimentary Tract Roentgenology,* pp. 923–962 (2nd ed.; St. Louis, C. V. Mosby Co., 1973).

Chapter 16

CONGENITAL LESIONS OF THE COLON

ATRESIA AND STENOSIS

Most intestinal atresias occur in the ileum (50%) and duodenum (23%). Isolated colon atresias are rare, occurring about once per 40,000 live births. Six of the 140 cases of intestinal atresia and one of 71 cases of intestinal stenosis reported by Gross were in the colon. The defect may occur in any portion of the colon and be in the form of a diaphragm or involve a longer segment. According to Bland-Sutton's classification there are three types: (1) complete obstruction of the intestinal lumen by a diaphragm; (2) an atretic cord joining proximal and distal segments of patent colon; and (3) complete separation of the proximal and distal segments of the colon with a V-shaped mesenteric defect corresponding to the missing area. In our experience, the most common form is atresia just distal to the hepatic flexure, with an atretic band extending to a patent lumen at the splenic flexure.

DEVELOPMENTAL ANATOMY. The development of atresia or stenosis of the colon is identical to that of similar lesions in other portions of the alimentary tract, i.e., focal ischemia secondary to intrauterine vascular insufficiency. Failure of recanalization of the solid cellular stage of colon development may account for some cases of colon atresia, but this is only theoretical. The majority of the stenotic lesions seen in infants are acquired and represent complications of necrotizing enterocolitis developing in the neonatal period.

SYMPTOMS. The symptoms and signs of colonic atresia resemble those of other forms of neonatal intestinal obstruction. Vomiting usually occurs soon after birth, but later than with higher obstructions, and abdominal distention is more extensive.

Obstipation is the rule, although one or several grossly normal meconium stools may be passed.

Surgical correction of atresia and stenosis of the colon has a somewhat poorer prognosis than that of similar lesions in the small intestine, but statistical evaluation of the difference is invalid because of the relatively fewer cases of the colonic lesions.

RADIOLOGIC EVALUATION. The abdominal scout film of a newborn infant with colonic atresia, especially if the lesion is in the ascending colon, is often indistinguishable from obstruction of the distal ileum. There is abnormal distention of small bowel loops similar to that described for low small bowel obstructions (Chapter 12). Air-fluid levels are noted on the upright and decubitus films and provide suggestive but inconclusive evidence that atresia, rather than meconium ileus, is present. The distended loops fill the entire abdomen and it is impossible to identify the colon distal to the obstruction. Even with atresias in the distal portions of the colon, accurate identification of the distended proximal colonic segment is often impossible because of the similarity of appearance to that of the distended small bowel. If the lateral view of the abdomen shows gas in the rectum, one may be certain that atresia or any other form of complete obstruction is not present, assuming that an enema has not been given. Atresia at the hepatic flexure or proximal transverse colon may produce a diagnostic gas pattern. The colon proximal to the atresia is dilated and readily appreciated in frontal and lateral projections (Fig. 16–1A, B, and C).

The administration of barium by mouth is contraindicated in a patient with any

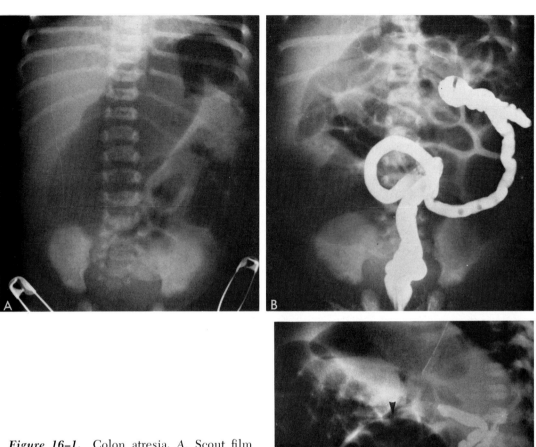

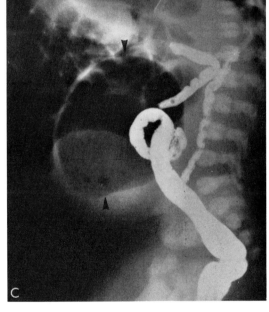

Figure 16–1. Colon atresia. *A*, Scout film shows distended loop of bowel in the midabdomen suggesting dilatation of the colon proximal to the splenic flexure area. *B*, Barium enema shows obstruction at the splenic flexure. *C*, Lateral view shows the area of atresia as well as the dilated colon (*arrows*). At surgery localized atresia was found at the distal portion of the transverse colon.

form of intestinal obstruction if the abdominal scout film does not definitely show whether the obstruction is in the colon or small intestine. Barium enema examination will accurately disclose the obstruction if the colon is the site. Barium studies in cases of colonic atresia show the colon distal to the obstruction to be abnormally small (microcolon) because it has not contained the normal quantity of intestinal contents. Obstruction to the retrograde flow of barium is met at the site of the atresia (Figs. 16–2A, B, and C, and 16–3A and B). If the obstruction is in the form of a diaphragm, the head of the barium enema may have a windsock configuration. In our experience membranous atresia of the descending colon does not show this configu-

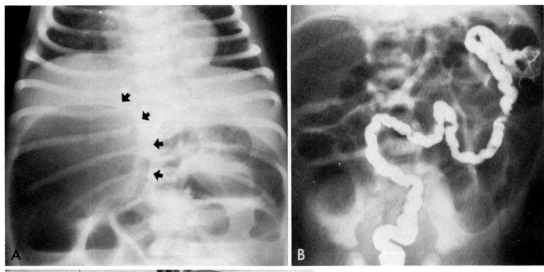

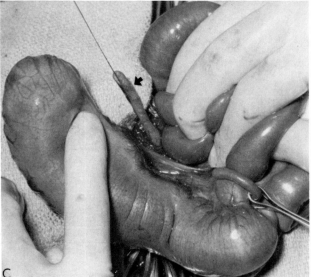

Figure 16–2. Atresia of colon. *A*, Abdominal scout film, showing gaseous distention of small bowel and right half of colon. Colon at site of atresia is rounded and distended (*arrows*). Multiple air-fluid levels are present. *B*, Barium enema shows abnormally small colon with complete obstruction to retrograde flow of contrast material proximal to splenic flexure. *C*, Photograph at operation showing atresia of nearly entire transverse portion of colon and marked distention of ascending colon. Arrow indicates distal colonic segment.

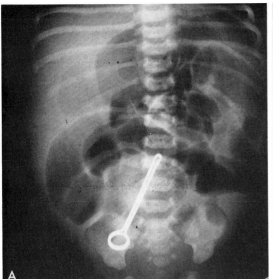
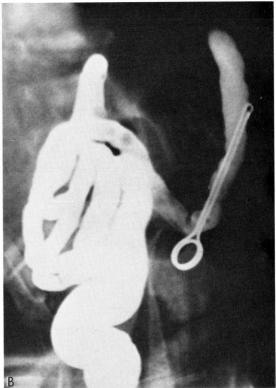

Figure 16–3. Colon atresia in patient with malrotation. *A,* Scout film shows distended loops of colon and small bowel. *B,* Barium shows coiling of loops of colon in the midabdomen and atresia in the left upper quadrant. At surgery the atresia was in the ascending portion of the colon which was in an abnormal position.

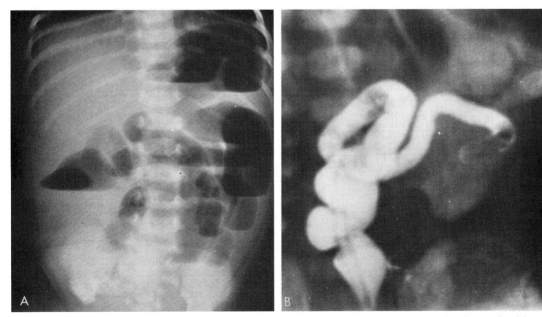

Figure 16–4. Atresia of the lower descending colon. *A,* Scout film shows multiple air-fluid levels within dilated bowel. *B,* Spot film made at the time of barium enema shows obstruction to the retrograde flow of barium in the lower descending portion of the colon. At surgery membranous atresia was found.

ration, perhaps due to the more solid consistency of meconium proximal to the obstruction (Fig. 16–4A and B).

The abdominal roentgenogram in colonic stenosis may appear normal or show varying degrees of small bowel and colonic distention, depending upon the severity of the obstruction (Fig. 16–5A and B). Gas may be identified in the sigmoid and rectum. Barium enema studies define the area of constriction. The normal anatomic constriction at the junction of the midgut and hindgut (Cannon's point), which may occasionally be identified in the distal portion of the hepatic flexure on barium enema examinations, should not be mistaken for a congenital stenosis.

ANORECTAL MALFORMATIONS

Because of the complexity of the embryologic development of the anorectal segment, many anomalies are possible. The commonest, and the type most responsible for neonatal alimentary tract obstruction, is imperforate anus or atresia of the anal canal. This condition occurs about once in every 5000 births. The formation of the anus and distal portion of the rectum is closely allied with the development of the urogenital sinus. Consequently, in approximately 70% of cases of anorectal malformations, fistulous tracts join the rectum with the urogenital structures or with the perineum. Associated anomalies, especially of the vertebra, kidneys, esophagus, or trachea, are present in nearly 40% of the cases. In order to remember the other areas to be checked radiographically when imperforate anus is found, use the mnemonic VATER: V—vertebrae; A—anorectal region; T—trachea; E—esophagus (atresia); and R—renal and radial areas. Some patients also have anomalies of the iris, congenital heart disease, and various defects of the forearms and hands.

DEVELOPMENTAL ANATOMY. The normal development of the urogenital sinus and anus has been described in Chapter 3. Imperforate anus is part of a complex set

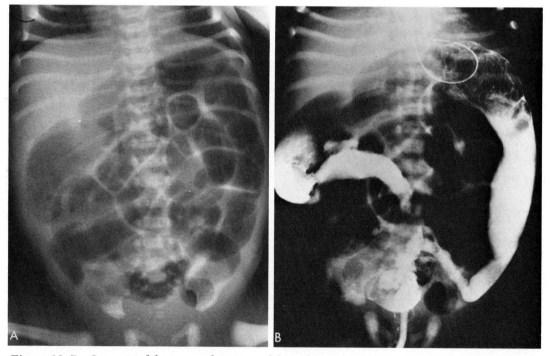

Figure 16–5. Stenosis of the sigmoid portion of the colon in a newborn infant. A, Abdominal scout film shows multiple distended loops of small bowel as well as gas within the colon proximal to the sigmoid. B, Barium enema shows stenotic segment of the sigmoid colon. Ganglion cells were present at biopsy and presumably this represents colonic stenosis secondary to intrauterine ischemic disease of the bowel.

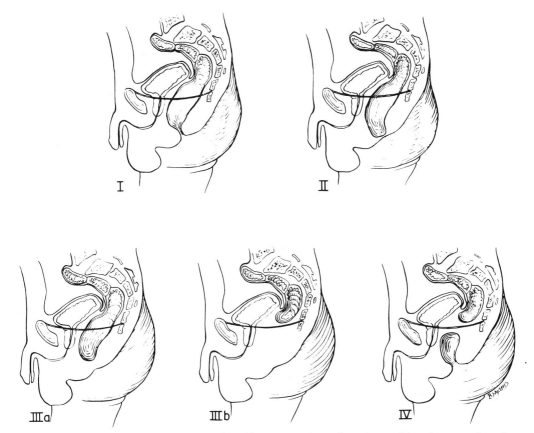

Figure 16–6. Classification of anorectal malformations based on the Ladd and Gross classification with Santulli's modification.

of abnormal embryologic events that occur after the fifth week of gestation, resulting in arrest of descent of the urorectal septum and failure of development of the proctodeum. Failure of the cloacal duct to close results in fistula between the rectum and genitourinary apparatus. Rectoperineal fistula occurs if the anterior part of the duct closes and the open posterior portion is displaced downward into the perineum. Any fistula between the rectum and urinary system is incorporated, in the female, into the genital system by the downward extension of the müllerian ducts at the expense of the posterior wall of the urogenital sinus. In the male the communication may be rectourethral, rectovesical, or rectoperineal. In the female the most common is rectovaginal, and next rectoperineal. Rectovesical fistula in the female is very rare.

Although many complex classifications of anorectal malformations are recognized,

for the sake of simplicity Ladd and Gross's classification of malformations of the anorectal segment, irrespective of associated fistulas, is as follows (Fig. 16–6).

TYPE I. Patent anus and rectum but with stenosis of the anal canal. This anomaly at the lower anal level is due to incomplete rupture of the anal membrane, whereas stenosis at a higher level is probably due to incomplete development of the bulbus terminalis.

TYPE II. Imperforate anus with the separating partition consisting of a thin septum. This anomaly represents persistence of the anal membrane.

TYPE III. The anus is imperforate and the rectum ends blindly. The pathogenesis is unknown but it perhaps represents resorption of the distal rectal segment concomitant with the normal degeneration of the tailgut. This important malformation has been subdivided by Santulli into a low obstruction (type III A) where the rectum terminates below the puborectalis sling (levator ani muscle) and high obstruction (type III B) where the obstruction is above the puborectalis sling. Type III constitutes approximately 90% of all anorectal malformations, and fistulas are common and frequently complex depending upon the sex of the infant and whether the obstruction is above (supralevator) or below (translevator) the puborectalis sling. This complex group of conditions is complicated by fistulas to many adjacent structures including the bladder, urethra, cloaca, vagina, vulva, or perineum. The intermediate lesion is a less common form where the obstruction is at or just below the puborectalis sling. A comprehensive study of these anomalies has been described by Stephens.

TYPE IV. The anus and lower portion of the rectum are normal, but separated from the upper rectal segment, which terminates as a closed pouch. This malformation is the result of obliteration at the proximal portion of the bulbus analis and is perhaps the result of localized ischemia occurring in intrauterine life.

CLINICAL PICTURE. The time of onset of symptoms depends upon the type of malformation. When the anus is imperforate the anomaly is usually discovered by inspection of the baby after birth. Rectal atresia with patency of the anus may not be detected at birth, but a presumptive diagnosis may be made from failure of a catheter to pass the anus. In the rare cases of imperforate anal membrane (type II) the dark meconium can be seen beneath the bulging thin membrane. In anal or rectal agenesis (type III), unless there is a fistula of adequate size connecting the atretic rectum to the urogenital system or to the perineum, symptoms and signs of intestinal obstruction develop within the first 24 hours.

If there is clinical evidence of a perineal fistula, the obstruction is obviously low. If there is no evidence of a perineal fistula the obstruction is probably high (supralevator) or intermediate. If meconium is in the urine, rectovesical or rectourethral fistula is present. Actually the fistulas in these anomalies represent the ectopic termination of the bowel. Radiographic studies are valuable in more accurately delineating the anatomy, both in regard to the level of the

obstruction and the presence or absence of fistulas. Obstructive findings may be present in severe cases of anorectal stenosis. In milder cases of anorectal stenosis, the only symptom may be chronic constipation and the anomaly may not be discovered until later life. When the atretic rectal segment communicates with the bladder, urethra, vagina, or perineum, meconium is passed at these sites.

RADIOLOGIC EVALUATION. Radiographs of the abdomen in cases of imperforate anus show gaseous distention of the colon and small intestine, the extent depending usually on the time interval since birth (Fig. 16–7). Air-fluid levels are present if films are made with the infant in an upright position. If there is a fistula between the atretic rectum and the genitourinary system or perineum large enough to allow the passage of adequate amounts of gas and meconium, the radiographic signs of obstruction are not present. Also, if there is associated esophageal atresia, as is frequently the case, the development of obstructive signs involving the lower bowel is prevented. A lateral exposure of the abdomen may disclose gas in the urinary bladder if a rectovesical or rectourethral fistula is present (Fig. 16–8).

Wangensteen and Rice first described the technic of obtaining films of the abdomen with the infant inverted. By this maneuver, the gas rises to the most caudal portion of the rectal pouch and, with a metallic marker on the skin at the site of the imperforate anus, the distance between the rectum and exterior can be ascertained. The lateral inverted view allows a more accurate estimate of the length of the atresia than the frontal projection because of the foreshortening effect obtained by the posterior direction of the rectum on anteroposterior views. The apparent distance may appear greater than it actually is found to be at the time of surgery, due to meconium filling the distal portion of the blind segment. The accuracy of the information gained from the inverted film is enhanced if the radiologic examination is prolonged sufficiently for air to permeate completely the terminal portion of the atresia, usually 12 to 24 hours after birth (Fig. 16–7). Maintaining the infant in an inverted position for five minutes or more before the exposure also helps to accomplish this.

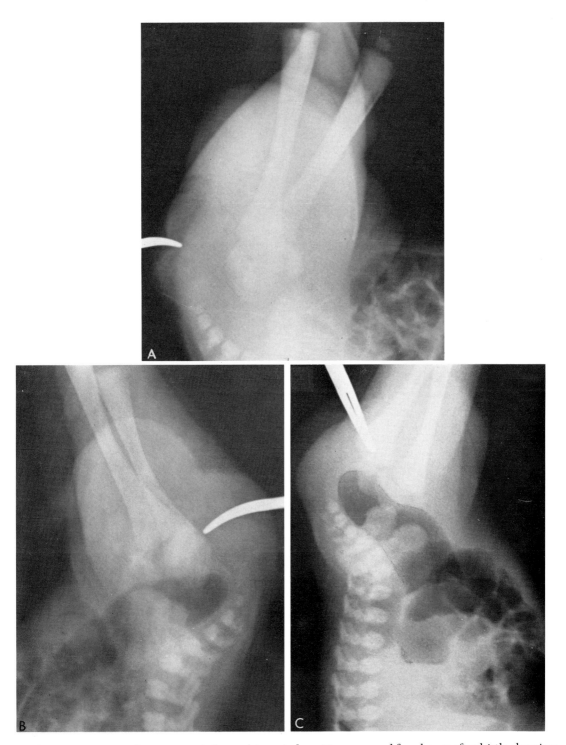

Figure 16–7. Imperforate anus. *A*, Lateral inverted position exposed four hours after birth, showing absence of gas in rectum or sigmoid. *B*, At eight hours, gas outlines the rectum. *C*, Repeat examination at twelve hours showing further progression of gas into atretic rectum and giving more accurate index of length of the atresia. A taped metallic marker at the anal dimple is preferable to the metallic probe shown in these illustrations.

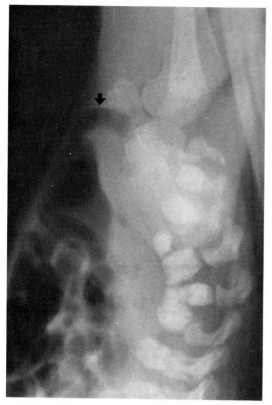

Figure 16–8. Imperforate anus with recto-vesical fistula. Lateral view of abdomen, showing gas in urinary bladder (*arrow*). Distal rectal segment is not clearly outlined, air having entered the bladder instead.

A more practical approach to the radiographic evaluation of imperforate anus and appropriate surgical correction has been proposed by Berdon, et al., the objective being to differentiate the high (supralevator) from the low (translevator) type of imperforate anus. These authors believe clinical evaluation is all that is necessary to determine the type of lesion present and thus the operative approach to be used, while others desire more positive preoperative verification of both the site of obstruction and origin of a fistula, if present. This clinical evaluation, although frequently accurate, can be documented and the anatomic defect more specifically delineated by appropriate radiographic studies. A lateral view of the pelvis will accurately show the pubococcygeal line, which is a line drawn from the upper border of the symphysis pubis to the sacrococcygeal junction and identifies the loca-

tion of the puborectalis sling (Fig. 16–9). This line bisects the upper one fourth and the lower three fourths of the ischium. In supralevator obstructions, sacral anomalies including agenesis are frequently present and consequently a line from the symphysis through the upper fourth of the ischium will serve to identify the puborectalis sling. The location of the gas-distended rectum at or above this line indicates a high obstruction; below this line, a low or possibly an intermediate obstruction.

In our experience, the injection of positive contrast medium under fluoroscopic guidance is a reliable method in delineating more clearly the location of the obstruction and in demonstrating small fistulas. Following preliminary supine and inverted films, the anal dimple is perforated with a 16-gauge Rochester needle, which is advanced until air and meconium are identified in the syringe. Following aspiration of as much air and meconium as possible, 3 to 5 ml of 20% Hypaque is introduced. Higher volumes are hygroscopic and may deplete plasma volume. Sometimes a fistula opacifies completely with this technic (Fig. 16–10). However, in many patients a beak-like deformity at the caudal end of the pouch identifies the site of the fistula (Fig. 16–11).

At some point in the patient's course, radiographic workup should always include cystourethrography and urography. Additional workup depends on whether there are other associated anomalies.

The radiographic diagnosis of rectal atresia with patency of the anus (type IV) is based on evidence of intestinal obstruction, as in cases of imperforate anus, and on the injection under fluoroscopy of a small amount of contrast material into the anus. The material fills only the anal segment and does not extend into the rectum. Following this, if films are made with the infant inverted, and not coughing or straining, the distance between gas in the atretic rectum and contrast material in the anal segment can be measured (Fig. 16–12).

In cases of anorectal stenosis, the abdominal radiographs may or may not show evidence of obstruction, depending on the narrowness of the stricture. Objective proof of the defect is obtained by the injection of contrast material through a small catheter inserted into the anus. It is important that

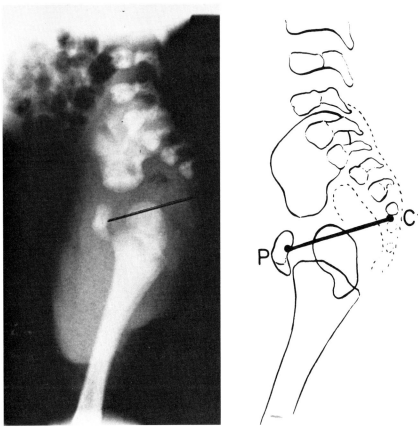

Figure 16-9. Lateral view of the pelvis showing location of the pubococcygeal line, which is the location of the puborectalis sling.

the tip of the catheter be inserted just past the anal sphincter in order to visualize the defective area (Fig. 16–13). The anorectal canal appears as a narrowed segment of variable diameter rather than having the oval shape of the normal rectum (Fig. 16–14).

Fistulas which communicate between the rectal atresia and the perineum or the urogenital system may be identified radiographically following injection of contrast material into the tract.

In some cases of rectal atresia (usually in males and high in location) with rectourinary fistula, calcified meconium may be seen within the lumen of the colon. Although the appearance may simulate meconium peritonitis, the calcifications are within the bowel and are more discrete and uniform (Figs. 16–15 and 16–16). These calcifications are apparently the result of the in-

teraction of fetal urine with meconium, possibly altering the pH or composition of the meconium.

An unusual form of anorectal malformation often considered as a form of imperforate anus is persistence of the cloaca in females. This lesion results from the lack of complete caudal descent of the urorectal septum, which normally divides the urogenital sinus from the anorectal canal. The severity of the lesion depends upon the degree of descent. If the urorectal septum is in near contact with the cloacal membrane the cloaca may be small, with the openings of the urinary, genital, and intestinal tracts close to the external orifice. On the contrary, the poorly formed urorectal septum provides for an elongated cloacal canal and fistulous communication at a considerable distance from the external orifice.

Text continued on page 316

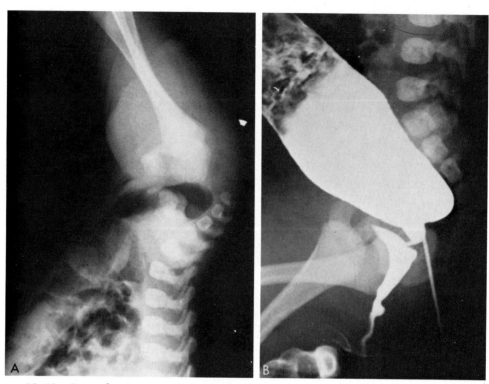

Figure 16–10. Imperforate anus. *A*, Lateral view of the lower abdomen and pelvis shows the slightly distended rectosigmoid with a long soft tissue gap between the anal dimple and the air-filled pouch. Note the small amount of air in the urinary bladder, indicating a fistula to the urinary tract. *B*, Slightly more than optimal amount of contrast medium injected into the rectum shows fistula to the vesicourethral junction and fills a dilated and deformed urethra. (Reprinted with permission from Wagner, M. L., Harberg, F. J., Kumar, M., and Singleton, E. B. The evaluation of imperforate anus utilizing percutaneous injection of water-soluble iodide contrast material, *Pediatr. Radiol.*, **1**:34, 1973.)

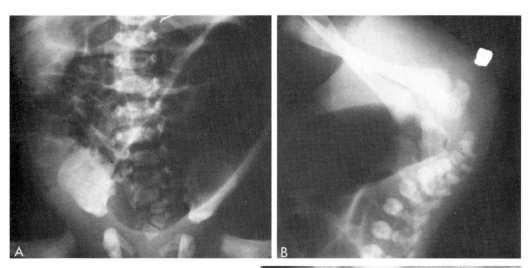

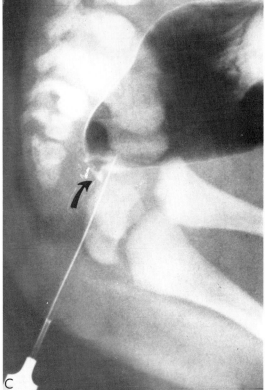

Figure 16–11. Imperforate anus. *A,* supine film of the abdomen shows dilated rectosigmoid colon with associated deformity of the sacrum. *B,* Lateral view shows the dilated rectosigmoid ending in a high position. *C,* Injection of contrast medium confirms the caudal extent of the distal pouch and shows a small beak (*arrow*) which is the origin of rectal fistula. (Reprinted with permission from Wagner, M. L., Harberg, F. J., Kumar, M., and Singleton, E. B. The evaluation of imperforate anus utilizing percutaneous injection of water-soluble iodide contrast material, *Pediatr. Radiol.,* **1**:34, 1973.)

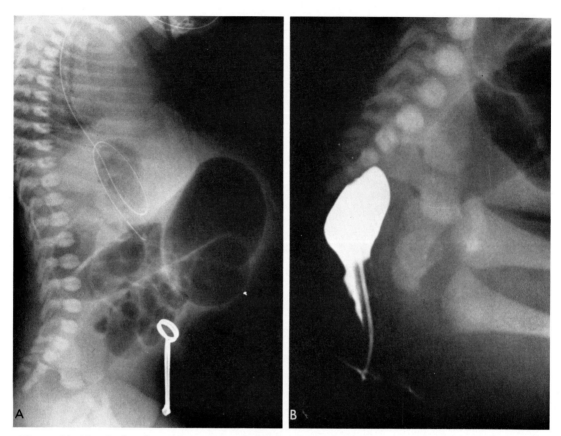

Figure 16–12. Isolated rectal atresia associated with omphalocele. *A,* Lateral view of the abdomen shows gas outlining the distal rectal segment proximal to the obstruction. *B,* Introduction of barium into the rectum shows more accurately the distance between the rectum and the distal anorectal pouch.

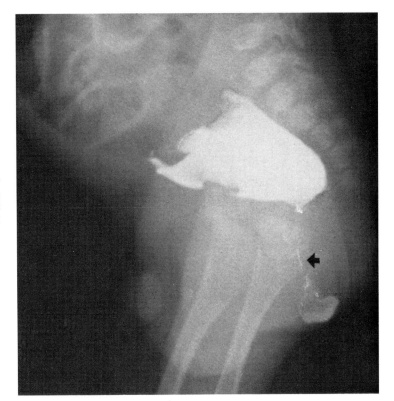

Figure 16–13. Anorectal stenosis in 1 month old infant. Anorectal stricture is outlined by a small amount of contrast material (*arrow*).

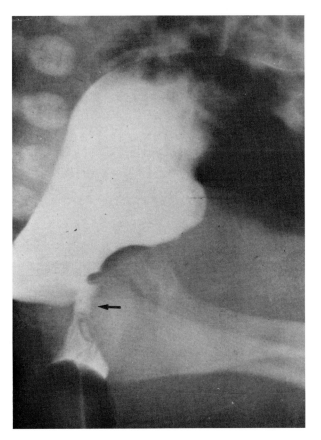

Figure 16–14. Anorectal stenosis. The tip of a Foley catheter has been inserted into the anal orifice and the inflated Foley bag pressed against the perineum to prevent loss of contrast medium. The stenotic segment is relatively short (*arrow*).

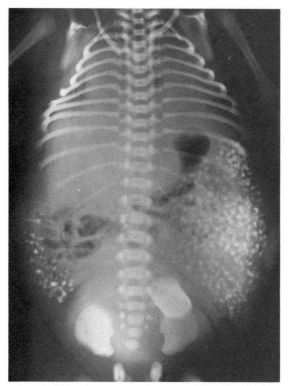

Figure 16–15. Imperforate anus with rectovesical fistula. Multiple discrete areas of calcification are seen within the lumen of the colon.

HIRSCHSPRUNG'S DISEASE: AGANGLIONOSIS

Congenital megacolon, or Hirschsprung's disease, was first described as a specific entity in 1887 by Harold Hirschsprung, a Copenhagen physician. He believed the disease to be a congenital defect, primarily affecting the distended portion of the colon, and made only casual mention of the normal-appearing rectosigmoid area in his patients. As early as 1901, Tittel noted scantiness of ganglion cells in the myenteric plexus of individuals with this condition. Among the various conflicting reports regarding the etiology which appeared in the succeeding years were several notable papers incriminating a deficiency in the ganglion cells of the rectum and the rectosigmoid areas as the causative factor. In 1948, the reports of Wilson and Zuelzer and of Whitehouse and Kernohan provided convincing evidence of the specific correla-

Clinically, there is a single orifice in the perineum without an anal dimple. Urine is discolored by meconium. Radiographically the lesion may be evaluated by flush technic of injecting the single orifice with contrast material to outline the vagina, bladder, and rectum entering the single canal (Fig. 16–17A and B), or if possible, catheterization of the individual elements as they enter the cloaca (Fig. 16–18). If there is stenosis of the vaginal orifice or narrowing of the urogenital sinus below the respective orifices, the structures draining into the cloaca may be markedly dilated, especially the vagina and/or uterus. These latter structures may fill with fluid or air and produce an enormous soft tissue density in the pelvis and abdomen, or an air-fluid level due to pneumovagina (Fig. 16–19). Associated anomalies of the urinary and genital systems are common, especially obstructive changes of the upper urinary tracts.

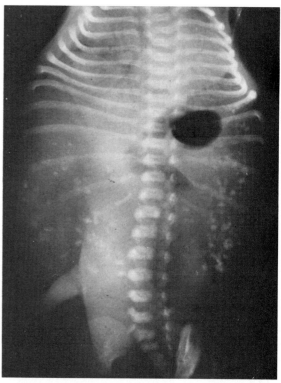

Figure 16–16. Imperforate anus with rectovesical fistula. Small discrete areas of calcification occupying the peripheral portion of the abdomen were found to be calcified intraluminal meconium at the time of autopsy.

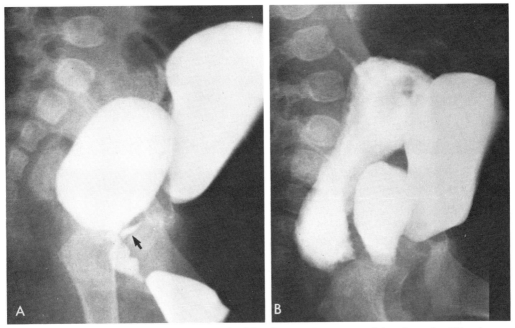

Figure 16–17. Cloacal anomaly in 9 month old infant. *A,* Injection of the cloacal orifice shows contrast medium entering dilated vagina and urinary bladder. The urethra (*arrow*) enters the common cloacal canal. *B,* Selective injection of the rectum shows this structure as well as the dilated vagina and bladder opacified with contrast medium.

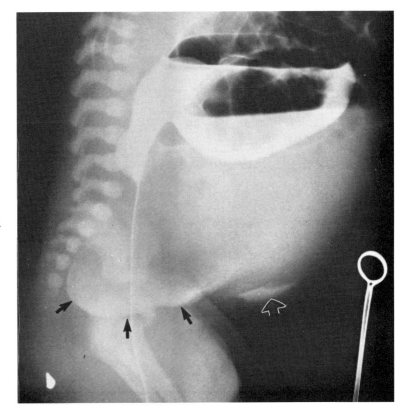

Figure 16–18. Common cloaca in newborn female with imperforate anus. Catheter extends through the cloaca into the rectum which has been compressed by the dilated hydrocolpos (*arrows*). A small amount of contrast medium is seen in the urinary bladder (*open arrow*).

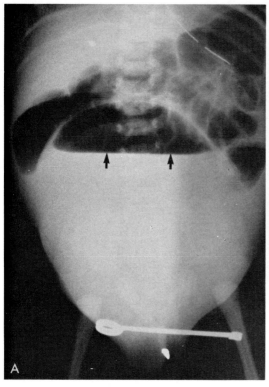

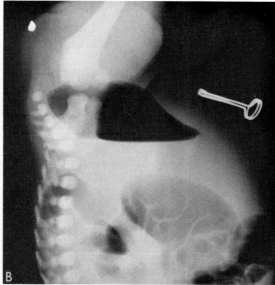

Figure 16–19. Cloacal anomaly in the newborn infant. *A*, Upright film shows air-fluid level in the dilated vagina (*arrows*). *B*, Lateral view made with the infant inverted shows collection of air in the hydrocolpos which extends posteriorly to the sacrum obstructing the rectum. Metallic marker identifies the anal dimple.

tion of aganglionosis and Hirschsprung's disease. This concept was verified in 1948 by Swenson and Bill who, by removing the segment which was neurologically deficient, provided the first satisfactory treatment. In the succeeding decade more articles were published on congenital megacolon than on any other single abnormality affecting the alimentary tract of infants and children.

It is now generally accepted that obstruction in Hirschsprung's disease is due to the inability of peristaltic action to pass the neurologically deficient segment, the hypertrophy of the proximal portions of the colon being compensatory to the obstruction. This is further complicated by absence of the normal defecation reflex. The reason for the deficiency of parasympathetic ganglion cells is unknown. Swenson considered it to represent a failure of development of the rectal and rectosigmoidal myenteric plexuses due to developmental fault in the extrinsic nerve supply, i.e., the pelvic parasympathetic system. This, however, does not explain cases in which a higher level of the colon is involved. Bo-

dian suggested that the primary defect is in the ganglion cells of Auerbach's and Meissner's plexuses and not related to the extrinsic innervation. At present, one of the more acceptable theories lies in the concept of ganglion cell migration from the neural crest. In Hirschsprung's disease there may be a diminished number of neural crest cells, or some defect in migration of the ganglion cells per se. Further investigation will undoubtedly establish the embryologic pathogenesis of aganglionosis.

In the classic form of Hirschsprung's disease, the aganglionic segment involves the rectum and distal sigmoid (Fig. 16–20). Atypical forms in which the deficient segment includes only the terminal portion of the rectum or extends cephalad to involve a long segment or all of the colon are occasionally encountered (see Fig. 12–38).

The condition usually is identified in the neonate or young infant and accounts for approximately 15 to 20% of the cases of neonatal bowel obstruction. The localized form of the disease is at least five times more common in males. The disease is frequently seen in families, although rare in parents of affected children. About 2% of patients with Hirschsprung's disease have Down's syndrome. Aganglionosis of the entire colon accounts for approximately 10% of patients, is equally common in girls, and may be familial. Localized or skipped areas of aganglionosis with normal distal myenteric plexuses are extremely rare. Most of the early suspected diagnoses of skipped aganglionosis were probably erroneous. Extremely low aganglionosis involving the anorectal junction is usually impossible to diagnose either histologically or by radiographic studies and presents the same clinical features as habit or functional constipation.

In Chagas' disease, the infectious organism (*Trypanosoma cruzi*) may destroy the rectal ganglion cells, producing megacolon radiographically identical to Hirschsprung's disease.

CLINICAL FINDINGS. Clinically, there is failure to pass meconium during the first 24 hours of life and the gradual development of abdominal distention and vomit-

ing. Cases of spontaneous rupture of the cecum or appendix have been reported. Alternating constipation and diarrhea may occur, the latter a result of periodic episodes of colitis. Occasionally, a compulsive mother can keep the colon decompressed by enemas so that the condition is not recognized until the first year or two of life, by which time the infant is usually undernourished, with a potbelly and wasted extremities.

The onset may be insidious and consist of progressive constipation beginning in the neonatal period, with gradual increase in size of the abdomen of an infant who is otherwise thriving. If the condition remains untreated, there is gradual increase in the degree of constipation and progressive distention of the abdomen during childhood. The outline of the colon and its enormous fecal content may be palpated and often visualized by its impression on the abdominal wall. Active peristaltic movements may also be seen traversing the distended segments. Manifestations of ob-

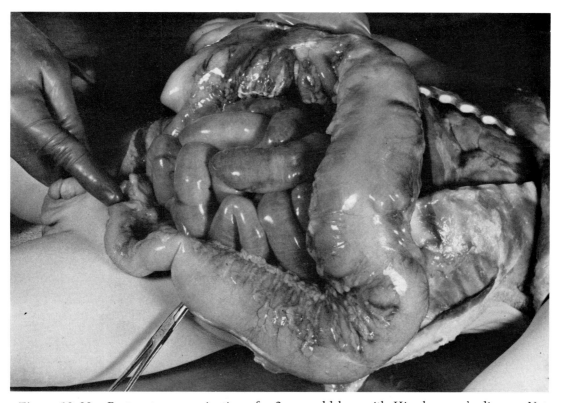

Figure 16–20. Postmortem examination of a 2 year old boy with Hirschsprung's disease. Note transition zone in sigmoid between normal-sized and dilated colon.

struction consisting of cramping, abdominal pain, and vomiting may occur periodically. Anorexia, lassitude, poor nutrition, and retardation of growth are often associated. Episodes of diarrhea are frequent, particularly in infancy, and blood in the stool may result from pressure necrosis and ulceration produced by the inspissated feces.

Digital rectal examination usually discloses an empty rectum or only a small amount of fecal material. Exceptions to this are the rare cases in which the aganglionic portion is limited to the anorectal junction, the rectum then taking part in the dilatation and containing a large quantity of fecal material.

Although patients with mild cases of congenital megacolon may be treated conservatively with daily enemas, mineral oil, appropriate diet, and parasympathomimetic drugs, the majority eventually require surgical intervention, the current procedure of choice being resection of the aganglionic segment. Following surgical correction (Swenson, Soave, or Duhamel procedures), there is a gradual reduction in the size of the abdomen, with return to normal size usually in six to eight months. Although the extensively hypertrophied and

dilated colon gradually becomes smaller, it seldom regresses to completely normal size.

RADIOLOGIC EVALUATION. The radiographic findings are, in part, the result of the inability of the aganglionic segment to partake in the peristaltic activity of fecal evacuation and, in part, attributable to the physiologic principle that denervated smooth muscle is abnormally sensitive to stimulation and tends to contract.

An abdominal scout film should precede the introduction of contrast material into the rectum. In the young infant with clinical evidence of obstruction, both upright and recumbent films are of value. In mild cases the scout film is frequently negative or may show slight excess of gas in the colon. In severe cases there is gaseous distention of the colon and the small bowel, often with air-fluid levels in the dilated loops. Gas is usually absent in the rectum, a lateral view usually being necessary to determine this (Fig. 16–21). However, the presence of some gas in the rectum does not exclude Hirschsprung's disease. In older infants the condition has been present long enough to cause dilatation of the colon, and the excessive accumulation of feces in the dilated bowel produces a

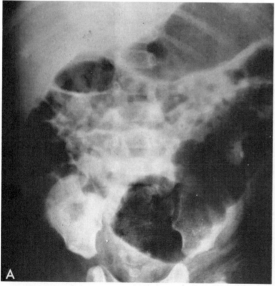 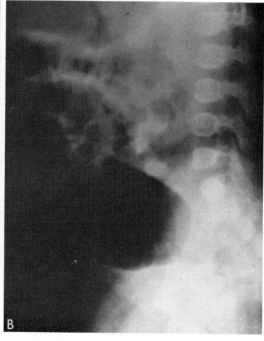

Figure 16–21. Hirschsprung's disease in 4 month old male infant. *A,* Abdominal scout film shows distention of the sigmoid. *B,* Lateral view shows disparity in the size and amount of gas in the rectum.

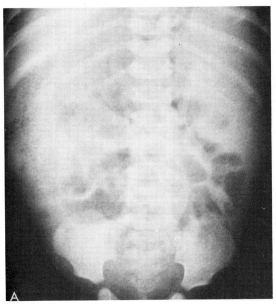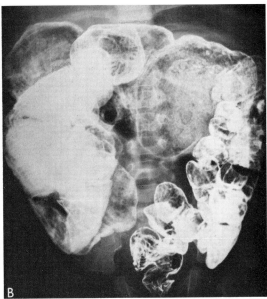

Figure 16–22. A, Hirschsprung's disease in 4 month old infant. The colon is dilated and filled with feces, producing a mottled appearance. Note also the flaring of the ilia, a common finding in young infants with ascites, abdominal masses, or other conditions producing increased intra-abdominal pressure. B, Barium enema shows long segment Hirschsprung's disease, the rectum and entire descending colon being aganglionic.

characteristic mottled appearance (Fig. 16–22A and B). Associated features, including calcified fecaloma, congenital heart disease, mongolism, pulmonary hypoplasia, and vertebral or rib abnormalities, may divert the radiologist's attention from the diagnosis. The pelvic configuration is often flared in infants with megacolon, resembling Down's syndrome. Other conditions producing an increase in intra-abdominal pressure may cause a similar pelvic configuration.

The examination is preferably carried out without attempts to cleanse the colon. Cathartics are definitely contraindicated, for they may cause serious complications in a condition in which the basic problem is one of obstruction. Preparatory enemas are also not advised because the constricted aganglionic segment may be sufficiently dilated by repeated cleansing enemas to conceal the junction between it and dilated bowel. In addition, the administration of water enemas to these patients is not without danger. A significant number of severe and fatal reactions have followed the administration of enemas to patients with megacolon. The cause of this "water intoxication" is unknown but apparently is re-

lated to rapid diffusion of water into the circulation due to the abnormally large absorbable surface and the high intraluminal pressure. The ensuing fall in electrolyte concentration and specific gravity may cause syncope and death. An alternate hypothesis is that the colonic stimulation produced by the introduction of fluid into an already distended colon causes reflex inhibition of the heart. Regardless of the mechanism of water intoxication, we have been sufficiently impressed by its danger to use only isotonic saline as the barium vehicle. This may be prepared by adding 2 level teaspoonfuls of sodium chloride (about 9 Gm) to 1 liter of fluid.

A small plastic enema tip is inserted just past the anal sphincter and secured by taping the buttocks and holding the infant's thighs straight and together as described on page 289. Care must be taken not to insert the enema tip past the aganglionic segment (Fig. 16–23). An inflated Foley catheter may completely obscure the lesion. It is important that the enema enter the rectum slowly in order for the fluoroscopist to follow the head of the barium column as it fills the rectum and passes into the sigmoid. Otherwise, the junction zone may be

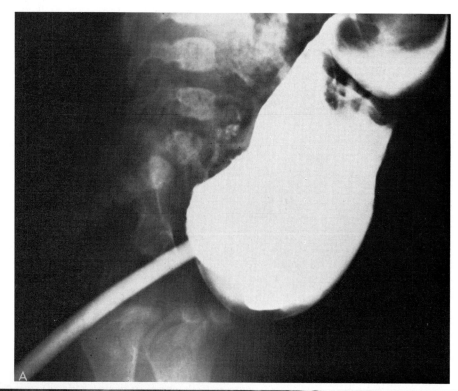

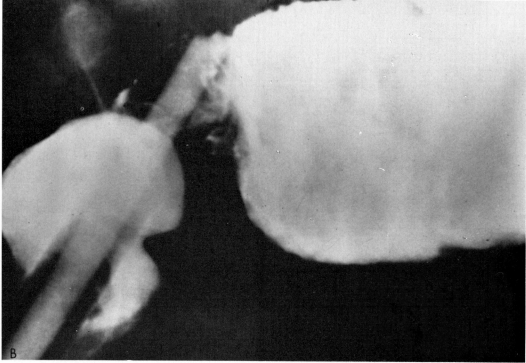

Figure 16–23. Hirschsprung's disease. *A*, Enema tip has been inserted past the area of aganglionosis into the dilated distal rectum. *B*, Reinjection with the tip withdrawn to a lower level shows the aganglionic segment and the transition zone more accurately.

obscured by redundancy of the rectosigmoid area. Also, the rapid passage of barium into the rectum may obscure a narrow segmental type of aganglionosis. By keeping the barium reservoir at a height of not more than 2 feet above the tabletop and by using a catheter or enema tip with a relatively small lumen, a slow rate of fill is assured. As the contrast material enters the superior portion of the rectum, the child is turned to a right anterior position in relation to the fluoroscopic screen in order to observe the fill of the sigmoid in profile. The normal slight constriction at the rectosigmoid flexure should not be mistaken for the transition zone of Hirschsprung's disease. Whether or not abnormality is noted, spot films should be taken of this area immediately, before there is additional fill of the sigmoid, the redundancy of which in the infant and young child will frequently obscure the rectosigmoid area (Fig. 16–24). If the transition zone between

narrow and dilated colon is encountered, as evidenced by barium suddenly entering the larger segment, the flow is discontinued. Because of the danger of inspissated barium producing complete obstruction, no attempt should be made to fill the rest of the colon. If enlargement of the colon is not encountered, the barium is allowed to continue to pass through the colon in an effort to locate a more proximal transition zone.

Anteroposterior and left posterior oblique radiographs are then obtained. If a transition zone is identified, as much of the enema as possible is siphoned off by lowering the reservoir below the level of the patient. The catheter is then removed and the patient encouraged to evacuate as much of the remaining barium as possible.

On rare occasions, a scybalum of feces may become so impacted as to produce obstruction within the aganglionic segment (Fig. 16–25).

The radiologic appearance of Hirsch-

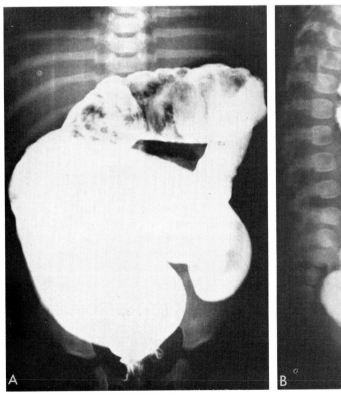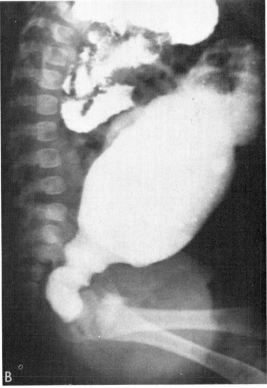

Figure 16-24. Hirschsprung's disease in a 6 month old infant with history of chronic constipation. A, Anteroposterior view, failing to show the narrow rectal segment because of overlying dilated sigmoid. B, Lateral view, showing more accurately the size of the rectum in relation to the megacolon. The amount of barium used in these illustrations is in excess of the optimal study.

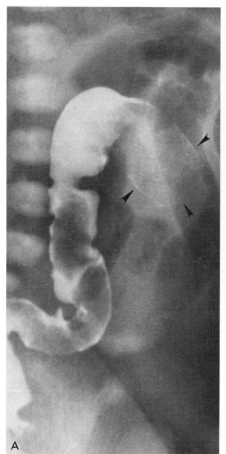

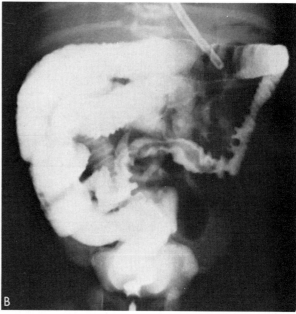

Figure 16–25. Hirschsprung's disease in 1 week old infant. *A,* Retrograde flow of barium is obstructed by fecal mass (*arrows*) in the distal sigmoid colon. *B,* Repeat examination two days later using Gastrografin enabled the colon to be visualized more completely. Biopsy of the rectum showed no evidence of ganglion cells.

sprung's disease depends largely upon the duration and severity of the obstruction. The distention of the bowel proximal to the segment of deficient innervation occurs gradually over a period of a few weeks to several months, according to the degree of obstruction. Therefore in the neonatal period it is usually impossible to detect a change in caliber of bowel at the junction with the aganglionic segment, and the diagnosis is based on the clinical findings and the completeness of evacuation of the barium enema. Many normal infants fail to show satisfactory evacuation on the immediate postevacuation film, but at 24 and 48 hours all of the mixture except a small amount in the cecum and rectum has been eliminated. Therefore, any infant suspected of having Hirschsprung's disease without radiologic evidence of megacolon should have delayed films one and two days after barium enema. If there is abnor-

mal retention of barium, Hirschsprung's disease is probably present (Figs. 16–26 and 16–27). Occasionally in the young infant the disproportion between the sizes of the rectum and the distended proximal colon will be appreciated (Fig. 16–28). Attempts to remove the contrast material by cleansing enemas are often unsuccessful if the aganglionosis is extensive and may force the material into the proximal portions of the small intestine (Fig. 16–29). This finding on delayed films is highly suggestive of total colon aganglionosis.

In the older child the disparity in size of the colon between the aganglionic segment and dilated bowel is readily apparent. The most common location of colonic aganglionosis is the rectum and distal portion of the sigmoid. In such cases barium studies show a rectum of normal or small size and the proximal portion of the defective segment located in the area where the colon becomes distended. This transition zone is usually abrupt but may be tapered (Fig. 16–30A, B, and C). A lateral view usually demonstrates the transition zone to better advantage (Fig. 16–31).

If associated colitis is present, the degree of colonic distention is increased and barium enema studies show evidence of irritability, increased serrations, and occasionally ulcerations (Fig. 16–32).

The aganglionic segment theoretically may be limited to the internal sphincter and the adjacent distal portion of the rectum. Such cases are virtually impossible to differentiate from habit-type constipation. The concept of the extremely low aganglionic segment localized to the anorectal junction is questionable and impossible to prove morphologically because of the normal absence of ganglion cells at this level.

Because a small percentage of patients with Hirschsprung's disease have abnormalities of the urinary tract, manifested by megaloureter and bladder dysfunction, excretory pyelograms and cystograms should be performed before surgical correction of the colonic defect is undertaken. More commonly, the distention of the sigmoid will displace the urinary bladder and partially obstruct the ureters (Fig. 16–33).

Follow-up barium enema studies after resection of the aganglionic segment are often disappointing. The colon may take many months to regress to normal size and may remain somewhat larger than normal indefinitely, depending upon the extent of the original dilatation (Fig. 16–34). However, in its evaluation one should keep in mind the relatively large size of the colon in young children. In all cases postoperatively the clinical results should take precedence over the radiologic evaluation. Frequently the clinical improvement is remarkable but the colon remains larger than normal. Consequently failure of complete resection of the aganglionic segment is more accurately estimated from the symptomatology than from the postoperative radiographic appearance of the colon (Fig. 16–35). In cases of incomplete resection clinical improvement does not occur and

Text continued on page 333

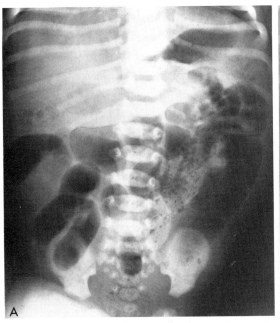
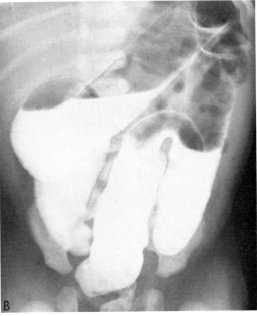

Figure 16–26. Hirschsprung's disease in newborn with progressive abdominal distention. *A,* Abdominal scout radiograph, showing gas in colon and gaseous distention of small intestine. Mottled pattern of gas and feces is identified in rectum and sigmoid. *B,* Radiograph exposed 48 hours after enema studies, at which time rectum and colon appeared normal, showing abnormal retention of contrast material.

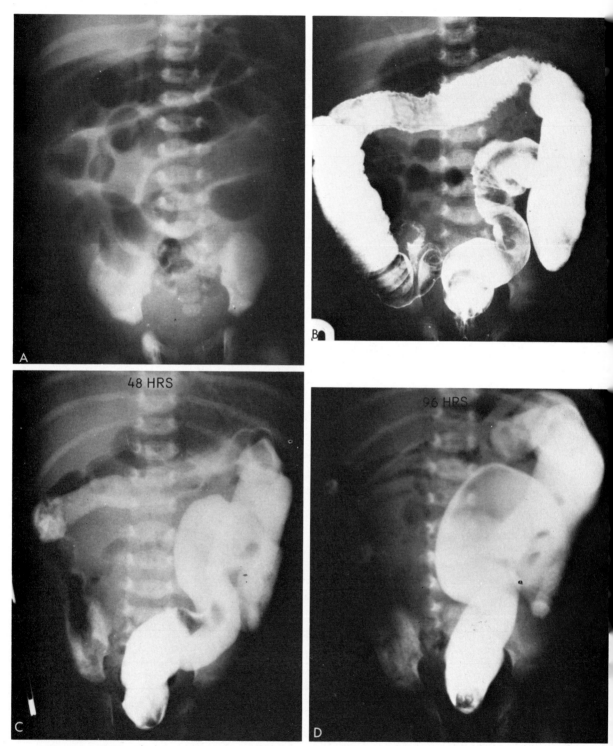

Figure 16–27. Hirschsprung's disease in 5 day old infant. *A*, Abdominal scout film shows multiple distended loops of small bowel. *B*, Barium enema examination shows normal caliber of the colon without radiographic evidence of a localized aganglionic segment. *C*, Radiograph made 48 hours after barium enema shows retained barium in the colon. *D*, Residual barium remains 96 hours following barium enema. Biopsy showed evidence of rectal aganglionosis.

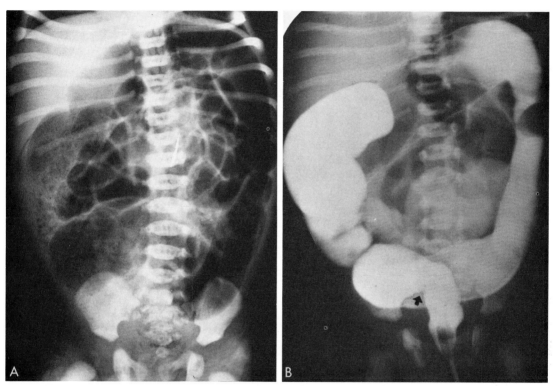

Figure 16–28. Hirschsprung's disease in 3 day old infant with abdominal distention and alternating diarrhea and constipation. *A*, Abdominal radiograph showing distention of colon and small intestine and extensive fecal accumulation in colon. *B*, Barium enema showing small rectum and dilated colon proximal to rectosigmoid junction (*arrow*).

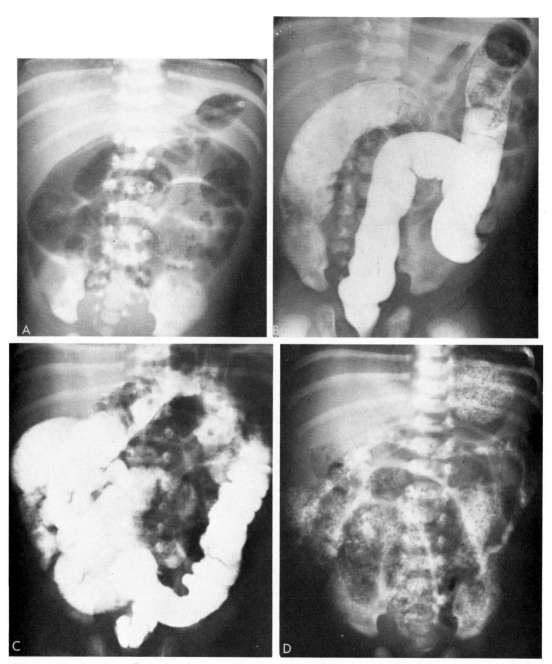

Figure 16–29. Aganglionosis of entire colon in 6 day old infant with signs of intestinal obstruction. *A*, Abdominal scout film showing mild gaseous distention of colon and small intestine. *B*, Barium enema showing no visible abnormality of colon. *C*, Film of abdomen exposed five days after *B* shows retention of contrast material in colon and some reflux into ileum. *D*, Attempts to remove contrast material by cleansing enemas for three days resulted in retrograde fill of small intestine and stomach. Specimen taken at operation shows entire colon aganglionic, with normal ganglion cells in terminal ileum.

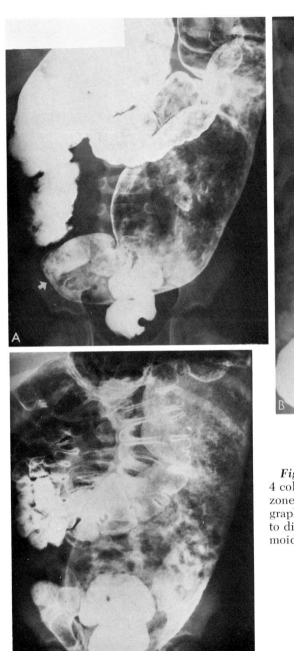

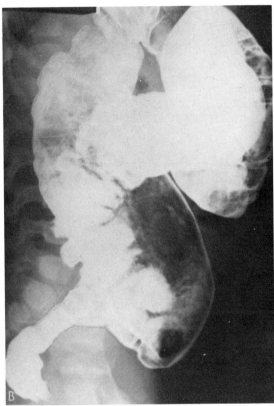

Figure 16–30. Hirschsprung's disease. *A*, At age 4 colon is already markedly dilated, with transition zone in the midsigmoid (*arrow*). *B*, Lateral radiograph emphasizes small size of rectum as compared to dilated sigmoid. *C*, At age 6 colon above midsigmoid level has continued to increase in size.

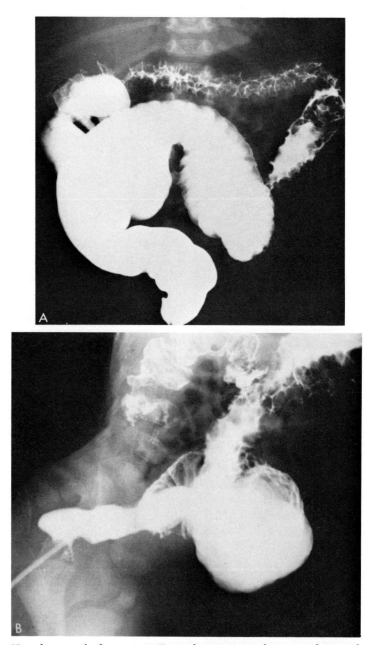

Figure 16–31. Hirschsprung's disease. A, Frontal projection shows evidence of megacolon but the transition zone between aganglionic rectal segment and the dilated sigmoid is not clearly delineated. B, Lateral view shows transition zone to better advantage.

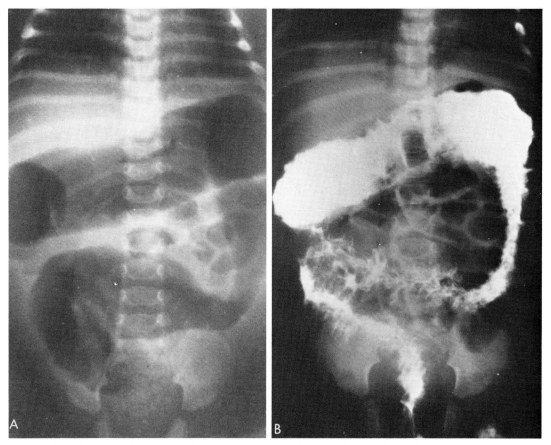

Figure 16–32. Hirschsprung's disease with associated colitis. *A,* Abdominal scout film shows an increased amount of gas in the colon. *B,* Barium enema study shows the colon to be irregular, with increased serrations and areas of ulceration.

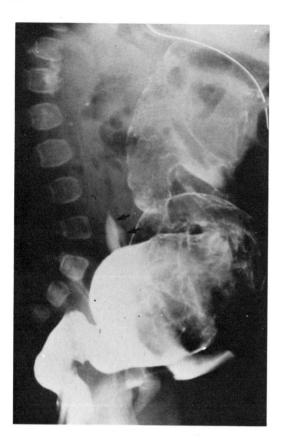

Figure 16–33. Hirschsprung's disease showing aganglionic rectum with distended sigmoid producing compression on the urinary bladder and partial obstruction of the ureters (*arrows*).

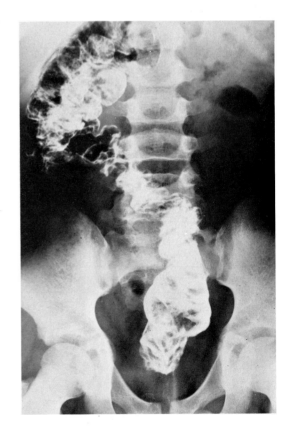

Figure 16–34. Postoperative study of Hirschsprung's disease (same patient shown in Fig. 16–30). Colon examination one year after resection of aganglionic segment shows satisfactory evacuation and enema. During fluoroscopy slight persistent enlargement of the distal colon was noted. Redundancy of sigmoid extending to right side of abdomen persists. Patient was asymptomatic and had shown excellent clinical improvement.

the radiographic appearance is frequently similar to the preoperative findings (Fig. 16–36). Rectal stricture may be another complication, especially if postoperative dilatations are neglected (Fig. 16–37A and B). However, in all successful resections the ability of the colon to evacuate its contents, as demonstrated in postevacuation radiographs, is markedly improved even though many months may pass before the colon regresses to a normal or nearly normal size.

HABIT OR FUNCTIONAL MEGACOLON

Although functional megacolon is an acquired condition, it is included here because of its clinical similarity to Hirschsprung's disease.

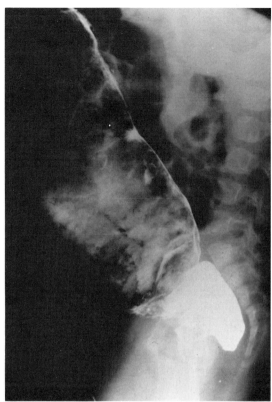

Figure 16–36. Incomplete resection of Hirschsprung's disease. Megacolon persists and the distal rectal segment was found to be aganglionic.

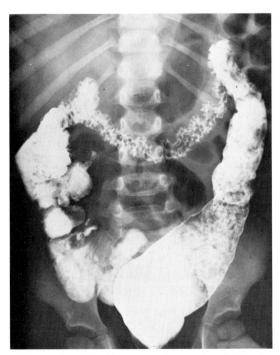

Figure 16–35. Postoperative study of Hirschsprung's disease (incomplete resection). Patient had resection of aganglionic segment three years previously. During the interim he had had chronic constipation and failed to show expected improvement. Biopsy of lower colon showed absence of ganglion cells, indicating incomplete resection.

Chronic constipation is the most common symptom leading to a request for barium enema as an initial study in the pediatric age group, the purpose usually being to determine if the cause is functional or due to Hirschsprung's disease. In most cases the cause is unknown and is presumed to be due to a suppression of the normal defecation urge at the age when bowel habits become established. Most examples of idiopathic megacolon are of this type. The attempts of an overzealous parent to establish strict bowel habits in the child or the use of too stringent disciplinary action following the infraction of these habits is believed to account for this type of constipation and the resulting megacolon. The term "functional" megacolon rather than psychogenic is preferable for this type, but unfortunately the former nomenclature has

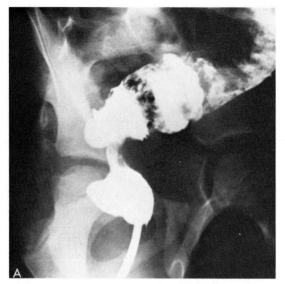
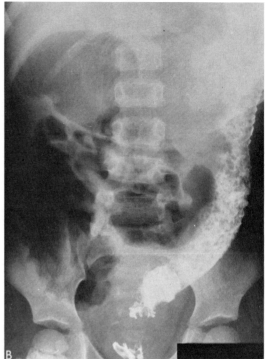

Figure 16–37. Postoperative rectal stricture following pull-through correction for Hirschsprung's disease in a 4 year old child. *A*, Oblique view shows the localized stricture. *B*, AP view shows marked irregularity of the sigmoid and descending portion of the colon as well as "thumbprinting" of the right half of the colon, representing associated edema and colitis.

become identified with the neuromuscular dysfunction of aganglionosis.

Usually, differentiation between Hirschsprung's disease and psychogenic megacolon is readily made from the history, physical examination, and radiologic studies. The distinguishing clinical features are listed below.

RADIOLOGIC EVALUATION. An abdominal scout film of a child with psychogenic megacolon may show an excessive amount of fecal material in the colon, including the rectum.

Under fluoroscopic observation, the contrast material is seen to pass into an abnormally large rectum rather than into the smaller, normal-sized rectum of Hirschsprung's disease (Fig. 16–38). The rectum is filled with feces and the rectosigmoid is dilated (Fig. 16–39). No attempt should be made to fill the entire colon with barium. This only complicates the initial problem and evacuation may be extremely difficult.

The sigmoid colon appears excessively long in children with functional constipation, suggesting that the etiology may in part be secondary to an abnormally long colon. However, this is usually considered to be the result of prolonged constipation rather than the cause of it.

It may be impossible to differentiate psychogenic megacolon from megacolon secondary to aganglionosis in the anorectal

PSYCHOGENIC MEGACOLON	HIRSCHSPRUNG'S DISEASE
1. Constipation begins at 2 to 3 years of age	1. Constipation starts from birth
2. Periodic voluminous stools	2. Scanty stools
3. Fecal soiling of diaper or underclothes	3. No fecal soiling
4. Physically well	4. Anorexia, lassitude, retarded growth
5. Usually no abdominal distention	5. Abdominal distention
6. Feces palpable in rectum	6. Rectum empty or contains only small amount of feces

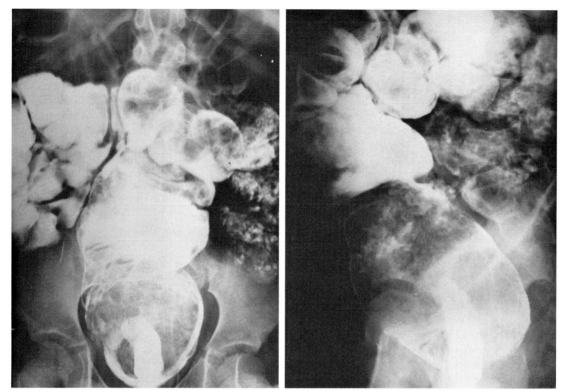

Figure 16–38. Psychogenic megacolon in 5 year old child. Constipation began at age 2. Dilatation of rectum extends to anus.

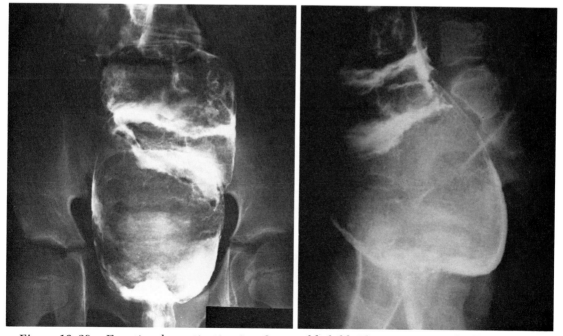

Figure 16–39. Functional constipation in a 9 year old child. The rectum is markedly dilated with fecal material.

area by radiologic methods alone. Both have fecal soiling and both have large amounts of feces palpable in the rectum. However, the other clinical features, especially the age of onset, may be helpful in differentiating these two forms of megacolon. Estimation of the thickness of the rectal wall by measuring the depth of the presacral tissues in lateral roentgenograms has been suggested as a possible means of differentiation, but in our experience is unreliable. Fortunately, in this type of aganglionosis, conservative medical measures usually are adequate and surgical intervention is not as necessary as for higher aganglionic segments.

MECONIUM PLUG SYNDROME

Meconium ileus, the meconium plug syndrome, and the small left colon syndrome are conditions which clinically and at times radiographically may be mistaken for Hirschsprung's disease. Meconium ileus has been described in Chapter 12.

Meconium plug syndrome is a common cause of obstipation in newborn infants but radiographic studies are seldom needed, the plug being dislodged by digital examination or by saline enemas. If the plug is not expelled within 12 to 24 hours after birth, abdominal distention may develop. In some cases the meconium plug lies in the more proximal portion of the colon and in such cases obstruction may become severe, associated with abdominal distention and vomiting. Barium enema studies in such cases will usually show a rectum and colon of normal size with inspissated meconium filling defects (Fig. 16–40). This finding helps distinguish meconium plug syndrome from meconium ileus where the colon distal to the obstruction is very small. However, in some cases of meconium plug syndrome, the colon distal to the obstruction is tapered and smaller than normal, resembling radiographic findings of the small left colon syndrome or Hirschsprung's disease. Study of trypsin in the available meconium is not reliable in differentiating meconium plug syndrome

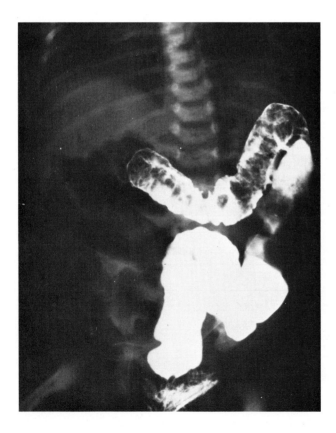

Figure 16–40. Meconium plug syndrome. Barium enema shows meconium filling the distal transverse portion of the colon and the proximal descending colon.

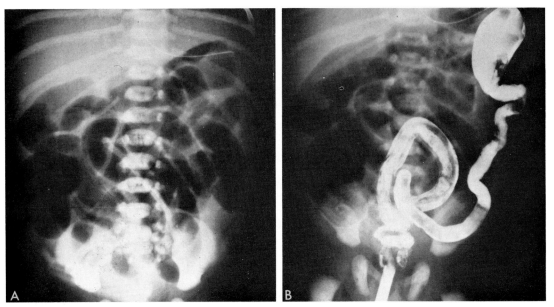

Figure 16–41. Small left colon syndrome in 2 day old infant. *A,* Abdominal scout film shows multiple distended loops of small bowel. *B,* Barium enema shows small left colon with transitional dilatation at the splenic flexure. The wall of the colon is smooth without segmental areas of contraction seen in Hirschsprung's disease. Recovery followed the barium enema.

from meconium ileus. The utilization of water-soluble iodide contrast solutions is of help in dislodging the plug. The hydrostatic effect of these solutions produces distention of the colon, with resulting dislodgement of the plug. However, these solutions must be used judiciously with an awareness that hypovolemia may develop. The meconium plug syndrome has been reported in newborn infants in whom hypermagnesemia has been etiologically implicated.

SMALL LEFT COLON SYNDROME

This is a relatively new entity in pediatric radiology described initially by Davis and characterized clinically by obstipation and abdominal distention. The clinical features may be identical to those seen in meconium ileus, the meconium plug syndrome, and Hirschsprung's disease. Characteristically most of the infants with the small left colon syndrome are mature infants, many of whom have a history of maternal diabetes.

The radiographic findings consist of a small left colon with dilatation of the colon proximal to the splenic flexure (Fig. 16–41A and B). The wall of the small distal colon is smooth and does not show the serrations usually seen in long segment Hirschsprung's disease (Fig. 16–42A, B, and C). Barium enema results in clinical improvement although this may have to be repeated more than once. Davis has also reported similar radiographic findings in asymptomatic babies of diabetic mothers.

In all probability the small left colon syndrome is due to immaturity of the neural plexuses. The normal maturing process of the neural plexuses of the alimentary tract occurs in a cephalad to caudal direction. Consequently in the small left colon syndrome there may be a failure of normal maturation of the neural tissues which become functional following the stimulation by barium enema.

One should guard against oversimplifying this condition because a competent differentiation between the small left colon syndrome and Hirschsprung's disease may not always be possible.

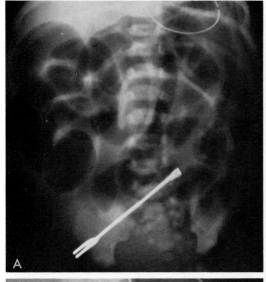

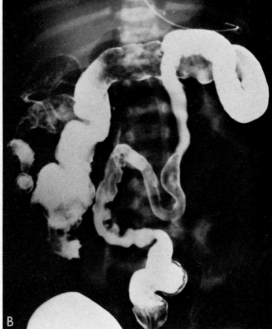

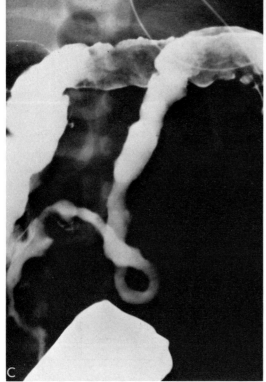

Figure 16–42. Hirschsprung's disease in a newborn simulating the small left colon syndrome. *A,* Abdominal scout film shows distended small bowel. *B,* Barium enema shows a small left colon with transitional dilatation at the splenic flexure. *C,* Spot film made at time of fluoroscopy shows segmental contractions of the narrow colon which help differentiate this condition from the small left colon syndrome. No ganglion cells were found at biopsy.

ABNORMALITIES OF COLON POSITION

The various types of anomalies of intestinal rotation, their embryologic development, and their roentgenologic appearance are discussed on page 181.

In *nonrotation*, the intestinal tract returns to the abdominal cavity without undergoing more than the initial 90-degree counterclockwise rotation. Consequently, the duodenum and upper jejunum lie in the right upper quadrant, and the colon, including the cecum, is in the left side of the abdomen, the ileum passing from right to left to enter the cecum (see p. 182).

Malrotation implies incomplete rotation of the intestine on its return from the umbilical cord into the abdomen. The degree of malrotation may be determined by the position of the cecum, which may be on the left side, higher than normal on the right side, or in an intermediate position.

In *reversed rotation,* the postarterial segment led by the cecum returns to the abdomen first, thereby reversing the normal relationship of the duodenum and colon to the superior mesenteric artery. The duodenum lies ventral to the artery and the transverse portion of the colon lies wedged under the superior mesenteric artery at its origin from the aorta. This situation produces partial or complete obstruction of the transverse colon, which may be determined by barium enema studies.

The failure of normal mesenteric peritoneal fusion of the ascending portion of the colon results in abnormal mobility of this structure and the cecum. This may be a significant finding during barium enema examination and suggests, if there are obstructive symptoms, that other abnormal mesenteric fixations are present and possibly volvulus of the midgut or an abnormal peritoneal band compressing some portion of the bowel. An abnormally mobile cecum is a potential site of volvulus formation. When this occurs, the cecum becomes markedly distended with gas and is displaced medially out of the right lower quadrant. The distended cecum may extend well across the midline, and multiple distended loops of small bowel are also present. The condition is relatively common in adults but for some reason is very rare in children.

In patients with left renal agenesis or ectopia, the splenic flexure of the colon is noted to lie in a more medial and posterior position than is normal. Any renal tissue (even dysplastic) in its normal position is the apparent stimulus to the formation of Gerota's retroperitoneal fascia. In the absence of this fascia, the splenic flexure swings medial to the stomach into the renal bed.

Radiographically the erect and prone films are helpful in delineating gas in the splenic flexure (Fig. 16–43) but a barium enema should be performed for confirmation.

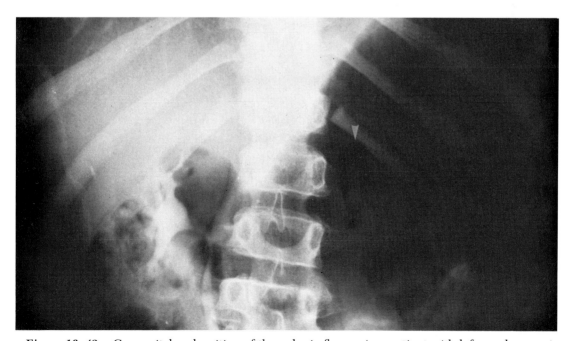

Figure 16–43. Congenital malposition of the splenic flexure in a patient with left renal agenesis.

DUPLICATIONS

Duplications of the colon are much less common than small bowel duplications. The largest series of cases has been reported by Gross, who found 13 of 68 alimentary tract duplications to be of colonic origin. They may be cystic or tubular in shape and may or may not communicate with the normal colon. Extensive duplica- tions of all or most of the colon are rarely seen. In such cases there is a high incidence of duplication of the bladder, urethra, and uterus. Triplication of the colon has also been reported.

DEVELOPMENTAL ANATOMY. The embryologic formation of colonic duplication is probably the same as for duplications elsewhere in the alimentary tract, discussed on page 197. Complete duplication

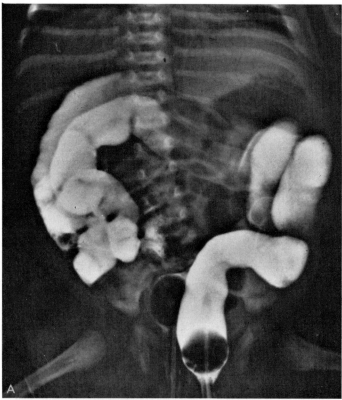

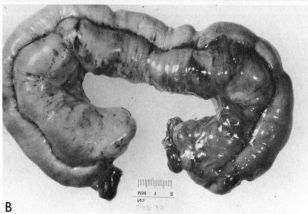

Figure 16–44. Complete duplication of the colon in a newborn infant. *A,* The infant had two anal openings and two vaginal openings. Separate injections of the anal openings show separate colons. *B,* Gross specimen. (Courtesy of Dr. L. J. Geppert, Wilford Hall, Lackland Air Force Base, San Antonio, Texas.)

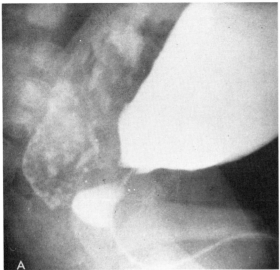

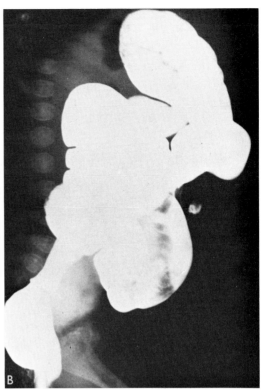

Figure 16–45. Rectal duplication in a male infant. *A*, Cystogram shows filling of bowel from a communication with the urethra. A posterior urethral valve is also present. *B*, Barium enema demonstrates the contrast material–filled duplication to be separate from the normal rectum. (Courtesy of Dr. G. Currarino, Dallas, Texas.)

of the colon associated with duplication of the urogenital structures probably represents a twinning process.

SYMPTOMS. Clinical evidence of colonic duplication, which may appear in infancy, childhood, or adulthood, results from obstruction of the normal colon by the enlarging duplication. The obstruction is usually partial, and there is commonly a long history of constipation, abdominal distress, and increasing abdominal distention. The duplication may be palpated through the abdominal wall. If there is an abdominal mass associated with duplication of a part or all of the genital tract, colonic duplication should be suspected.

RADIOLOGIC EVALUATION. Ordinarily, the duplication cannot be visualized directly on plain films. However, it may be suspected from the displacement of adjacent gas-filled loops of bowel. A colonic duplication in the pelvis may be indistinguishable from a distended urinary bladder or hydrometrocolpos. If the lumen of the duplication communicates with the colon, it may become distended by gas and reach

an enormous size. The complete colonic duplication reported in an adult by Weber and Dixon contained material of amorphous density which they ascribed to calcium excreted into the closed lumen.

Barium enema studies will opacify the duplication if there is communication between the normal colon and the duplicated segment or if there are two anal openings (Fig. 16–44). If not, the duplication may be accurately localized by the displacement it produces on the barium-filled colon. Occasionally the duplication will communicate with the urinary tract (Fig. 16–45). Complete duplication of the colon may be filled with barium if its distal portion communicates with the rectum or sigmoid. If communication is only in the proximal portion, the normal colon fills before the duplication. Oral barium administration is more successful than enema in identifying this type.

Diverticula

True diverticula of the colon are analogous to cystic duplications, and possibly most cases reported as diverticula are actually duplication anomalies. The adult form of diverticulosis, i.e., pseudodiverticula with protrusion of mucosa and submucosa between the muscular fibers of the colonic wall, is unknown in infants but was reported by Bearse in a 12 year old child. The abnormality is detected only by barium enema, the barium-filled diverticula appearing as pear-shaped areas of density projecting beyond the wall of the colon.

REFERENCES

Atresia and Stenosis

Arendt, J. The significance of Cannon's point in the normal and abnormal function of the colon, *Am. J. Roentgenol., 54*:149, 1946.

Barnard, C. N., and Louw, J. H. The genesis of intestinal atresia, *Minn. Med., 39*:745, 1956.

Bell, M. J., Ternberg, J. L., Askin, F. B., McAlister, W., and Shackelford, G. Intestinal stricture in necrotizing enterocolitis, *J. Pediatr. Surg., 11*:319, 1976.

Benson, C. D., Lotfi, M. W., and Brough, A. J. Congenital atresia and stenosis of the colon, *J. Pediatr. Surg., 3*:253, 1968.

Bland-Sutton, J. D. Imperforate ileum, *Am. J. Med. Sci., 98*:457, 1889.

Blank, E., Afshani, E., Girdany, B. R., and Pappas, A. "Windsock sign" of congenital membranous atresia of the colon, *Am. J. Roentgenol., 120*:330, 1974.

Bley, W. R., and Franken, E. A., Jr. Roentgenology of colon atresia, *Pediatr. Radiol., 1*:105, 1973.

Gross, R. E. *The Surgery of Infancy and Childhood* (Philadelphia: W. B. Saunders, 1953).

Harbour, M. J., Altman, D. H., and Gilbert, M. Congenital atresia of the colon, *Radiology, 84*:19, 1965.

Krasna, I. H., Becker, J. M., and Schneider, K. M., et al. Colonic stenosis following necrotizing enterocolitis of the newborn, *J. Pediatr. Surg., 5*:200, 1970.

Lloyd, D. A., and Cywes, S. Intestinal stenosis and enterocyst formation as late complications of neonatal necrotizing enterocolitis, *J. Pediatr. Surg., 8*:479, 1973.

Louw, J. H. Congenital intestinal atresia and stenosis in the newborn: Observations on its pathogenesis and treatment, *Ann. R. Coll. Surg. Engl., 25*:209, 1959.

Rabinowitz, J. G., Wolf, B. S., Feller, M. R., and Krasna, R. Colonic changes following necrotizing enterocolitis in the newborn, *Am. J. Roentgenol., 103*:359, 1968.

Anorectal Malformations

Berdon, W. E., Baker, D. H., Santulli, T. V., and Amoury, R. The radiologic evaluation of imperforate anus: An approach correlated with current surgical concepts, *Radiology, 90*:466, 1968.

Berdon, W. E., Baker, D. H., Wigger, H. J., Mitsudo, S. M., Williams, H., Kaufmann, H. J., and Shapiro, L. Calcified intraluminal meconium in newborn males with imperforate anus: Enterolithiasis in the newborn, *Am. J. Roentgenol., 125*:449, 1975.

Berdon, W. E., Hochberg, B., Baker, D. H., Grossman, H., and Santulli, T. V. The association of lumbosacral spine and genitourinary anomalies with imperforate anus, *Am. J. Roentgenol., 98*:181, 1966.

Cheng, G. K., Fisher, J. H., O'Hare, K. H., Retik, A. B., and Darling, D. B. Anomaly of the persistent cloaca in female patients. *Am. J. Roentgenol., 120*:413, 1974.

Gross, R. E. *The Surgery of Infancy and Childhood* (Philadelphia: W. B. Saunders, 1953).

Kurlander, G. J. Roentgenology of imperforate anus, *Am. J. Roentgenol., 100*:190, 1967.

Ladd, W. E., and Gross, R. E. Congenital malformations of the anus and rectum: A report of 162 cases, *Am. J. Surg., 23*:167, 1934.

Quan, L., and Smith, D. W. The VATER association, *J. Pediatr., 82*:104, 1973.

Robertson, D. A. R., Samuel, E., and MacLeod, W. Radiologic assessment of imperforate anus, *Br. J. Radiol., 38*:444, 1965.

Santulli, T. V. *Pediatric Surgery* (2nd ed.; Chicago: Year Book Medical Publishers, 1969), pp. 938–1007.

Santulli, T. V., Kiesewetter, W. B., and Bill, A. H., Jr. Anorectal anomalies: A suggested international classification, *J. Pediatr. Surg., 5*:281, 1970.

Santulli, T. V., Schullinger, J. N., Kiesewetter, W. B., and Bill, A. H., Jr. Imperforate anus: A survey from the members of the Surgical Society of the American Academy of Pediatrics, *J. Pediatr. Surg., 6*:484, 1971.

Smith, E. D. Urinary anomalies and complications in imperforate anus and rectum, *J. Pediatr. Surg., 3*:337, 1968.

Stephens, F. D., and Smith, E. D. *Ano-Rectal Malformations in Children* (Chicago: Year Book Medical Publishers, 1971).

Wagner, M. L., Harberg, F. J., Kumar, A. P. M., and Singleton, E. B. The evaluation of imperforate anus utilizing percutaneous injection of water-soluble iodide contrast material, *Pediatr. Radiol., 1*:34, 1973.

Wangensteen, O. H., and Rice, C. O. Imperforate anus—a method of determining the surgical approach, *Ann. Surg., 92*:77, 1930.

Winslow, O., Litt, R., and Altman, D. Imperforate anus from a roentgenologic standpoint, *Am. J. Roentgenol., 85*:718, 1961.

Hirschsprung's Disease: Aganglionosis

Ajayi, O. O. A., Solanke, T. F., Seriki, O., and Bohrer, S. P. Hirschsprung's disease in the neonate presenting as cecal perforation, *Pediatrics, 43*:102, 1969.

Berdon, W. E., and Baker, D. H. The roentgenographic diagnosis of Hirschsprung's disease in infancy, *Am. J. Roentgenol., 93*:432, 1965.

Berdon, W. E., Koontz, P., and Baker, D. H. The diagnosis of colonic and terminal ileum aganglionosis, *Am. J. Roentgenol., 91*:680, 1964.

Bill, A. H., Jr., and Chapman, N. D. The enterocolitis of Hirschsprung's disease: Its natural history and treatment, *Am. J. Surg., 103*:70, 1962.

Bodian, M., and Carter, C. O. A family study of Hirschsprung's disease, *Ann. Hum. Genet.*, 26:261, 1963.

Bodian, M., Stephens, F. D., and Ward, B. C. H. Hirschsprung's disease, *Lancet*, 1:19, 1950.

Chandler, N. W., and Zwiren, G. T. Complete reflux of the small bowel in total colon Hirschsprung's disease, *Radiology*, 94:335, 1970.

Davis, W. S., and Allen, R. P. Conditioning value of the plain film examination in the diagnosis of neonatal Hirschsprung's disease, *Radiology*, 93:129, 1969.

Duhamel, B. A new operation for the treatment of Hirschsprung's disease, *Arch. Dis. Child.*, 35:38, 1960.

Ehrenpreis, T. *Hirschsprung's Disease* (Chicago: Year Book Medical Publishers, 1970).

Ferriera-Santos, R., and Carrill, C. F. Acquired megacolon in Chagas disease, *Proc. R. Soc. Med.*, 54:1047, 1961.

Frech, R. S. Aganglionosis involving the entire colon and a variable length of small bowel, *Radiology*, 90:249, 1968.

Grewal, R. S., et al. Congenital megacolon, *J. Int. Coll. Surg.*, 43:61, 1965.

Hiatt, R. B. The pathologic physiology of congenital megacolon, *Ann. Surg.*, 133:313, 1951.

Hirschsprung, H. Stuhltragheit Neugehorener in Folge von Dilatation und Hypertrophie des Colons, *Jahrb. Kinderh.*, 27:1, 1887.

Hope, J. W., Borns, P. F., and Berg, P. K. Roentgenologic manifestations of Hirschsprung's disease in infancy, *Am. J. Roentgenol.*, 95:217, 1965.

Kilcoyne, R. F., and Taybi, H. Conditions associated with congenital megacolon, *Am. J. Roentgenol.*, 108:615, 1970.

Martin, L. W., and Perrin, E. V. Neonatal perforation of the appendix in association with Hirschsprung's disease, *Ann. Surg.*, 166:799, 1967.

Moseley, P. K., and Segar, W. E. Fluid and serum electrolyte disturbances as a complication of enemas in Hirschsprung's disease, *Am. J. Dis. Child.*, 115:714, 1968.

Nissan, S., and Bar-Maor, J. A. Further experience in the diagnosis and surgical treatment of short-segment Hirschsprung's disease and idiopathic megacolon, *J. Pediatr. Surg.*, 7:738, 1971.

Okamoto, E., and Ueda, T. Embryogenesis of the intramural ganglia of the gut and its relation to Hirschsprung's disease, *J. Pediatr. Surg.*, 2:437, 1967.

Reeder, M. M., and Hamilton, L. C. Tropical disease of the colon, *Sem. Roentgenol.* 3:62, 1968.

Schey, W. L., and White, H. Hirschsprung's disease: Problems in the roentgen interpretation, *Am. J. Roentgenol.*, 112:105, 1971.

Shopfner, C. E. Urinary tract pathology associated with constipation, *Radiology*, 90:865, 1968.

Soave, F. A new surgical technique for the treatment of Hirschsprung's disease, *Surgery*, 56:1007, 1964.

Sprinz, H., et al. Hirschsprung's disease with skip area, *Ann. Surg.*, 153:143, 1961.

Swenson, O. A new concept of the pathology of megaloureters, *Surgery*, 32:367, 1952.

Swenson, O. Congenital megacolon, *Pediatr. Clin. North Am.*, 14:187, 1967.

Swenson, O. Medical progress: Hirschsprung's disease (aganglionic megacolon), *N. Engl. J. Med.*, 260:972, 1969.

Swenson, O., and Bill, A. H., Jr. Resection of rectum and rectosigmoid with preservation of the sphincter for benign spastic lesions producing megacolon, *Surgery*, 24:212, 1948.

Swenson, O., and Davidson, F. Z. Similarities of mechanical intestinal obstruction and aganglionic megacolon in the newborn infant. A review of 64 cases, *N. Engl. J. Med.*, 262:64, 1960.

Swenson, O., Fisher, J. H., and MacMahon, H. E. Rectal biopsy as an aid in the diagnosis of Hirschsprung's disease, *N. Engl. J. Med.*, 253:632, 1955.

Swenson, O., Neuhauser, E. B. D., and Pickett, L. K. New concepts of the etiology, diagnosis and treatment of congenital megacolon (Hirschsprung's disease), *Pediatrics*, 4:201, 1949.

Swenson, O., Sherman, J. O., and Fisher, J. H. Diagnosis of congenital megacolon: An analysis of 501 patients, *J. Pediatr. Surg.*, 8:587, 1973.

Tittel, K. Über eine angeborene Missbildung des Dickdarmes, *Wien. Klin. Wochenschr.*, 14:903, 1901.

Whitehouse, F. R., and Kernohan, J. W. Myenteric plexus in congenital megacolon, *Arch. Intern. Med.*, 82:75, 1948.

Winkelman, J., Co-existent megacolon and megaureter, *Pediatrics*, 39:258, 1967.

Ziskind, A., and Gellis, S. S. Water intoxication following tap-water enemas, *Am. J. Dis. Child.*, 96:699, 1958.

Zuelzer, W. W., and Wilson, J. L. Functional intestinal obstruction on a congenital neurogenic basis in infancy, *Am. J. Dis. Child.*, 75:40, 1948.

Habit or Functional Megacolon

Davidson, M., Kugler, M. M., and Bauer, C. H. Diagnosis and management in children with severe and protracted constipation and obstipation, *J. Pediatr.*, 62:261, 1963.

Garrard, S. D., and Richmond, J. B. Psychogenic megacolon manifested by fecal soiling, *Pediatrics*, 10:474, 1952.

Kottmeier, P. K., and Clatworthy, H. W., Jr. Aganglionic and functional megacolon in children—a diagnostic dilemma, *Pediatrics*, 36:572, 1965.

Mercer, R. D. Constipation, *Pediatr. Clin. North Am.*, 14:175, 1967.

Santulli, T. V. Constipation, in Benson, C. C., Mustard, W. T., and Ravitch, M. M., et al., editors, *Pediatric Surgery* (2nd ed.; Chicago: Year Book Medical Publishers, 1969), pp. 1012–1015.

Meconium Plug Syndrome and Small Left Colon Syndrome

Clatworthy, H. W., Jr., Howard, W. H. R., and Lloyd, J. Meconium plug syndrome, *Surgery*, 39:131, 1956.

Davis, W. S., Allen, R. P., Favara, B. E., and Slovis, T. L. Neonatal small left colon syndrome, *Am. J. Roentgenol.*, 120:322, 1974.

Ellis, D. G., and Clatworthy, H. W., Jr. Meconium plug syndrome revisited, *J. Pediatr. Surg.*, 1:54, 1966.

Gillis, D. A., and Grantmyre, E. B. Meconium plug syndrome in Hirschsprung's disease, *Can. Med. Assoc. J.*, 92:225, 1965.

Mikity, V. G., Hodgman, J. E., and Paciulli, J. Meconium blockage syndrome, *Radiology*, 88:740, 1967.

Pochaczevsky, R., and Leonidas, J. C. The meconium plug syndrome. Roentgen evaluation and differentiation from Hirschsprung's disease and other pathologic states, *Am. J. Roentgenol.*, *120*: 342, 1974.

Sokal, M. M., Koenigsberger, M. R., Rose, J. S., Berdon, W. E., and Santulli, T. V. Neonatal hypermagnesemia and the meconium plug syndrome, *N. Engl. J. Med.*, *286*:823, 1972.

Swischuk, L. E. Meconium plug syndrome, a cause of neonatal intestinal obstruction, *Am. J. Roentgenol.*, *103*:339, 1968.

Taybi, H., and Patterson, J. Plain film diagnosis of meconium plug syndrome: Presacral mass, *Radiology*, *104*:113, 1972.

Tucker, A. S., and Izant, R. J., Jr. Problems with meconium, *Am. J. Roentgenol.*, *112*:135, 1971.

Van Leeuwen, G., Riley, W. C., Glenn, L., and Woodruff, C. Meconium plug syndrome with aganglionosis, *Pediatrics*, *40*:665, 1967.

Abnormalities of Colon Position

Berdon, W. E., Baker, D. H., Bull, S., and Santulli, T. V. Midgut malrotation and volvulus. Which films are most helpful? *Radiology*, *96*:375, 1970.

Estrada, R. L. *Anomalies of Intestinal Rotation and Fixation* (Springfield, Ill.: Charles C Thomas, 1958).

Gross, R. E. *The Surgery of Infancy and Childhood* (Philadelphia: W. B. Saunders, 1953), pp. 192–203.

Houston, C. S., and Wittenborg, M. H. Roentgen evaluation of anomalies of rotation and fixation of the bowel in children, *Radiology*, *84*:1, 1965.

Mascatello, V., and Lebowitz, R. L. Malposition of the colon in left renal agenesis and ectopia, *Radiology*, *120*:371, 1976.

Simpson, A. J., Leonidas, J. C., Krasna, I. H., Becker, J. M., and Schneider, K. M. Roentgen diagnosis of midgut malrotation: Value of upper gastrointestinal radiographic study, *J. Pediatr. Surg.*, 7:243, 1972.

Singleton, E. B. Radiologic evaluation of intestinal obstruction in the newborn, *Radiol. Clin. North Am.*, *1*:571, 1963.

Duplications

Beach, P. D., Brascho, D. J., Hein, W. R., Nichol, W. W., and Geppert, L. J. Duplication of the primitive hindgut of human beings, *Surgery*, *49*:779, 1961.

Bearse, C. Diverticulosis and diverticulitis of colon in young people, *J.A.M.A.*, *132*:371, 1946.

Bremer, J. L. Diverticula and duplications of the intestinal tract, *Arch. Pathol.*, *38*:132, 1944.

Gray, A. W. Triplication of large intestine, *Arch. Pathol.*, *30*:1215, 1940.

Gross, R. E. *The Surgery of Infancy and Childhood* (Philadelphia: W. B. Saunders, 1953), pp. 221–245.

Gross, R. E., Holcomb, G. W., and Farber, S. Duplications of the alimentary tract, *Pediatrics*, 9:449, 1952.

Kottra, J. J., and Dodds, W. J. Duplication of the large bowel, *Am. J. Roentgenol.*, *113*:310, 1971.

Ravitch, M. M. Hindgut duplication, doubling of colon and genitourinary tracts, *Ann. Surg.*, *137*:588, 1953.

Ravitch, M. M., and Scott, W. W. Duplication of entire colon, bladder and urethra, *Surgery*, *38*:843, 1953.

Van Zwalenberg, B. R. Double colon: Differentiation of cases into two groups with case report, *Am. J. Roentgenol.*, *68*:22, 1952.

Weber, H. M., and Dixon, C. F. Duplication of entire large intestine (colon duplex), *Am. J. Roentgenol.*, *55*:319, 1946.

Chapter 17

ACQUIRED LESIONS OF THE COLON

CHRONIC ULCERATIVE COLITIS

Although chronic ulcerative colitis is relatively rarer in children than in adults, many cases in the pediatric age group have been reported. The condition is more common in older children but may affect even young infants.

The etiology is unknown; apparently there is no specific infectious agent. There is suggestive evidence that the pathogenic mechanism is spasm of the colonic musculature with compression of the intramural blood vessels followed by localized ischemia and necrosis of the mucosa. The high incidence of emotional and psychogenic problems in children with ulcerative colitis suggests that they are at least partially responsible for the chronicity of the disease, and possibly play an important role in its initial development.

The inflammatory process usually begins in the rectum and extends proximally to involve the rectosigmoid and descending portions of the colon. If the disease remains unchecked it may eventually involve the entire colon, through a series of exacerbations and remissions. The earliest pathologic findings are edema, hyperemia, and granularity of the mucosa with multiple small punctate hemorrhages. This picture is followed by ulceration of the mucosa with extension into the muscularis. The submucosal coalescence of the ulcerations undermines the mucous membrane and denudes the mucosa, leaving only a number of polyp-like islands of edematous mucosa. Fibrosis of the damaged musculature results in shortening and rigidity of the colon and loss of the haustral markings.

CLINICAL PICTURE. The onset may be sudden, resembling acute enteritis, but more often is gradual with first an increase in the number of formed stools, followed by looser bowel movements containing blood, mucus, and pus accompanied by abdominal cramps. Fever, lassitude, loss of weight, debility, and growth retardation are common, and in severe cases death may occur from dehydration, hemorrhage, or perforation and peritonitis. The disease apparently predisposes young individuals to carcinoma of the colon. Although this complication generally occurs in adulthood, it has been reported in late childhood. Recent statistical studies in children indicate a 5% risk of cancer after ten years of the disease. This increased to 25% after 20 years, and by 20% each decade thereafter. Total colonic involvement increases the cancer risk over those with disease limited to the rectum.

RADIOLOGIC EVALUATION. The roentgenologic diagnosis of ulcerative colitis at any age depends on the demonstration by barium studies of the alteration in the mucosal pattern, evidence of ulceration, or changes in the length of the colon and of its haustral markings. Vigorous catharsis should not be used in preparation of the colon for barium studies. Mild laxatives may be given, but we prefer to use only isotonic saline enemas. When the disease has an acute and abrupt onset, the radiographic changes appear earlier than in the more common insidious form. In the earliest stages, there are no roentgen changes except perhaps colonic irritability manifested by frequent recurrent spastic contractions of the involved colon noted during fluoroscopy. This in itself is difficult to evaluate and is seen occasionally in the normal colon in response to pressure by the enema. At this stage of the disease proctoscopic findings are more diagnostic. Substitution of thickened mucosal markings for the normal crinkly mucosal pattern on the postevacuation film is one of the earliest radiographic features and results from edema and thickening of the mucous membrane. Ulcerations appear as irregularities in the colonic wall with barium niches extending beyond the confines of the lumen. Only a few ulcers may be present, or there may be multiple ulcerations involving long segments of the colon producing a serrated configuration (Fig. 17–1). In more advanced stages, the extension of the basilar portion of the ulcer beneath the mucous membrane produces the typical collar-button configuration (Fig. 17–2). As the disease progresses, the destruction of the mucous membrane leaves islands of thickened mucosa which appear radiographically as polyps, the pseudopolyposis of ulcerative colitis (Fig. 17–3). Chronicity results in shortening and rigidity of the colon and obliteration of the haustral markings. Haustrations are often poorly defined in the ascending and descending colon of normal individuals, but their absence in the transverse portion usually indicates that the colon is or has been the site of a chronic inflammatory process (Fig. 17–4).

The pathologic changes, and consequently the radiographic findings, are usually most severe and often localized in the distal portions of the colon. Occasionally, however, the process involves the proximal segments. In such cases proctoscopic findings are lacking and additional reliance must be placed on the roentgenologic impression.

If perforation occurs, pneumoperitoneum may be identified on upright or decubitus films. Barium enema studies naturally should not be performed if this complication develops in a patient suspected of having ulcerative colitis.

A dreaded complication of ulcerative co-

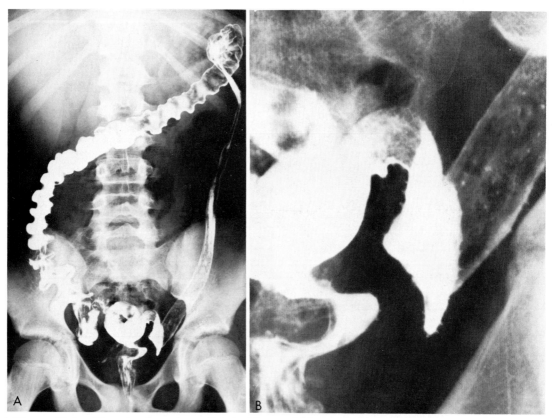

Figure 17–1. Chronic ulcerative colitis in 11 year old boy. *A*, Postevacuation film showing absence of normal mucosal pattern in descending and sigmoid portions of colon. *B*, Enlargement of sigmoid segment showing multiple minute ulcers projecting beyond confines of lumen.

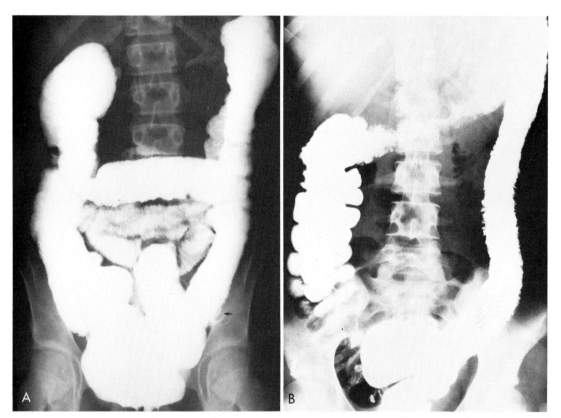

Figure 17–2. Chronic ulcerative colitis in a 10 year old child. Barium-filled colon shows absence of normal mucosal pattern, absence of normal haustrations in the transverse portion of the colon, multiple serrations of the entire colonic wall, and early deep penetrating ulcerations (*arrow*). *B*, More extensive submucosal ulceration in a 15 year old girl with long-standing ulcerative colitis.

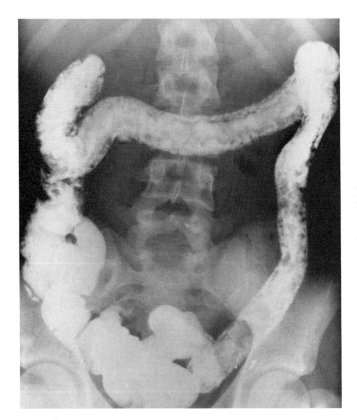

Figure 17–3. Chronic ulcerative colitis in a 15 year old boy. There is loss of normal mucosal pattern, loss of haustral markings, and multiple pseudopolyps occupying all segments of the colon. The terminal ileum is normal.

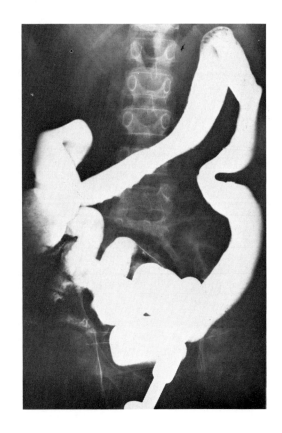

Figure 17–4. Chronic ulcerative colitis in 6 year old girl. Disease is more advanced than in Figure 17–1. Haustral markings are absent from transverse portion of colon and entire structure has rigid appearance with fairly constant caliber involving all segments.

litis is toxic dilatation of the colon (toxic megacolon). This condition is considerably more common in adults and generally occurs during the more chronic phase of the disease. The etiology is unknown. There is a sudden onset of abdominal distention, tenderness, and absence of bowel sounds. Clinical features of systemic toxicity are usually present. The abdominal radiographs demonstrate either diffuse or segmental dilatation of the colon, which may become enormous. Fluid levels are common and, although few in number, are long, denoting their colonic location. A barium enema examination is unnecessary for diagnosis and, in fact, is contraindicated because of the high incidence of spontaneous perforation.

GRANULOMATOUS COLITIS

Granulomatous colitis or Crohn's disease of the colon is slightly more common in the pediatric age group than chronic ulcerative colitis. It is usually characterized by fever, abdominal cramps, and diarrhea. However, unlike ulcerative colitis, gross blood in the stool is less common. Fistulas are common in granulomatous colitis, especially in the perianal regions. Perianal ulceration as the only early clinical manifestation of the disease may precede any clinical or radiographic evidence of colon involvement.

RADIOGRAPHIC FINDINGS. The radiographic findings early in the course of the disease may be very subtle and consist only of an increase in the prominence of the haustral markings. As the condition progresses, ulcerations are identified and some of these may appear in the advanced stages as longitudinal ulcerations within the bowel wall (Fig. 17–5). Denudement of mucosa, narrowing and stricture formations, and pseudopolypoid changes are additional findings occurring with the progression of the disease. The lesions may be

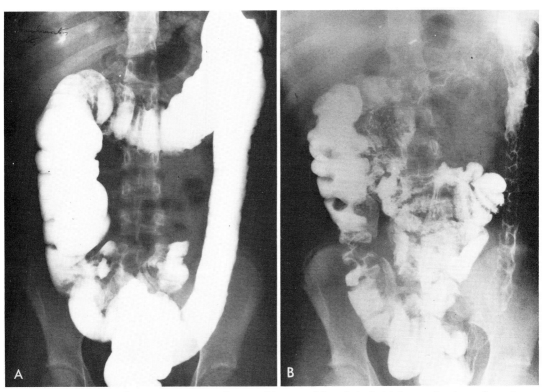

Figure 17–5. Granulomatous enterocolitis in 10 year old girl. *A,* Initial examination when the patient was having symptoms suggestive of Crohn's disease shows mild constriction of terminal ileum. The colon was thought to be normal. *B,* Examination one month later shows involvement of the transverse and descending colon with horizontal ulcers and transverse fissures.

eccentric and skip areas are common. These findings help differentiate radiographically this condition from chronic ulcerative colitis (Fig. 17–6). Involvement is most common in the right side of the colon and when the terminal ileum is also affected the condition is more appropriately called granulomatous enterocolitis (Fig. 17–7). Later in the course of the disease, pericolonic abscesses, sinus tract formation, or fistulas extending to other loops of bowel may occur (Fig. 17–8). These features further help distinguish this disease from ulcerative colitis.

Ulcerative colitis with involvement of the terminal ileum (backwash ileitis) should be differentiated from granulomatous ileocolitis. In the former condition, there is continuous involvement of bowel without skip areas, the mucosa has a granular appearance, and sinuses and fistulas do not occur (Fig. 17–9). However, clear differentiation between the two conditions is not possible in 20 to 30 per cent of the cases.

Patients with Crohn's disease are usually best managed on supportive medical programs as long as possible. Surgical intervention is mandatory in the presence of complications of abscess and fistula formation.

INFECTIOUS COLITIS

The most common acute infectious colitis in our experience is due to salmonella organisms. The onset is acute, characterized by diarrhea which often is grossly bloody. Radiographically there is spasm in the area of involvement, usually the sigmoid and descending portions of the colon (Fig. 17–10). Ulcerations may be identified, suggesting early ulcerative colitis. However, a recovery of salmonella organisms in the stools is diagnostic and differentiates this condition from the acute onset of the more chronic forms of colitis.

AMOEBIC AND TUBERCULOUS COLITIS

Amoebic and tuberculous colitis usually involve primarily the cecum and ascending

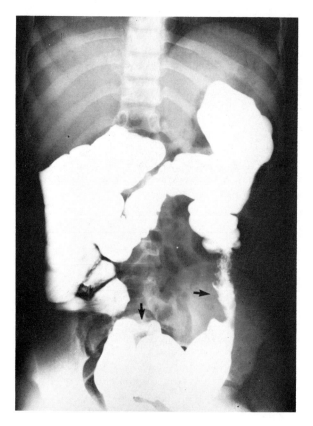

Figure 17–6. Granulomatous colitis in 15 year old girl showing skip areas of involvement of the descending and sigmoid colon (*arrows*).

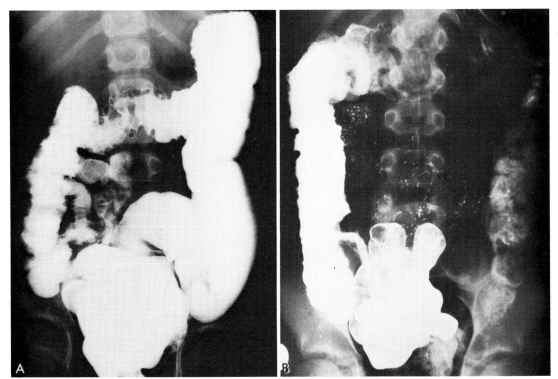

Figure 17–7. Granulomatous enterocolitis in two children, each 11 years of age. *A*, The mucosa of the ascending and proximal portions of the colon is irregular and nodular and there is selective involvement of the terminal ileum near the ileocecal valve. *B*, More advanced changes of granulomatous enterocolitis showing constriction of the terminal ileum, edema of the ileocecal valve, and irregular nodular changes in the mucosa of the ascending colon. The transverse and descending portions of the colon are normal.

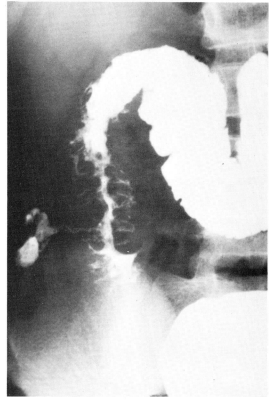

Figure 17–8. Regional enteritis in a 4 year old child. Colon examination showing irregularity of ascending colon and extension of contrast material into pericecal abscess.

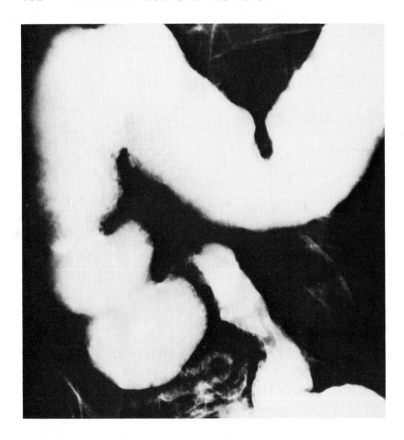

Figure 17–9. Chronic ulcerative colitis with "backwash" ileitis in 16 year old boy. There is loss of normal mucosal pattern of the cecum, ascending colon, and terminal ileum, with a diffuse granular pattern. There is minimal involvement of the terminal ileum and there are no identifiable skip areas.

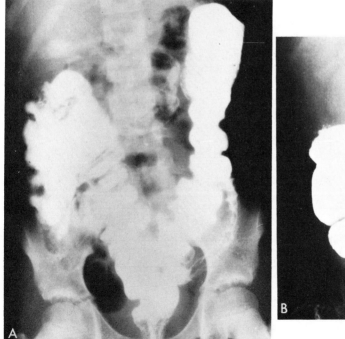

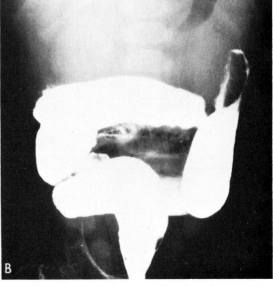

Figure 17–10. Infectious colitis. *A*, Salmonella colitis involving the sigmoid and descending colon in an 8 year old child. Marked irregularity of the mucosa of the sigmoid portion of the colon is noted. The colon returned to normal after appropriate treatment. *B*, Shigella colitis in an 18 month old infant. There is loss of normal mucosal pattern as well as marked spasm of the splenic flexure.

portions of the colon, but occasionally the former may show rectal ulcerations. Pain and tenderness localized in the right lower abdomen and bacteriologic and parasitologic studies help differentiate these conditions from granulomatous and chronic ulcerative colitis. In both conditions there is hyperirritability of the cecum, with spastic constriction of this structure and the involved portion of the ascending colon. Barium studies fail to distend the cecum and recurrent contractions prevent adequate filling. The cecal tip is usually affected and the resulting deformity may give the cecum a conical configuration (see Fig. 13–26). Colonic perforation is an occasional complication of amebiasis. Differentiation of an inflammatory lesion of the cecum from a carcinoma does not present the problem in children that it does in adults.

Inflammatory lesions of the colon associated with ischemic bowel disease have been presented in the previous chapter.

TYPHLITIS

Typhlitis is a complication of terminal leukemia or aplastic anemia in children who are agranulocytic. Pathologically there is severe hemorrhagic necrosis of the cecum. The etiology is unknown but, in all probability, the mucosal integrity of the gastrointestinal tract has been affected by either the disease itself, the therapy utilized, or a combination of both. The reason for the localization of the necrotic process to the cecum has not been explained.

Clinically the patient develops spiking fever, abdominal distention, and pain during the terminal period of his illness. Although a feeling of fullness involving the right lower quadrant may be detected, a palpable mass is usually not present. Radiographically there is a lack of bowel gas in the right lower quadrant with progressive distention of the small bowel and diminution of colonic gas (Fig. 17–11). The radiographic features are similar to those of advanced gangrenous appendicitis with pericecal abscess.

MISCELLANEOUS FORMS OF COLITIS

There are several systemic diseases which may present with symptoms and radiologic findings suggesting an inflammatory process of the colon. One of these is

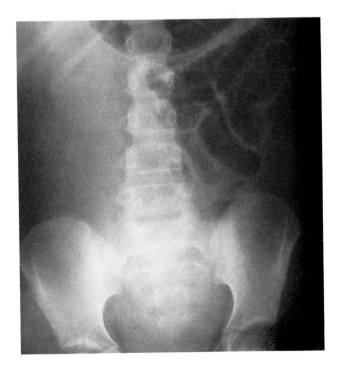

Figure 17–11. Radiograph of the abdomen of a 9 year old girl with aplastic anemia made one day prior to death shows features of typhlitis consisting of large soft tissue density in the right side of the abdomen with dilated small bowel gas and negligible colon gas. (Reprinted with permission from Wagner, M. L., Rosenberg, H. S., Fernbach, D. J., and Singleton, E. B. Typhlitis: A complication of leukemia in childhood, *Am. J. Roentgenol.*, **109**:341, 1970.)

the hemolytic uremic syndrome, in which abdominal pain and bloody diarrhea may be the initial clinical features. A number of these cases have simulated acute ulcerative colitis, especially in the older child, only to be followed by microangiopathic hemolytic anemia, thrombocytopenia, and nephropathy—the diagnostic findings of this syndrome. Radiographically the colon may show spasm, submucosal edema, and "thumbprinting" (Fig. 17–12). The x-ray appearance returns to normal, usually by two weeks. The histologic findings show edema and submucosal hemorrhage, but no ulceration or inflammation.

Other entities which may produce similar radiographic findings include Henoch-Schönlein purpura and the Kasabach-Merritt syndrome (giant hemangioma with platelet trapping).

TUMORS

Colonic Polyposis

Colonic polyps are not uncommon in children and may be found at any age, but are rare in infants under 1 year. The most common of these lesions is the juvenile polyp, which may occur as a single lesion or as several polyps in an isolated area or scattered throughout the colon. The juvenile polyp probably begins as a retention cyst secondary to obstruction of the orifice of a colonic mucous gland. This is complicated by hyperplasia of the mucous gland with superimposed infection.

Colonic polyps are more common in males than in females, although the difference in sex incidence is not great. The rectum is by far the most common site of involvement and next, the sigmoid. The polyp may vary from a few millimeters to several centimeters in size and may be attached to the colonic wall on a broad base or by a long pedicle.

CLINICAL PICTURE. Painless rectal bleeding is the usual symptom of rectal or colonic polyps. If the polyp is situated low in the rectum the stool may be streaked with blood; if the polyp is in a more proximal location the blood may be intimately interspersed with the stool. Prolapse of a rectal polyp through the anus occasionally

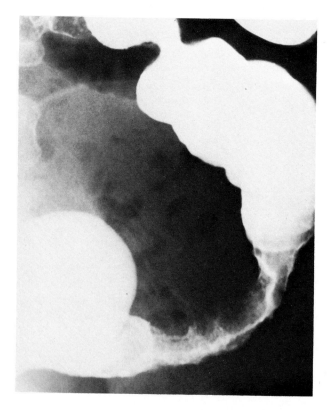

Figure 17–12. Hemolytic uremic syndrome in a 9 year old female. Colon examination for bloody diarrhea demonstrates "thumbprinting" and spasm of the sigmoid colon due to intramural hemorrhage.

occurs if the polyp is low enough and is pedunculated. Radiologic studies are necessary to search for additional polyps, for approximately a third of these children will have additional lesions. A variety of less specific clinical symptoms may be present, such as abdominal pain, constipation, diarrhea, and signs of intussusception.

RADIOLOGIC EVALUATION. Radiographic identification of colonic polyps is impossible unless the colon is completely cleared of fecal particles before barium enema studies are begun (see Chapter 14).

Barium is allowed to enter the rectum slowly and is followed fluoroscopically through all portions of the colon. Any filling defects observed should be palpated in an effort to displace them into higher or lower portions of the colon. In this way fecal particles and air bubbles may be distinguished from polyps. Although a pedunculated polyp also can be displaced over a distance of a few centimeters, the extent is limited by the length of its stalk (Fig. 17–13). Care should be taken to avoid filling the ileum because of retention of barium in this segment after evacuation. The residual barium in the small bowel overlaps the sigmoid and obscures detail of this area, particularly on the air studies.

Before the child is allowed to evacuate, an anteroposterior film of the abdomen is obtained. A large polyp may be identified as a filling defect in the barium column, but as a rule the excess contrast material in the colon obscures the polypoid lesion. The child is then allowed to evacuate as much of the barium as possible and films in both anteroposterior and posteroanterior positions are obtained. The latter position produces pressure on the colon and helps to flatten out the redundant sigmoid, affording a more complete view of this area. In the anteroposterior position, any liquid barium left in the colon changes its distribution, permitting inspection of the mucosa which may have been obscured in the posteroanterior view. The postevacuation films are invaluable in the identification of polyps. The colon is in a contracted state, and the overlapping and redundancy of the various segments are less pronounced than in the distended colon. A polyp is identified as a filling defect or circular area of radiolucency within the irregular mucosal folds (Fig. 17–14).

If a polyp has not been identified by conventional routine and spot films, air is injected into the rectum under fluoroscopic control. Lateral or oblique spot films of the rectum and rectosigmoid segments are routinely made, and films of any suspicious area seen during fluoroscopy. An alternate method of double-contrast study is given in Chapter 14. In the double-contrast studies, the barium adherent to the polyp produces

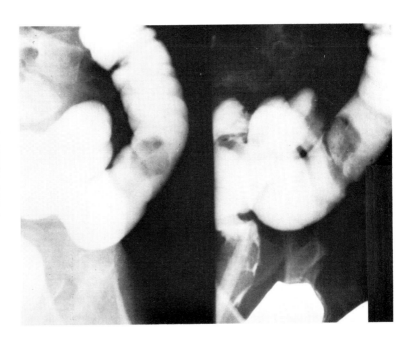

Figure 17–13. Pedunculated juvenile polyp. Spot films of the distal sigmoid show change in position of the pedunculated polyp with the pressure by the gloved hand. The stalk is well delineated.

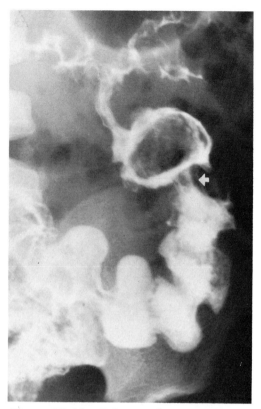

Figure 17-14. Colonic polyp in a 2 year old boy. Postevacuation radiograph shows filling defect in proximal sigmoid. Arrow indicates stalk of attachment.

a ring-shaped area of barium density (Fig. 17-15A and B). Occasionally a polyp will have an unusually long stalk, as shown in Figure 17-16.

Before the patient leaves the x-ray department, all films are examined. If a polyp is questionably identified, the patient is returned to the fluoroscopy room and barium is again introduced into the colon and spot films made of the suspicious region. The differentiation between fecal particles and polyps is often impossible on a single examination; consequently, we prefer to reexamine these patients immediately rather than subject them to a repetition of scheduling and preparation with cathartics and enemas. Because spontaneous extrusion of the polyp usually occurs and because malignancy is not a consideration in the juvenile polyp, repeated examinations in an effort to find a suspected polyp are not justified unless bleeding is excessive.

The utilization of the flexible fiberoptic colonoscope by an experienced physician has proved to be a safe and practical method of polyp resection in any part of the colon.

Familial polyposis is an autosomal dominant condition with high penetrance. The polyps in this condition are adenomatous polyps with a natural history to the development of carcinoma in more than 90% by the fifth decade.

Gardner's syndrome is characterized by gastrointestinal polyps, osteomas of bone, generally the skull and mandible, and benign soft tissue masses. This syndrome is inherited as an autosomal dominant condition with a strong tendency toward malignant changes in the polyps. The bowel lesions are located mainly within the colon, although occasionally stomach and small bowel polyps may be present.

The lesions of the *Peutz-Jeghers syndrome* are multiple hamartomas involving the small bowel and frequently the stomach and colon. These patients have melanin deposits on the lips and buccal mucosa (see Fig. 13-53). The abnormality is frequently discovered after intussusception has been produced by the polyp. Although the usual Peutz-Jeghers hamartomatous polyp is benign, occasional instances of malignant degeneration of these polyps have been reported.

Other forms of inherited gastrointestinal polyposis include generalized juvenile polyposis, an autosomal dominant condition in which the lesions are hamartomas, and Turcot syndrome, an autosomal recessive lesion in which the polyps are adenomatous. Neurofibromatosis, an autosomal dominant condition, may on occasion produce polypoid-like gastrointestinal lesions.

The Cronkhite-Canada syndrome, which consists of alopecia, skin hyperpigmentation and nail dystrophy, is a nongenetic cause of gastrointestinal polyposis.

Histiocytic Fibroma

Histiocytic fibroma may be found in any part of the body, including the gastrointestinal tract. The lesion is composed of histiocytes which have the capacity to produce collagen. It is usually benign but must be differentiated from a malignant sarcoma. Abdominal pain and bowel obstruction

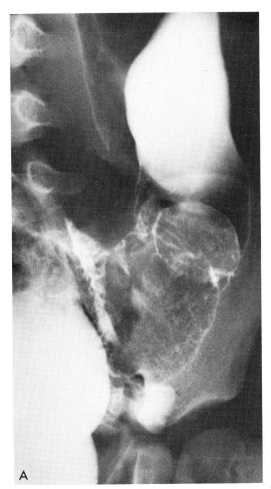

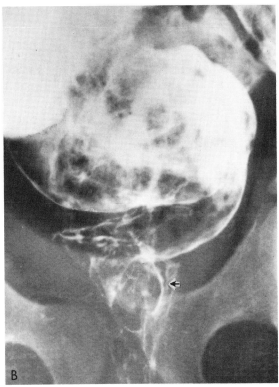

Figure 17–15. Juvenile polyps of the colon. *A,* Air contrast study showing large polyp as filling defect in sigmoid. *B,* Two year old girl with history of rectal bleeding. Double contrast study showing small polyp (*arrow*) in distal portion of rectum.

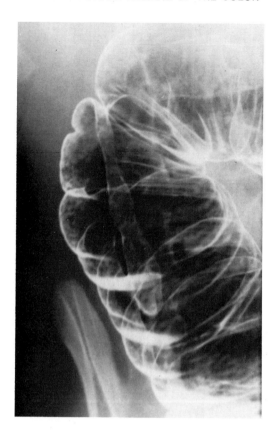

Figure 17–16. Juvenile polyp in the ascending colon in a 10 year old boy. Air contrast studies clearly demonstrate the length of the polyp, which was successfully removed by colonoscopy.

Figure 17–17. Histiocytic fibroma in a 1 month old infant. The barium enema disclosed an irreducible intussusception at the lower end of the descending colon. (Reprinted with permission from Singleton, E. B., and Johnson, F. Localized lesions of the colon in infants and children, *Semin. Roentgenol.*, 11:111, 1976.)

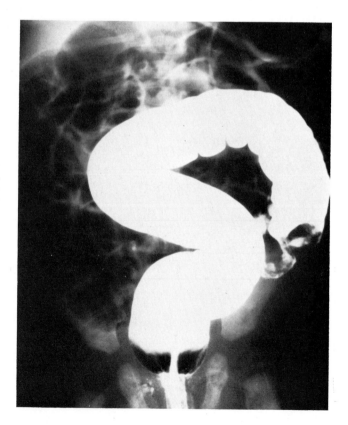

may be the clinical presentations (Fig. 17–17).

Hemangioma

Hemangiomas of the colon are uncommon lesions in children and are often associated with hemangiomas in other parts of the body such as the skin. They may occur as an isolated entity or in an associated underlying genetic abnormality such as the Osler-Weber-Rendu syndrome, Turner's syndrome, or Peutz-Jeghers syndrome. The clinical presentation may be in the form of gastrointestinal bleeding or mechanical bowel obstruction.

Radiographically there is little to distinguish a hemangioma from other forms of intramural filling defects (Fig. 17–18). However, a presumptive diagnosis of hemangioma may be raised if the patient has other hemangiomas. Although gastrointestinal examination is useful in determining the extent and location of the lesions, angiography is of greater value in determining the character of these abnormalities (Fig. 17–19).

Lymphoid Hyperplasia

Lymphoid hyperplasia of the intestinal tract is a condition commonly seen in children. These lesions may present in two forms: in the *focal* type, an aggregate of benign lymphoid tissue is found in an isolated area, and in the *diffuse nodular* form, lymphoid hyperplasia is found throughout much of the gastrointestinal tract, especially the colon. Diffuse nodular hyperplasia may be seen in children with gastrointestinal bleeding and perhaps represents lymphoid reaction to an unidentified infection. However, in our experience the diffuse form is frequently found in normal children who have nonspecific abdominal complaints, and probably is a reflection of the normal abundance of lymphoid tissue in this age group.

Radiographically the lesions are demonstrated to best advantage utilizing the double-contrast colon examination. Although the submucosal nodules are fairly evenly distributed throughout the colon, they are best demonstrated on the left side,

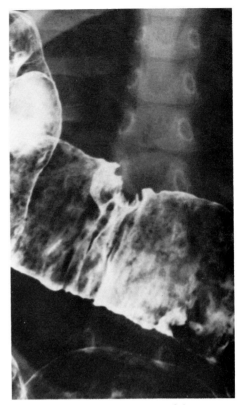

Figure 17–18. Hemangioma of the transverse colon in a 2 year old child. An irregularly shaped sessile filling defect is identified on the superior wall of the transverse colon. Proved at operation. (Reprinted with permission from Singleton, E. B. and Johnson, F. Localized lesions of the colon in infants and children, *Semin. Roentgenol.*, **11**:111, 1976.)

especially in the rectum and sigmoid. Small radiolucent filling defects are identified which are of uniform size and typically show a small umbilication within the center (Fig. 17–20). This entity should not be confused with multiple colonic polyps for obvious reasons.

MISCELLANEOUS BENIGN NEOPLASMS

Involvement of the rectum by a benign neoplasm arising in the pelvis may produce obstruction by extrinsic pressure. Teratomas are the most common of these lesions and are usually identified from teeth or osseous structures in the neoplasm. Pelvic hemangiomas are rare but when they occur may encroach on the rectum. Phleb-

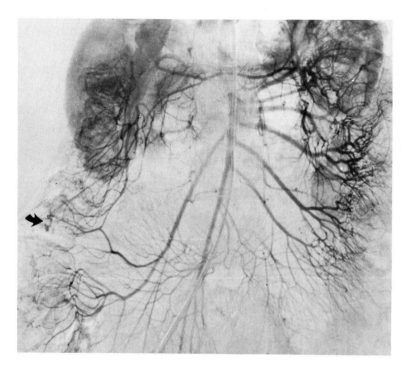

Figure 17-19. Small arteriovenous malformation in the ascending colon (*arrow*) demonstrated by superior mesenteric arteriography. Confirmed at operation. (Reprinted with permission from Singleton, E. B., and Johnson, F. Localized lesions of the colon in infants and children, *Semin. Roentgenol.,* **11**:111, 1976.)

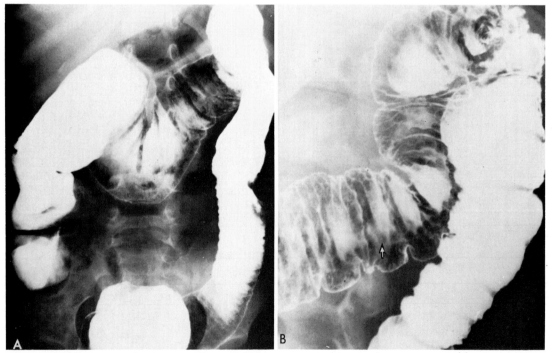

Figure 17-20. Lymphoid hyperplasia of the colon. *A,* Barium enema and air contrast studies demonstrate multiple filling defects in the sigmoid and transverse portions of the colon in a 2 year old child with diarrhea. *B,* Spot film of the splenic flexure in a 10 year old. Multiple filling defects are noted with barium trapped in the central umbilications (*arrow*).

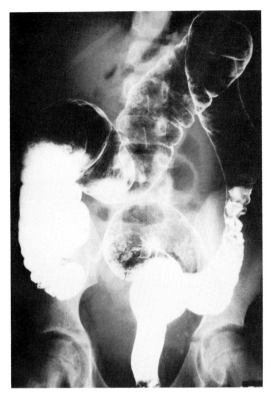

Figure 17-21. Pelvic hemangioma in a 9 year old girl with anemia and occasionally painful bowel movements. Barium enema shows straightening of the rectum circled by the hemangioma. Multiple phleboliths are identified in the left side of the pelvis.

oliths can usually be identified in such cases (Fig. 17-21).

MALIGNANT NEOPLASMS

Malignancies of the colon are rare in children. The majority of the malignant intestinal tumors encountered in early life are sarcomatous, and lymphosarcoma is the most frequent of this group.

The clinical features are often of short duration and include anemia, weight loss, abdominal pain, and frequently a palpable mass. Radiographically a soft tissue density may be present or occasionally bowel obstruction secondary to intussusception (Fig. 17-22). Barium studies may show coarse, nodular folds of the colon (Fig. 17-23), and spreading of contiguous small bowel loops denotes spread to the mesentery. Occasionally fistulous tracts from the bowel to the surrounding soft tissue mass are present.

The clinical and radiographic features of lymphoma and Crohn's disease may be similar, but the marked nodularity and large soft tissue mass in the former help to make the differentiation.

Malignancies of the colon may result from direct extension of adjacent abdominal tumors in the retroperitoneal structures (Figs. 17-24, 17-25, and 17-26).

Another lesion that is unexpected in children is carcinoma of the colon. Less than 200 cases have been reported in the Western world since 1900. The colonic sites are the same as in adults.

The most common symptom is abdominal discomfort, followed by rectal bleeding and change in bowel habits, usually constipation. Pathologically, there is a preponderance of colloid (mucin-producing) adenocarcinoma in childhood. The prognosis is usually poor, with most children

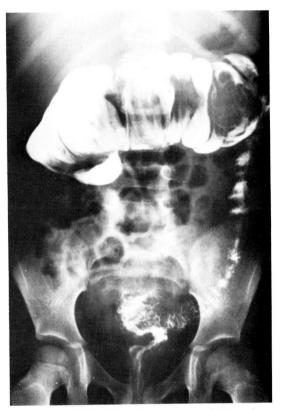

Figure 17-22. Lymphosarcoma of the colon producing intussusception in a 4 year old child. Postevacuation barium enema radiograph shows barium trapped within the intussusception. At operation primary lymphosarcoma was found to be responsible for the intussusception.

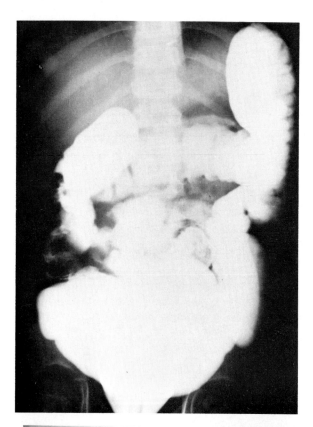

Figure 17–23. Reticulum cell sarcoma of the cecum in ascending colon in a 5 year old boy. There is deformity of the cecum and ascending colon with coarse nodular pattern replacing normal mucosal markings.

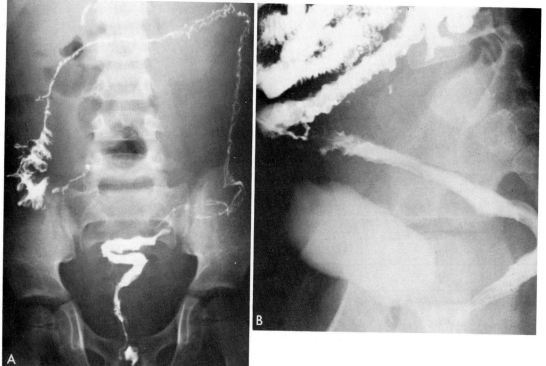

Figure 17–24. Malignant neoplasms of the colon. *A*, Boy, aged 5, with extensive invasion of entire colon by abdominal lymphosarcoma. *B*, Child, aged 3, with invasion of rectum by lymphoma which apparently had its origin retroperitoneally.

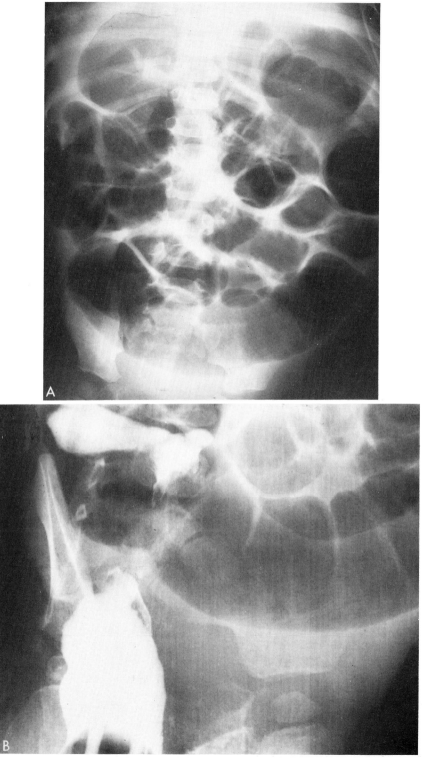

Figure 17–25. Malignant neoplasm of colon in a 2½ year old child with Wilms' tumor of the right kidney and metastasis to retroperitoneal structures producing obstruction at rectosigmoid junction. *A,* Abdominal scout film shows distention of small bowel and colon. *B,* Barium enema shows concentric obstruction in the retrosigmoid area secondary to extensive metastatic disease in the cul de sac.

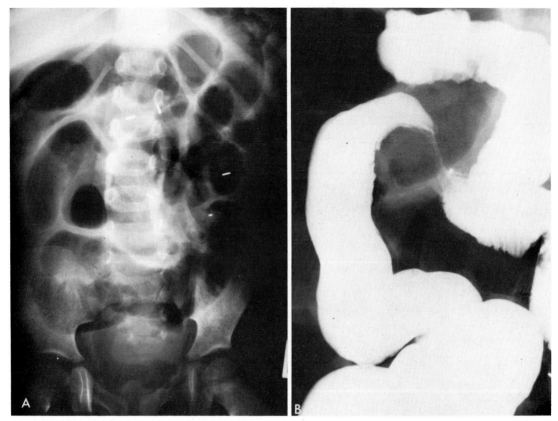

Figure 17–26. Three year old boy with metastatic neuroblastoma. *A*, Abdominal scout film shows distention of the colon and small bowel. *B*, Barium enema shows localized stricture in the rectosigmoid junction which at laparotomy was found to be a combination of adhesions, radiation fibrosis, and tumor implants.

dying within a year. The radiographic findings are similar to those in the adult (Fig. 17–27).

INSPISSATED MILK SYNDROME

Although the formation of a lactobezoar (inspissated milk syndrome) is more common in the stomach (see p. 143), it may produce obstruction in the distal small bowel or colon (Fig. 17–28).

CHILAIDITI'S SYNDROME

In this condition there is interposition of the hepatic flexure of the colon between the diaphragm and liver. Theoretically, when associated with aerophagia this condition can produce diurnal abdominal distention and pain and a palpable liver. Radiographs of the abdomen show gas-distended colon between the right hemidiaphragm and liver (Fig. 17–29). However, interposition of the hepatic flexure between the liver and diaphragm is occasionally seen in normal children and its validity as a syndrome is questionable.

VOLVULUS

Although volvulus of the cecum and sigmoid is much less common in the pediatric age group than in the adult it may occasionally occur. Because of the marked redundancy of the sigmoid colon in the pediatric age group it is surprising that sigmoid volvulus is not more common. The obstructive symptoms are usually acute, and abdominal scout films followed by barium enema are helpful in confirming the diagnosis (Fig. 17–30).

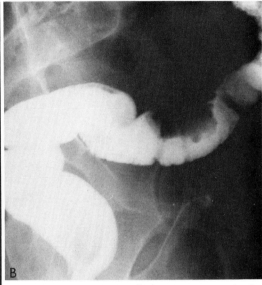

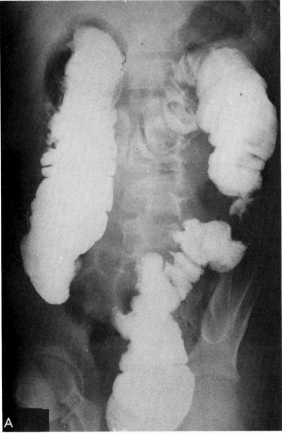

Figure 17–27. Adenocarcinoma of the colon. *A*, Boy, aged 15, with annular constricting adenocarcinoma of the lower descending colon. *B*, 17 year old rodeo cowboy with filling defect in the distal sigmoid which at laparotomy was found to be an adenocarcinoma (*A* reprinted by permission from Singleton, E. B., and Johnson, F. Localized lesions of the colon in children, *Semin. Roentgenol.*, 11:111, 1976.)

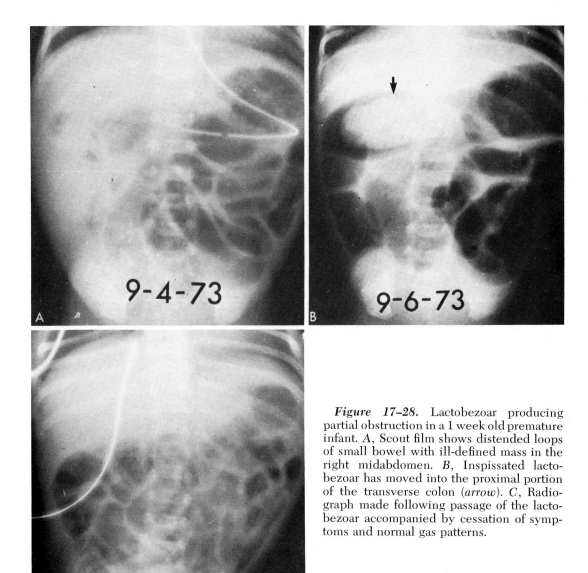

Figure 17–28. Lactobezoar producing partial obstruction in a 1 week old premature infant. *A,* Scout film shows distended loops of small bowel with ill-defined mass in the right midabdomen. *B,* Inspissated lactobezoar has moved into the proximal portion of the transverse colon (*arrow*). *C,* Radiograph made following passage of the lactobezoar accompanied by cessation of symptoms and normal gas patterns.

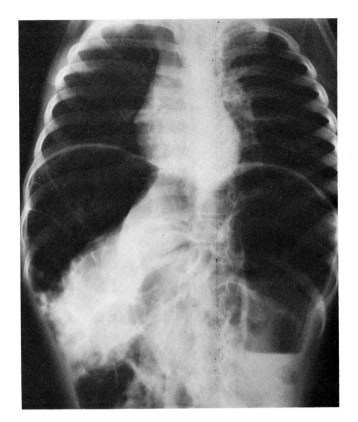

Figure 17–29. Questionable Chilaiditi syndrome in a young child. There is distention of the colon with interposition of the hepatic flexure between the diaphragm and liver.

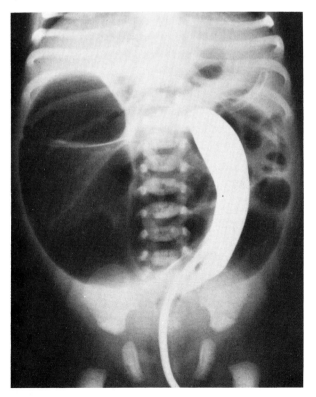

Figure 17–30. Sigmoid volvulus in 1 day old infant. There is marked distention of the colon proximal to the obstruction in the sigmoid colon.

APPENDICITIS

Appendicitis is common in older children but very rare before age 2 and a distinct rarity in infants less than 1 year of age. The youngest patients recorded, to our knowledge, were discovered by Potter at postmortem examination of infants 6 and 23 days old. The difficulty of diagnosis of appendicitis in infancy is due to the necessity of depending mainly on objective findings and the vagaries of symptoms—vomiting, refusal to take nourishment, fretfulness, and diarrhea or constipation. Rupture, appendiceal abscess, and peritonitis occur in about 70% of cases and are due to the failure of early diagnosis and to the deficiency in the omentum, which is an effective barrier against the spread of infection in older children and adults.

It is generally accepted that inflammation of the appendix follows blockage of the lumen by a fecalith, inspissated material, or a foreign body. The accumulation of secretory products in the obstructed appendix then leads to ischemia and necrosis of the appendiceal wall. Because of the funnel-shaped cecum and appendix commonly seen in young infants, blockage of the lumen is not easily accomplished, and this probably explains the rarity of appendicitis in the infant.

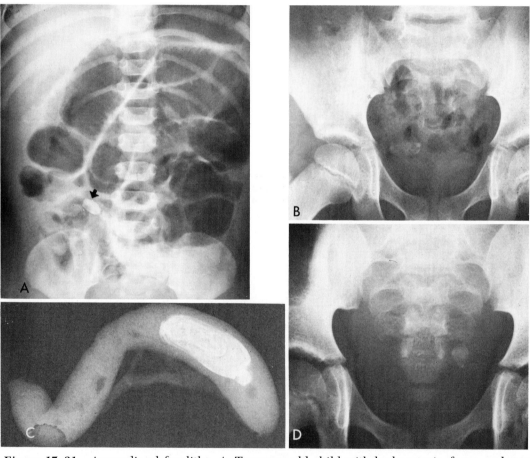

Figure 17–31. Appendiceal fecaliths. *A*, Two year old child with leukocytosis, fever, and acute condition of abdomen. Anteroposterior film of abdomen shows oval area of calcific density (*arrow*) above crest of ileum and moderate distention of small bowel. Laparotomy disclosed acute perforated appendicitis with appendiceal fecalith. *B*, Six year old child with history of vague intermittent right lower quadrant pain. Abdominal radiograph shows typical laminated appendiceal fecalith. *C*, Radiograph of appendix removed from patient in *B*. *D*, Seven year old boy with signs and symptoms of perforated appendix. Pear-shaped fecalith is present in the left side of the pelvis. At laparotomy appendix was found ruptured and fecalith extended into opposite side of pelvis.

RADIOLOGIC EVALUATION. X-ray diagnosis in most cases of appendicitis, whether in infants, children or adults, is seldom possible. However, certain findings on the abdominal scout film of individuals with appendicitis may be helpful. Appendiceal fecaliths which contain sufficient calcium salts to be detected radiographically appear as laminated concretions in the right lower quadrant. Their identification in the presence of signs and symptoms suggestive of appendicitis confirms the diagnosis. The incidence of ruptured appendix associated with fecaliths is extremely high, and most authorities believe that a fecalith will ultimately lead to acute appendicitis. Consequently, the radiographic identification of a fecalith, even in the asymptomatic individual, is believed by many to be sufficient reason for appendectomy. Their laminated appearance differentiates them from ureteral calculi and calcified mesenteric lymph nodes (Figs. 17–31 and 17–32). Other helpful signs are areas of deficient bowel gas in the right lower quadrant, especially with air-fluid levels in the cecum and/or terminal ileum suggesting localized ileus. These findings, however, may occur with inflammatory lesions in this area other than appendicitis. Barium enema examination has been found by some to be useful in the diagnosis of acute appendicitis, but our experience has been that clinical and plain film findings are adequate.

Periappendiceal abscesses of sufficient size will displace the cecum from its normal position. Occasionally gas may be identified in the inflammatory mass and there is obliteration of the adjacent preperitoneal fat line (Fig. 17–33). Accompanying signs of mechanical obstruction involving the ileocecal region are frequently encountered in children with ruptured appendix (Fig. 17–34). This is probably the result of either mechanical obstruction by the inflammatory process or localized paralytic ileus involving this region. Generalized peritonitis is characterized by distention of stomach, small bowel, and colon—i.e., paralytic type of ileus. The distended loops are separated an abnormal distance from each other by the accumulation of exudate in the peritoneal cavity.

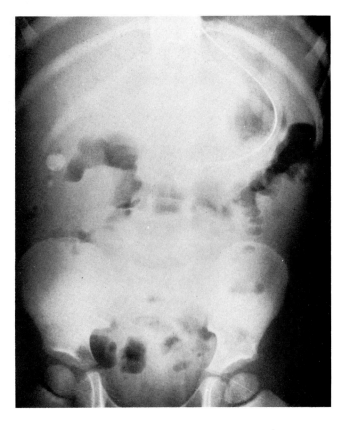

Figure 17–32. Appendiceal fecaliths in retrocecal appendix in a 2 year old boy. The fecaliths are usually high in position because of the retrocecal position of the appendix. In addition there is surrounding soft tissue abscess within which are small air bubbles.

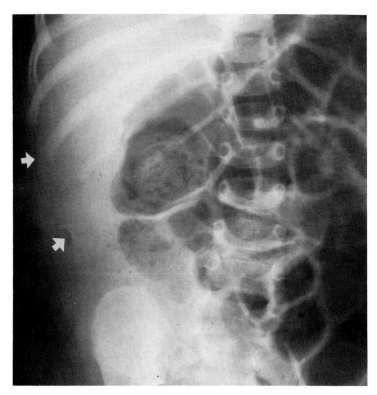

Figure 17–33. Periappendiceal abscess. Infant, aged 16 months, with leukocytosis, abdominal pain, and distention. Abdominal radiograph shows displacement of cecum to left. Upper arrow points to preperitoneal fat line which is abruptly obliterated inferior to this; lower arrow, to collection of gas in pericecal abscess.

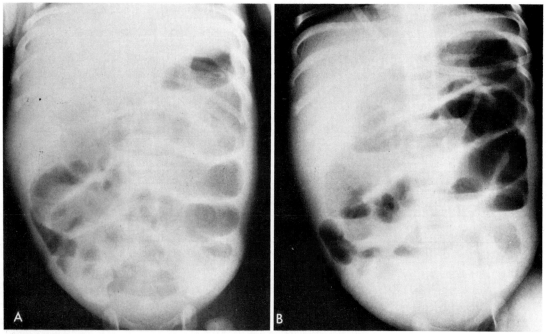

Figure 17–34. Ruptured appendix in 3 week old infant presenting with clinical and radiographic findings of small bowel obstruction.

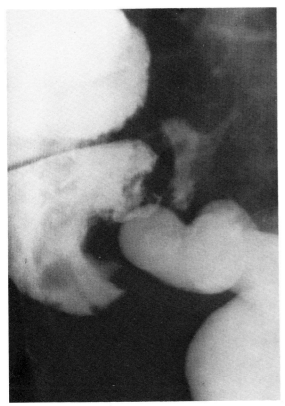

Figure 17–35. Invaginated appendiceal stump. Inverted stump is identified as a filling defect in cecal tip.

After appendectomy and invagination of the appendiceal stump, a filling defect may be noted at the tip of the cecum in barium enema studies (Fig. 17–35). This possibility should always be considered before suggesting that a cecal neoplasm is present. A fecal fistula may persist following drainage of a periappendiceal abscess. The injection of contrast material into the external sinus may aid in outlining the tract. The passage of a small polyethylene catheter into the sinus often facilitates the procedures; then, under fluoroscopy, the contrast material is injected and its passage followed into the bowel (Fig. 17–36).

FOREIGN BODIES

Foreign bodies enter the colon after ingestion or less commonly may be inserted through the anus (Figs. 17–37 and 17–38). Ingested foreign bodies which reach the colon usually are evacuated without difficulty. Occasionally sharp-pointed objects become lodged in the colon, and this should be suspected if the object is not passed within several days and reexamination shows its position to be unchanged. A small or elongated object which remains in the right lower quadrant should be suspected of being within the appendix. Barium enema examination will help to determine this.

Geophagia (dirt-eating) should be suspected when abnormally opaque material or gravel is identified in the colon and there is no history of an examination of the upper or lower intestinal tract with contrast material or of medication with an opaque substance such as bismuth (Fig. 17–39).

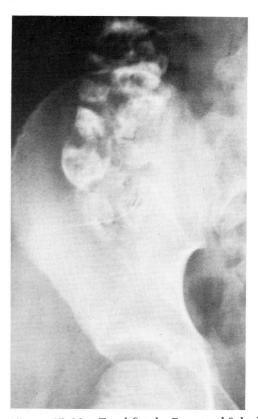

Figure 17–36. Fecal fistula. Boy, aged 6, had had draining sinus since removal of perforated appendix six months previously. A small catheter was passed into the sinus and water-soluble contrast medium injected. Contrast material passed through a minute tract into cecum.

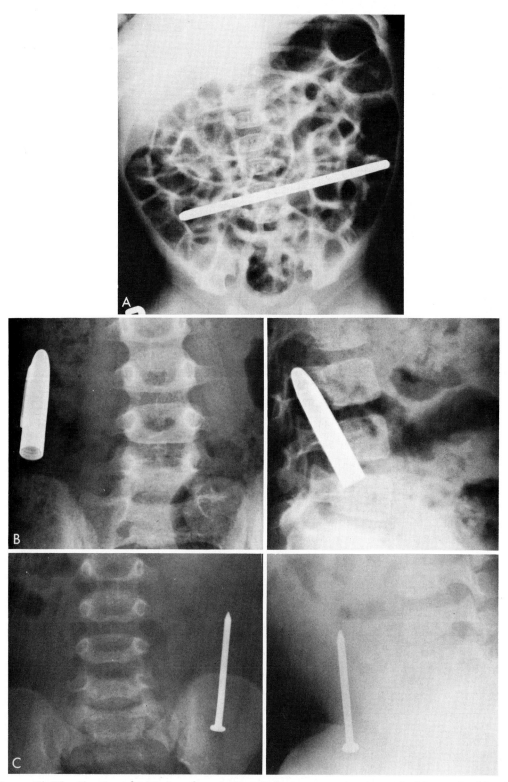

Figure 17–37. Foreign objects in colon. *A,* Rectal thermometer in sigmoid of 6 month old infant. Object passed spontaneously after 6 days. *B,* Fountain pen cap in ascending colon, passed spontaneously. *C,* Nail in descending colon, passed one day later.

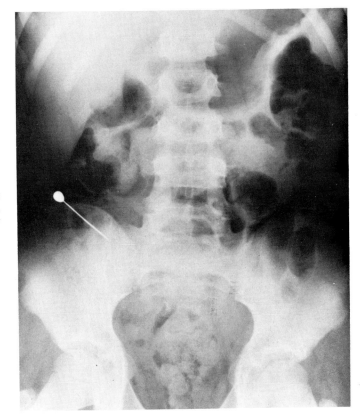

Figure 17–38. Ingested hat pin within the cecum of a 10 year old. The object passed spontaneously without complications.

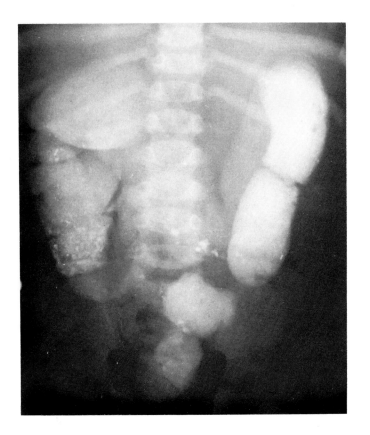

Figure 17–39. Geophagia in a 1 year old child. Opaque material fills the colon. There was no previous history of gastrointestinal examination.

REFERENCES

Ulcerative and Granulomatous Colitis

Ament, M. E., and Ochs, H. D. Gastrointestinal manifestations of chronic granulomatous disease, N. Engl. J. Med., 288:382, 1973.

Berger, L. A., and Wilkinson, D. The investigation of colitis in infancy, Pediatr. Radiol., 2:145, 1974.

Berger, M., Gribetz, D., and Korelitz, B. I. Growth retardation in children with ulcerative colitis: The effect of medical and surgical therapy, Pediatrics, 55:459, 1975.

Broberger, O., and Lagercrantz, R. Ulcerative colitis in childhood and adolescence, Adv. Pediatr., 14:9, 1966.

Davidson, M., Bloom, A. A., and Kugler, M. D. Chronic ulcerative colitis of childhood. An evaluative review, J. Pediatr., 67:471, 1965.

DeVroede, G. J., Taylor, W. F., Sauer, W. G., Jackman, R. J., and Stickler, G. B. Cancer risk and life expectancy of children with ulcerative colitis, N. Engl. J. Med., 285:17, 1971.

Ein, S. H., Lynch, M. J., and Stephens, C. A. Ulcerative colitis in children under 1 year: A 20-year review, J. Pediatr. Surg., 6:264, 1971.

Enzer, N. B., and Hijmans, J. C. Ulcerative colitis beginning in infancy, J. Pediatr., 63:437, 1963.

Guttman, F. M. Granulomatous enterocolitis in childhood and adolescence, J. Pediatr. Surg., 9:115, 1974.

Hijmans, J. C., and Enzer, N. B. Ulcerative colitis in childhood. A study of 43 cases, Pediatrics, 29:389, 1962.

Lassrich, M. A. Crohn's disease: Granulomatous enteropathy, Progr. Pediatr. Radiol., 2:317, 1969.

Lium, R. Observations on etiology of ulcerative colitis, Am. J. Med. Sci., 197:841, 1939.

Margulis, A. R. Radiology of ulcerative colitis, Radiology, 105:251, 1972.

Margulis, A. R., Goldberg, H. I., Lawson, T. L., Montgomery, C. K., Rambo, O. N., Noonan, C. D., and Amberg, J. R. The overlapping spectrum of ulcerative and granulomatous colitis: A roentgenographic-pathologic study, Am. J. Roentgenol., 113:325, 1971.

Marshak, R. H., and Lindner, A. E. Ulcerative and granulomatous colitis, J. Mt. Sinai Hosp. (New York), 33:444, 1966.

Marshak, R. H., and Lindner, A. E. Granulomatous colitis, Sem. Roentgenol., 3:27, 1968.

Marshak, R. H., and Lindner, A. E. Ulcerative and granulomatous colitis, in Margulis, A. R., and Burhenne, H. J., editors, Alimentary Tract Roentgenology (2nd ed.; St. Louis: C. V. Mosby, 1973), pp. 963–1013.

McCaffery, T. D., Nasr, K., Lawrence, A. M., and Kirsner, J. B. Severe growth retardation in children with inflammatory bowel disease, Pediatrics, 45:386, 1970.

Rudhe, U., and Keats, T. Granulomatous colitis in children, Radiology, 84:24, 1965.

Stanley, P., Fry, I. K., Dawson, A. M., and Dyer, N. Radiological signs of ulcerative colitis and Crohn's disease of the colon, Clin. Radiol., 22:434, 1971.

Stein, G. N., Roy, R. H., and Finkelstein, A. K. Roentgen changes in ulcerative colitis, Sem. Roentgenol., 3:3, 1968.

Wright, R. Ulcerative colitis, Gastroenterology, 58:875, 1970.

Infectious Colitis

Farman, J., Rabinowitz, J. G., and Meyers, M. A. Roentgenology of infectious colitis, Am. J. Roentgenol., 119:375, 1973.

Amoebic and Tuberculous Colitis

Abrams, J. S., and Holden, W. D. Tuberculosis of the gastrointestinal tract, Arch. Surg., 89:282, 1964.

Anscombe, A. R., Keddie, N. C., and Schofield, P. F. Cecal tuberculosis, Gut, 8:337, 1967.

Bentley, G., and Webster, J. H. M. Gastro-intestinal tuberculosis. A 10-year review, Br. J. Surg., 54:90, 1967.

Brenner, S. M., Annes, G., and Parker, J. G. Tuberculous colitis simulating nonspecific granulomatous disease of the colon, Am. J. Dig. Dis., 15:85, 1970.

Brombart, M., and Massion, J. Radiologic differences between ileo-caecal tuberculosis and Crohn's disease, Am. J. Dig. Dis., 6:589, 1961.

Gershon-Cohen, J., and Kremens, V. X-ray studies of the ileocecal valve in ileocecal tuberculosis, Radiology, 62:251, 1954.

Hill, M. C., and Goldberg, H. I. Roentgen diagnosis of intestinal amebiasis, Am. J. Roentgenol., 99:77, 1967.

Pittman, F., El-Hashimi, W., and Pittman, J. C. Studies of human amebiasis, Gastroenterology, 65:581, 1973.

Weinfeld, A. The roentgen appearance of intestinal amebiasis, Am. J. Roentgenol., 96:311, 1966.

Typhlitis and Miscellaneous Forms of Colitis

Amromin, G. D., and Solomon, R. D. Necrotizing enteropathy; complication of treated leukemia or lymphoma patients, J.A.M.A., 192:23, 1962.

Bar-Ziv, J., Ayoub, J. I. G., and Fletcher, B. D. Hemolytic uremic syndrome: A case presenting with acute colitis, Pediatr. Radiol., 2:203, 1974.

Berman, W., Jr. The hemolytic-uremic syndrome: Initial clinical presentation mimicking ulcerative colitis, J. Pediatr. 81:275, 1972.

Grossman, H., Berdon, W. E., and Baker, D. H. Reversible gastrointestinal signs of hemorrhage and edema in the pediatric age group, Radiology, 84:33, 1965.

Handel, J., and Schwartz, S. Gastrointestinal manifestations of the Schönlein-Henoch syndrome, Am. J. Roentgenol., 78:643, 1957.

Johnson, W., and Borella, L. Acute appendicitis in childhood leukemia, J. Pediatr., 67:595, 1965.

Kasabach, H. H., and Merritt, K. K. Capillary hemangioma with extensive purpura: Report of a case, Am. J. Dis. Child., 59:1063, 1940.

Lieberman, E. Hemolytic-uremic syndrome, J. Pediatr., 80:1, 1972.

Prolla, J. C., and Krischner, J. B. Gastrointestinal lesions and complications of leukemias, Ann. Intern. Med., 61:1084, 1964.

Rodriguez-Erdmann, F., and Levitan, R. Gastrointestinal and roentgenological manifestations of

Henoch-Schönlein purpura, *Gastroenterology*, 54:260, 1968.

Siegal, D. L., and Bernstein, W. C. Gastrointestinal complications of leukemias, *Dis. Colon Rectum*, 8:377, 1965.

Wagner, M. L., Rosenberg, H. S., Fernbach, D. J., and Singleton, E. B. Typhlitis: A complication of leukemia in childhood, *Am. J. Roentgenol.*, 109:341, 1970.

Tumors

Andren, L., and Frieberg, S. Spontaneous regression of polyps of colon, *Acta Radiol. (Stockholm)*, 46:507, 1956.

Capitanio, M. A., and Kirkpatrick, J. A. Lymphoid hyperplasia of the colon in children: Roentgen observations, *Radiology*, 94:323, 1970.

Collins, J. O., Falk, M., and Guibone, R. Benign lymphoid polyposis of the colon: Case report, *Pediatrics*, 38:897, 1966.

Cremin, B. J., and Louw, J. H. Polyps in the large bowel in children, *Clin. Radiol.*, 21:195, 1970.

Cronkhite, L. W., Jr., and Canada, W. J. Generalized gastrointestinal polyposis: An unusual syndrome of pigmentation, alopecia, and onychotrophia, *N. Engl. J. Med.*, 252:1011, 1955.

Dolan, K. D., Seibert, J., and Seibert, R. W. Gardner's syndrome. A model for correlative radiology, *Am. J. Roentgenol.*, 119:359, 1973.

Duhamel, J., and Bauche, P. Polyps of the colon beyond the reach of the sigmoidoscope, *Arch. Dis. Child.*, 40:173, 1965.

Erbe, R. W. Inherited gastrointestinal-polyposis syndrome, *N. Engl. J. Med.*, 294:1101, 1976.

Fragoyannis, S. G., and Anagnostopulos, G. Hemangiolymphomatous hamartoma of the mesentery, *Am. J. Dis. Child.*, 128:233, 1974.

Franken, E. A., Jr. Lymphoid hyperplasia of the colon, *Radiology*, 94:329, 1970.

Franklin, R., and McSwain, B. Juvenile polyps of the colon and rectum, *Ann. Surg.*, 175:887, 1972.

Gardner, E. J. Genetic and clinical study of intestinal polyposis: Predisposing factor for carcinoma of the colon and rectum, *Am. J. Hum. Genet.*, 3:167, 1951.

Godard, J. E., Dodds, W. J., Phillips, J. C., and Scanlon, P. T. Peutz-Jeghers syndrome: Clinical and roentgenographic features, *Am. J. Roentgenol.*, 113:316, 1971.

Grossman, H., Berdon, W. E., and Baker, D. H. Reversible gastrointestinal signs of hemorrhage and edema in the pediatric age group, *Radiology*, 84:33, 1965.

Holden, K. R., and Alexander, F. Diffuse neonatal hemangiomatosis, *Pediatrics*, 46:411, 1970.

Holgerson, L. O., Miller, R. E., and Zintel, H. A. Juvenile polyps of the colon, *Surgery*, 69:288, 1971.

Jeghers, H., et al. Generalized intestinal polyposis and melanin spots of the oral mucosa, lips, and digits: Syndrome of diagnostic significance, *N. Engl. J. Med.*, 241:993, 1949.

Koehler, P. R., Kyaw, M. M., and Fenlon, J. W. Diffuse gastrointestinal polyposis with ectodermal changes. Cronkhite-Canada syndrome, *Radiology*, 103:589, 1972.

MacKenzie, D. H. *The Differential Diagnosis of Fibroblastic Disorders*, (Oxford: Blackwell Scientific Publications, 1970), pp. 107–113.

Marshak, R. H., Moseley, J. E., and Wolf, B. S. The roentgen findings in familial polyposis with special emphasis on differential diagnosis, *Radiology*, 80:374, 1963.

McKusick, V. A., Genetic factors in intestinal polyposis, *J.A.M.A.*, 182:271, 1962.

Reid, J. D. Intestinal carcinoma in the Peutz-Jeghers syndrome, *J.A.M.A.*, 229:833, 1974.

Silverberg, S. G. "Juvenile" retention polyps of the colon and rectum, *Am. J. Dig. Dis.*, 15:617, 1970.

Singleton, E. B., and Johnson, F. Localized lesions of the colon in infants and children, *Sem. Roentgenol.*, 11:111, 1976.

Toccalino, H., Gustavino, E., DePinni, F., O'Donnell, J., and Williams, M. Juvenile polyps of the rectum and colon, *Acta Paediatr. Scand.*, 62:337, 1973.

Todd, I. P. Juvenile polyps, *Arch. Dis. Child.*, 39:106, 1964.

Turcot, J., et al. Malignant tumors of the central nervous system associated with familial polyposis of the colon: Report of 2 cases, *Dis. Colon Rectum*, 2:465, 1959.

Veale, A.M.O. *Intestinal Polyposis* (Cambridge: Cambridge University Press, 1965).

Veale, A. M. O., McColl, I., Bussey, H. J., and Morson, B. C. Juvenile polyposis coli, *J. Med. Genet.*, 3:5, 1966.

Wiot, J. F., and Felson, B. Solitary benign colon tumors, *Sem. Roentgenol.*, 11:123, 1976.

Wolfson, J. J., Goldstein, G., Krivit, W., and Hong, R. Lymphoid hyperplasia of the large intestine associated with dysgammaglobulinemia: Report of a case, *Am. J. Roentgenol.*, 108:610, 1970.

Zitler, M. H. Roentgenographic findings in Gardner's syndrome, *J.A.M.A.*, 192:158, 1965.

Malignant Neoplasms

Bartram, C., and Chrispin, A. R. Primary lymphosarcoma of the ileum and caecum, *Pediatr. Radiol.*, 1:28, 1973.

Donaldson, M. H., Taylor, P., Rawitscher, R., and Sewell, J. B. Colon carcinoma in childhood, *Pediatrics*, 48:307, 1971.

Middelkamp, J. N., and Haffner, H. Carcinoma of the colon in children, *Pediatrics*, 32:558, 1963.

Pickett, L. K., and Briggs, H. C. Cancer of the gastrointestinal tract in childhood, *Pediatr. Clin. North Am.*, 14:223, 1967.

Chilaiditi's Syndrome

Behlke, F. M. Hepatodiaphragmatic interposition in children, *Am. J. Roentgenol.*, 91:669, 1964.

Chilaiditi, D. Zur Frage der Hepatoptose im allgemeinen Anschluss an drei Falle von temporärer partieller Leberverlagerung, *Fortschr. Röntgenstr.*, 16:173, 1910.

Jackson, A. D. M., and Hodson, C. J. Interposition of the colon between liver and diaphragm (Chilaiditi's syndrome) in children, *Arch. Dis. Child.*, 32:151, 1957.

Volvulus

Hunter, J. G., Jr., and Keats, T. E. Sigmoid volvulus in children: A case report, *Am. J. Roentgenol.*, 108:621, 1970.

Lillard, R. L., Allen, R. P., and Nordstrom, J. E. Sigmoid volvulus in children: Case report, *Am. J. Roentgenol.,* 97:223, 1966.

Appendicitis

Benson, C. D., et al. Acute appendicitis in infants: Fifteen year study, *Arch. Surg., 64*:561, 1952.

Felson, B., and Bernhard, C. M. The roentgenologic diagnosis of appendiceal calculi, *Radiology, 49*:178, 1947.

Neuhauser, E. B. D. Acute appendicitis: The x-ray examination, *Postgrad. Med., 45*:64, 1969.

Potter, E. L., and Craig, J. M. *Pathology of the Fetus and Infant* (3rd ed.; Chicago: Year Book Medical Publishers, 1975), p. 367.

Schey, W. L. Use of barium in the diagnosis of appendicitis in children, *Am. J. Roentgenol., 118*:95, 1973.

Snyder, W. H., and Chaffin, L. Appendicitis during first two years of life. Report on 21 cases and review of 447 cases from literature, *Arch. Surg., 64*:549, 1952.

Soter, C. S. The contribution of the radiologist to the diagnosis of acute appendicitis, *Sem. Roentgenol.,* 8:375, 1973.

Weber, H. M., and Good, A., Jr. Invaginated appendiceal stumps roentgenologically simulating polypoid neoplasms, *Radiology, 34*:440, 1940.

Wilkinson, R. H., Bartlett, R. H., and Eraklis, A. J. Diagnosis of appendicitis in infancy: The value of abdominal radiographs, *Am. J. Dis. Child., 118*:687, 1969.

Williams, H. J. Coproliths in children: Recognition and significance, *Pediatrics, 34*:372, 1964.

Foreign Bodies

Alexander, W. J., Kadish, J. A., and Dunbar, J. S. Ingested foreign bodies in children, *Progr. Pediatr. Radiol., 2*:256, 1969.

Clayton, R. S., and Goodman, P. H. The roentgenographic diagnosis of geophagia (dirt eating), *Am. J. Roentgenol., 73*:203, 1955.

Chapter 18

CONGENITAL DIAPHRAGMATIC HERNIA

Congenital diaphragmatic hernias arise from developmental defects in the diaphragm and are often clearly evident on ordinary radiographs of the child's chest and abdomen. Traumatic diaphragmatic hernias are rare in the child but, when present, are readily diagnosed by correlation of the history and the radiographic evidence of abdominal viscera within the thorax.

Several types of congenital diaphragmatic hernias are recognized:

1. Pleuroperitoneal (foramen of Bochdalek) hernia
2. Hiatus hernia with normal esophagus
3. Retrosternal (foramen of Morgagni) hernia
4. Eventration of the diaphragm
5. Localized absence of the diaphragm
6. Peritoneopericardial hernia

An understanding of the various forms of diaphragmatic hernia depends upon a knowledge of the normal development of the diaphragm and the deficiencies in this development which result in herniation of abdominal contents into the thorax.

DEVELOPMENTAL ANATOMY. Because of the complexity of the formation of the diaphragm and the number of components entering into its formation, defects are not unusual. The ventral portion of the diaphragm is formed by the septum transversum, an unsplit mass of mesoderm which extends dorsally from the ventral body wall beneath the pericardium. The septum is joined posteriorly by a portion of the mesoesophagus of the dorsal mesentery, forming a bridge between the ventral and dorsal surfaces of the celomic cavity. Lateral and posterior to this central mass are the pleuroperitoneal foramina, communications between the thoracic and abdominal cavities. These canals eventually become closed by ingrowth of a double-layered membrane composed of pleura and peritoneum, the pleuroperitoneal membrane. Incomplete closure of the pleuroperitoneal foramina results in a defect in the posterolateral portion of the diaphragm (the foramen of Bochdalek) which allows herniation of abdominal viscera into the thorax (Fig. 18–1). Normally, striated muscle develops between these serous membranes, forming a functional muscular component. The failure of this process results in a flaccid inefficient septum known as eventration, which succeeds in maintaining the intra-abdominal structures in the abdomen but bulges into the thorax because of intra-abdominal pressure. The entire hemidiaphragm may be deficient in musculature, or only a localized segment may be involved.

Normally there is a small, comparatively weak area at the attachment of the diaphragm to each parasternal portion of the anterior chest wall (Larrey's spaces). Rarely, there is an actual defect at this site, known as the foramen of Morgagni, resulting in communication between the abdomen and the thorax. This defect may be to the right or left of the sternum or, if the diaphragmatic attachment at the sternum is also inadequate, may be retrosternal. In such cases the abdominal contents herniate into the thorax through the retrosternal or parasternal area.

Hiatus hernia, in which a small portion of the stomach lies above the diaphragm, with an associated short esophagus, is discussed in Chapter 5. Large congenital defects in the region of the esophageal hiatus allow a large part or all of the stomach to herniate into the thorax. Similarly, a failure of normal development in areas other than the foramina already mentioned results in localized defects of various sizes through

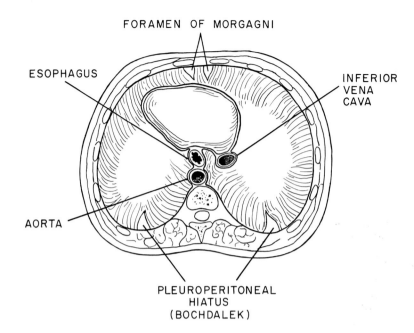

Figure 18–1. Cross section of diaphragm showing usual sites of diaphragmatic hernias. (Redrawn from Caffey, J. *Pediatric X-Ray Diagnosis* (6th ed.; Chicago: Year Book Medical Publishers, 1972), p. 290.

which one or several intra-abdominal structures may herniate.

PLEUROPERITONEAL (FORAMEN OF BOCHDALEK) HERNIA

Incomplete closure of the pleuroperitoneal communication is the most common type of diaphragmatic hernia due solely to faulty development of the diaphragm. However, it is relatively rarer than esophageal hiatal hernia.

Symptoms consisting of cyanosis and difficulty in breathing appear soon after birth, and death may be sudden as a result of the cardiac and respiratory embarrassment produced by the large hernia.

Usually the diaphragmatic defect involves the left pleuroperitoneal foramen, with herniation of most of the stomach, small intestine, and colon into the left hemithorax. Solid viscera, the liver and spleen, may also be incorporated in the hernia. A hernial sac is usually not present, although smaller hernias covered by a thin sac of parietal pleura and parietal peritoneum do occur. The latter type is actually a form of eventration probably developing later in embryonic life after the pleuroperi-

toneal canals have closed, but before ingrowth of the muscular components. If a hernial sac is present, it must be removed surgically, because recurrence may develop or the sac may fill with fluid or even become infected.

RADIOLOGIC EVALUATION. Radiographs of the chest and abdomen are diagnostic. One side of the chest, usually the left, contains multiple gas-filled segments of bowel that give the entire hemithorax a cystic appearance (Fig. 18–2). Multiple air-fluid levels are often present. Vague areas of increased density representing a combination of the fluid content of the bowel and herniated solid structures are also apparent. The lung on the side of the hernia is hypoplastic, the severity of which depends upon the time of herniation in utero. The function of the opposite lung is severely limited by the displacement of mediastinal structures. Although the diaphragmatic defect is in the posterior lateral portion, this is seldom apparent in either frontal or lateral views because of the large size of the hernia which usually fills the entire hemithorax. If there is mechanical obstruction in the herniated bowel, the loops may be markedly dilated. The abdominal cavity is small and holds few gas-containing structures. Usually a small amount of gas is identified in the descend-

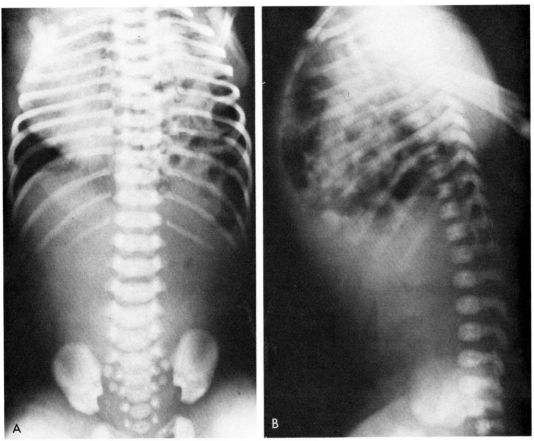

Figure 18–2. Left posterolateral (foramen of Bochdalek) hernia. *A*, Anteroposterior roentgenogram shows entire left hemithorax filled with poorly defined areas of opacity and radiolucency, the latter representing loops of bowel. Mediastinal structures are markedly displaced to right. *B*, Lateral view further emphasizes extent of hernia and shows, as does *A*, nearly complete absence of gas-containing bowel in abdomen. At operation, much of the small intestine, ascending and transverse portions of colon and distal portions of the stomach and spleen were found in the left hemithorax.

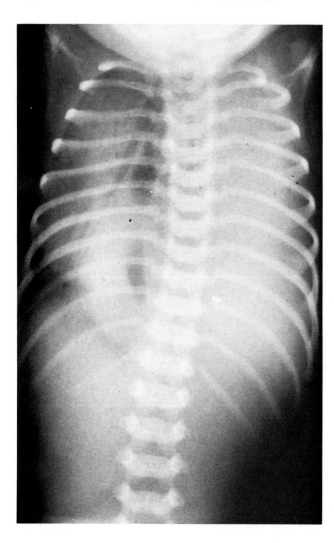

Figure 18–3. Foramen of Bochdalek hernia. The left hemithorax is opaque and there is absence of intestinal gas in the abdomen and in the herniated bowel. The examination was made in the first few minutes of life before ingested air had entered the gastrointestinal tract. (Reprinted with permission from Singleton, E. B., and Wagner, M. L. *Radiologic Atlas of Pulmonary Abnormalities in Children*, (Philadelphia: W. B. Saunders, 1971), p. 81.

ing colon and in the unherniated part of the stomach. The use of contrast material either orally or by enema is unnecessary and should be considered contraindicated because it delays the surgery which is usually urgently required. Occasionally the affected hemithorax is opaque, simulating a mass lesion or pleural effusion. This form of presentation occurs before the infant has swallowed air (Fig. 18–3). In such an instance, the instillation of a small amount of air into the stomach through a nasogastric tube followed by serial films will provide the diagnosis.

Herniation of abdominal viscera through the pleuroperitoneal foramen may develop after birth. When this occurs it is invariably on the right and is associated with a progressive respiratory distress, increased density in the right lower thorax, and mediastinal shift to the left. The hernia usually contains liver. Confirmation may be made by injecting air into the peritoneal cavity and identifying it in the right pleural space above the herniated viscera (Fig. 18–4). Umbilical venography and isotope studies are additional methods of identifying the position of the liver. Occasionally foramen of Bochdalek hernia may not produce symptoms until later in life (Fig. 18–5).

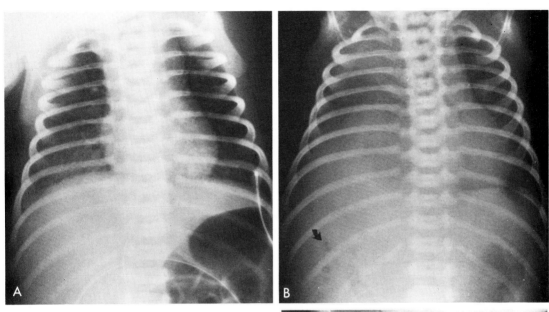

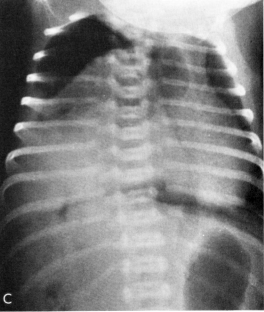

Figure 18-4. Foramen of Bochdalek hernia developing in the neonatal period. *A,* Radiograph made because of mild respiratory distress at 2 days of age shows questionable infiltrate in the right lower lobe. *B,* Repeat examination one week later shows opacification of the right hemithorax, atelectasis of the right upper lobe, and displacement of mediastinal structures to the left. There is also elevation of the hepatic flexure (*arrow*). *C,* Chest radiograph made following intraperitoneal instillation of air shows pneumoperitoneum as well as extension of air into the right pleural space above the herniated liver.

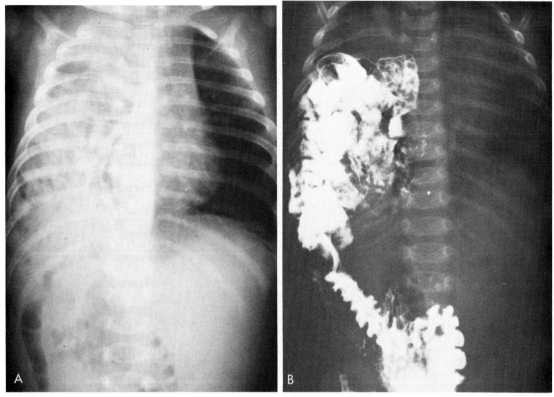

Figure 18–5. Foramen of Bochdalek hernia. *A*, Loops of bowel are seen within the right hemithorax. *B*, Upper gastrointestinal tract examination outlines the herniated intestinal tract. The entire small bowel and most of the colon are in the right hemithorax. (Reprinted with permission from Singleton, E. B., and Wagner, M. L., *Radiologic Atlas of Pulmonary Abnormalities in Children* (Philadelphia: W. B. Saunders, 1971), p. 80.

HIATUS HERNIA WITH NORMAL ESOPHAGUS

The small hiatus hernias associated with gastroesophageal incompetence and a short esophagus are discussed elsewhere. A less common form of hiatus hernia is due to a congenital defect involving the central tendon of the diaphragm in the region of the esophageal hiatus. Although uncommon, it is second in frequency to the posterolateral type of congenital diaphragmatic hernia. The stomach is usually the only intra-abdominal structure which is herniated, and the extent of the herniation varies from time to time because of its sliding characteristics. A hernial sac limits the extent of the herniation. In the paraesophageal type the cardioesophageal junction remains below the diaphragm and only the fundus is in the thorax, lying in a paraesophageal location behind the heart and often extending into the right hemithorax. In the large, sliding type of hiatus hernia the major portion of the stomach may be in the chest, with the fundus posterior to the heart, the body and antrum lying over the right hemidiaphragm, and the pylorus and duodenum extending medially and inferiorly into the abdomen.

Symptoms usually develop after infancy or may not appear until adulthood. They include varying degrees of upper gastrointestinal distress, dyspepsia, and vomiting. Only rarely are there signs of respiratory interference. If there is significant gastroesophageal reflux, esophagitis and subsequent stricture of the esophagus may develop.

RADIOLOGIC EVALUATION. Hiatus hernia may be identified on chest roentgenograms, the appearance depending upon the size of the hernia. In the paraesophageal type, posteroanterior films may show a collection of gas in the right cardiophrenic sulcus. If the hernia is small, it does not extend far enough to the right to be visible in the frontal view but may be identified with heavily penetrated films as a loculus of radiolucency superimposed upon the cardiac image. In either instance lateral roentgenograms will show the air-filled pouch in the retrocardiac area. Upright films frequently disclose an air-fluid level in the hernia, and if radiographs are exposed with the patient supine, the fluid content of the stomach may opacify the hernia, giving it a solid appearance. The extent of the hernia is visible only after the ingestion of contrast material. The fundus is identified posterior to the heart, with the body and antrum of the stomach lying in the abdomen. Constriction of the stomach at the level of the diaphragmatic defect is often recognizable.

With larger hernias in which nearly the entire stomach is in the chest, the appearance on chest roentgenograms is similar to that just described but more extensive. The loculus of gas representing the inverted antrum is identified in the right cardiophrenic area and may extend to the chest wall. A similar loculus representing the fundus may be seen to the left of the heart. The esophagus is of normal length and consequently has a redundant configuration, since the cardia is above its normal position either in the chest or at the level of the diaphragmatic defect. With contrast material in the stomach the body and proximal portions of the antrum are identified to the right of the esophagus, and the distal portion of the antrum projects medially and inferiorly through the diaphragmatic defect (Fig. 18–6). Variations of these two extremes may occur, not only in different cases but in the same patient, from time to time. Rarely, distal portions of the intestinal tract are herniated into the chest through the hiatal defect; interval studies,

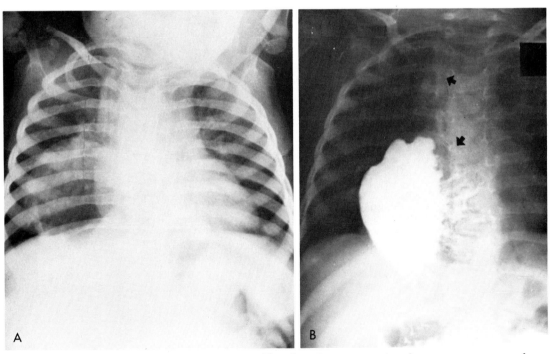

Figure 18–6. Large hiatus hernia in 2 year old girl. *A,* Posteroanterior chest roentgenogram showing loculus of gas occupying right cardiophrenic angle. *B,* Barium studies showing fundus and cardia of stomach within thorax. The redundant esophagus is faintly outlined by barium *(arrows)*. At operation a large hiatus hernia was found and repaired.

the purpose of which is to follow the course of barium through the small bowel and colon, will readily disclose this.

RETROSTERNAL (FORAMEN OF MORGAGNI) HERNIA

This is the third most common type of hernia associated with faulty development of the diaphragm. The defect usually extends to the right of the sternum because of the more intimate pericardial attachment on the left. A hernial sac is usually present and, consequently, with the relatively small size of the defect, limits the size of the hernia. The content of the hernia is usually limited to omentum, although transverse colon, distal portion of stomach, or the small bowel may also be herniated through the defect.

Symptoms do not appear until later life, if at all, and consist of vague digestive disturbances.

RADIOLOGIC EVALUATION. The appearance of the hernia on roentgenograms of the chest depends on the hiatal contents. If only omentum is in the sac, a small area of density is identified in the right cardiophrenic angle, and a lateral view will show this to be against the anterior wall. The appearance in such cases may be identical to an ordinary fat pad, which is commonly seen in this area in adults. If gas-containing bowel is in the hernia, a loculus of gas is identified in the right costophrenic angle. Its retrosternal location in lateral projection readily differentiates it from a hiatus hernia (Fig. 18–7). Gastrointestinal studies made after ingestion of contrast material will reveal which portion of the intestinal tract is herniated and, in the case of omental herniation, may show upward traction of the transverse colon.

EVENTRATION OF THE DIAPHRAGM

In cases of diaphragmatic eventration there is either congenital failure of formation of the muscular components of the diaphragm or degeneration due to phrenic paralysis. Consequently the diaphragm at the site of involvement consists of a thin, ineffectual amyotonic structure which allows

protrusion of intra-abdominal contents into the thorax. The eventration may be bilateral, involve an entire hemidiaphragm, or involve only a small segment. The cases of foramen of Bochdalek hernia which have a hernia sac of parietal pleura and parietal peritoneum are probably extreme types of eventration which are formed after closure of the posterolateral canal but before ingrowth of the muscular elements.

In mild localized forms of eventration symptoms are generally absent and the condition is an incidental finding on routine chest roentgenograms. In extreme forms, affecting an entire hemidiaphragm, dyspnea may be severe, requiring surgical correction.

RADIOLOGIC EVALUATION. Chest roentgenograms disclose elevation of a portion of the diaphragm or of one entire side (Fig. 18–8). On fluoroscopy, motion is seen to be restricted; in cases of extreme involvement paradoxical motion is present. In a localized area of eventration, movement of the eventrated portion shows only a lag during inspiration, without true paradoxical movement, as compared with the adjacent normal muscle. In eventration of the left hemidiaphragm the stomach may be inverted with the antrum higher than the fundus, the so-called upside-down stomach; the splenic flexure and spleen may also be in an abnormally high position. On the right, the liver usually lies beneath the eventration. Differentiation between an eventration and a true hernia may at times be impossible without pneumoperitoneum. Injection of air into the peritoneal cavity will delineate the diaphragm and thereby differentiate it from true hernia.

LOCALIZED ABSENCE OF THE DIAPHRAGM

In this rare form of diaphragmatic hernia the congenital defect may involve either the muscular or the tendinous portions. Symptoms depend on the degree of herniation.

Chest roentgenograms rarely show the defect but reveal abnormal densities in the chest, representing herniated abdominal structures (Figs. 18–9, 18–10, and 18–11). Usually the size of the defect limits the extent of the hernia and only one intra-ab-

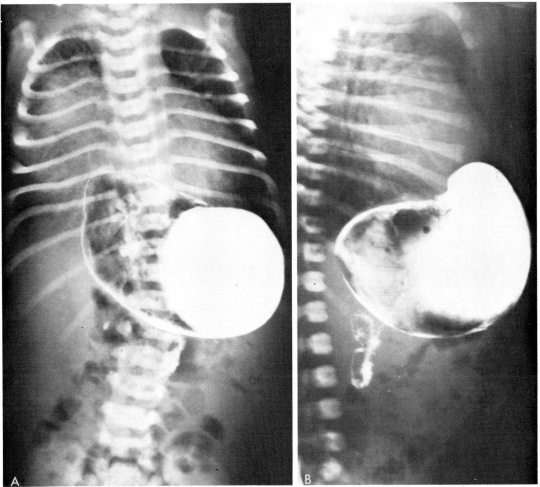

Figure 18-7. Foramen of Morgagni hernia. Infant of 3 months with history of vomiting. *A,* Upper gastrointestinal tract examination showing stomach partially inverted, with antrum extending into medial basilar portion of right hemithorax. Density in right lung represents extensive aspiration pneumonia. *B,* Lateral view shows hernia occupying retrosternal position.

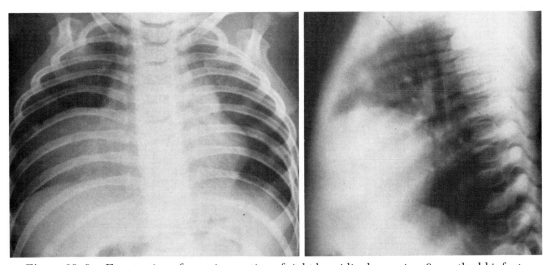

Figure 18-8. Eventration of anterior portion of right hemidiaphragm in a 6 month old infant.

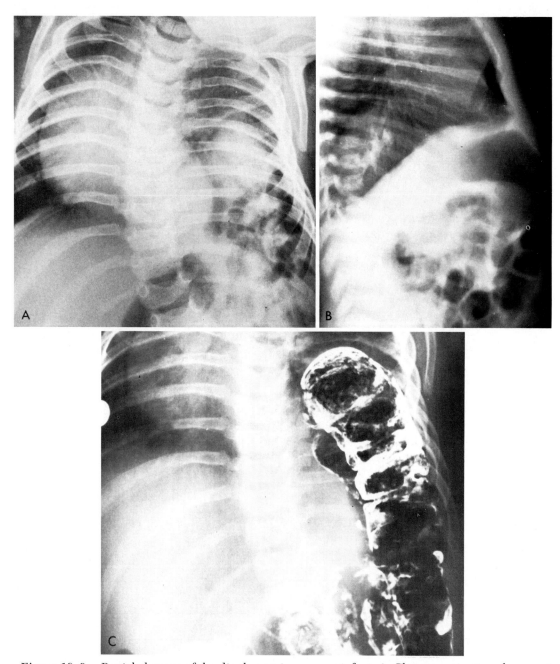

Figure 18–9. Partial absence of the diaphragm in a young infant. *A,* Chest examination shows evidence suggesting diaphragmatic hernia in the left hemithorax. *B,* IV pyelogram shows herniated left kidney. *C,* Colon studies show herniation of the splenic flexure.

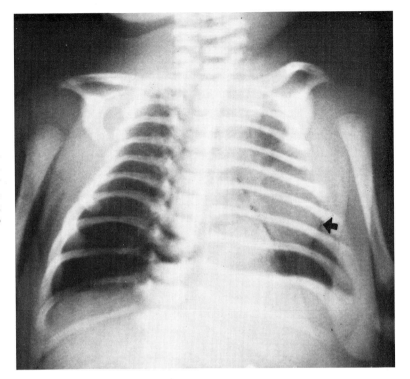

Figure 18–10. Herniation of spleen through congenital defect in posteromedial portion of left hemidiaphragm. At operation, mass (*arrow*) in left hemithorax was found to be spleen.

dominal structure, such as the spleen, kidney, or a portion of the liver, may be identified. In such cases correct diagnosis is usually made at the time of thoracotomy or investigation of an abnormal intrathoracic mass utilizing angiography or a liver-spleen scan. Herniation of a portion of the intestinal tract may also occur and is identified by its gas content. Differentiation in this case from the other forms of diaphrag-

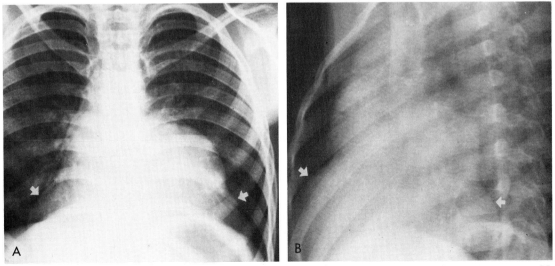

Figure 18–11. Congenital absence of central tendon of diaphragm in an asymptomatic 6 year old boy. A, Posteroanterior chest roentgenogram showing elevation of heart by large mass (*arrows*). B, Oblique view, confirming subcardiac location of mass. At operation central tendon of the diaphragm was proved to be absent with herniation of liver through defect.

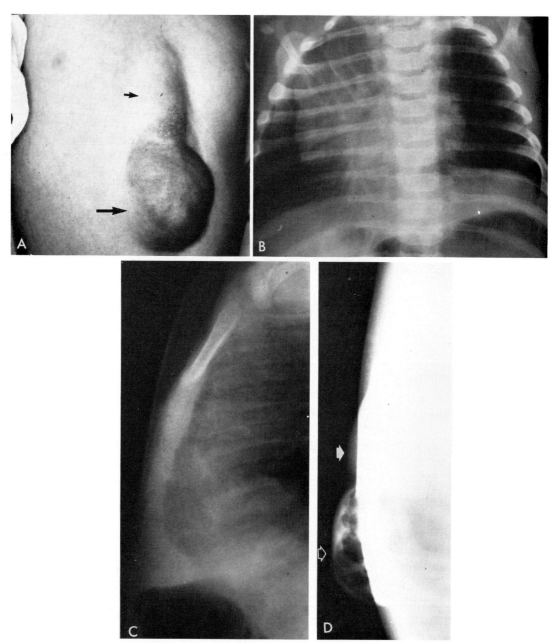

Figure 18–12. A, 3 month old baby with congenital left ventricular diverticulum and associated thoracic and abdominal defects. Note the epigastric mass (left ventricular diverticulum – *small arrow*) and omphalocele (*large arrow*). B, Frontal chest roentgenogram demonstrates slight cardiac enlargement with dextrocardia. Note diminished vasculature supplying the left lung. C, Lateral view shows ossification only of the manubrium of the sternum with tapering of its posteroinferior aspect. D, Lateral view of the lower thoracic and upper abdominal region demonstrates the omphalocele (*open arrow*). Note small soft tissue density just superior to the omphalocele representing the diverticulum (*closed arrow*). (Reprinted with permission from Wagner, M. L., Singleton, E. B., and Leachman, R. D. Congenital left ventricular diverticulum, *Am. J. Roentgenol.*, **122**:137, 1974.)

matic hernia in which bowel is incorporated in the chest is usually impossible.

PERITONEOPERICARDIAL HERNIA

This rare form of diaphragmatic hernia is associated with multiple congenital anomalies involving the sternum and anterior aspect of the upper abdominal wall. A syndrome exists in which there is a defect in the anterior diaphragm due to faulty development of the septum transversum and deficiency of the diaphragmatic pericardium in this area. Other associated features of the syndrome include a defect of the lower sternum, supraumbilical and midline abnormalities such as umbilical hernias, and omphalocele. Cardiac abnormalities are commonly present and include dextrocardia with varying types of congenital heart disease and congenital left diverticula. The diverticulum protrudes through the pericardial defect, lies just above the hernia, and presents clinically as a pulsatile midline upper abdominal mass (Fig. 18–12A, B, C, and D).

On occasion, intra-abdominal contents such as bowel or omentum may protrude into the pericardial cavity through the anterior diaphragmatic and pericardial defects.

REFERENCES

Arey, L. B. *Developmental Anatomy: A Textbook and Laboratory Manual of Embryology* (7th ed.; Philadelphia: W. B. Saunders, 1974).

Astley, R. *Radiology of the Alimentary Tract in Infancy* (Baltimore: Williams & Wilkins, 1956).

Avnet, N. L. Roentgenologic features of congenital bilateral anterior diaphragmatic eventration, *Am. J. Roentgenol.*, 88:743, 1962.

Baffes, T. G. Diaphragmatic hernia, in Mustard, W. T., Ravitch, M. M., et al., editors, *Pediatric Surgery* (2nd ed.; Chicago: Year Book Medical Publishers, 1969), pp. 342–356.

Baran, E. M., Houston, H. E., Lynn, H. B., and O'Connell, E. J. Foramen of Morgagni hernias in children, *Surgery*, 62:1076, 1967.

Berdon, W. E., Baker, D. H., and Amoury, R. The role of pulmonary hypoplasia in the prognosis of newborn infants with diaphragmatic hernia and eventration, *Am. J. Roentgenol.*, 103:413, 1968.

Bremer, J. L., The diaphragm and diaphragmatic hernia, *Arch. Pathol.*, 36:539, 1943.

Burke, E. C., Wenzl, J. E., and Utz, D. C. The intrathoracic kidney: Report of a case, *Am. J. Dis. Child.*, 113:487, 1967.

Canino, C. W., Eichman, J., Rominger, C. J., and Ryan, J. J. Congenital right diaphragmatic hernia, *Radiology*, 82:249, 1964.

Cantrell, G. R., Haller, J. A., and Ravitch, M. M. Syndrome of congenital defects involving abdominal wall, sternum, diaphragm, pericardium and heart., *Surg. Gynecol. Obstet.*, 107:602, 1958.

Gross, R. E., *The Surgery of Infancy and Childhood* (Philadelphia: W. B. Saunders, 1953).

Kirchner, S. G., Burko, H., O'Neill, J. A., Jr., and Stahlman, M. Delayed radiographic presentation of congenital right diaphragmatic hernia, *Radiology*, 115:155, 1975.

Lundstrom, C. H., and Allen, R. P. Bilateral eventration of the diaphragm: Case report with roentgen manifestations, *Am. J. Roentgenol.*, 97:216, 1966.

Potts, W. J., DeBoer, A., and Johnson, F. R. Congenital diverticulum of left ventricle: Case report, *Surgery*, 33:301, 1953.

Reed, J. O., and Lang, E. F. Diaphragmatic hernia in infancy, *Am. J. Roentgenol.*, 82:437, 1959.

Sagel, S. S., and Ablow, R. C. The use of umbilical venography for the diagnosis of congenital right-sided diaphragmatic hernia, *Radiology*, 91:797, 1968.

Spencer, R. P., Spackman, T. J., and Pearson, H. A. Diagnosis of right diaphragmatic eventration by means of liver scan, *Radiology*, 99:375, 1971.

Thomsen, G., Vesterdal, J., and Wenkel-Smith, C. C. Diaphragmatic hernia into the pericardium, *Acta Paediatr.*, 43:485, 1954.

Wagner, M. L., Singleton, E. B., and Leachman, R. D. Congenital left ventricular diverticulum, *Am. J. Roentgenol.*, 122:137, 1974.

Wayne, E. R., Campbell, J. B., Burrington, J. D., and Davis, W. S. Eventration of the diaphragm, *J. Pediatr. Surg.*, 9:643, 1974.

Wilson, A. K., Rumel, W. R., and Ross, O. L. Peritoneopericardial diaphragmatic hernia: Report of a case in a newborn infant, *Am. J. Roentgenol.*, 57:42, 1947.

Chapter 19

THE LIVER, GALLBLADDER AND PANCREAS

INTRODUCTION

The liver, gallbladder and pancreas are closely related embryologically and anatomically, sharing interrelated physiologic and pathologic processes. The embryologic development has been fully described in Chapter 3. Many of the congenital, inflammatory, metabolic, and neoplastic diseases involving one of these organ systems may secondarily affect the other; and jaundice, abdominal pain, and a palpable mass are common clinical findings. Consequently an intimate correlation of clinical and radiologic data is necessary in any given circumstance.

CONGENITAL ANOMALIES OF THE LIVER AND GALLBLADDER

An understanding of the embryology of the vitelline and umbilical veins is necessary in relating to certain clinical problems which result from alterations of the embryologic process. The paired vitelline veins are arranged like a ladder around the duodenum, with the middle anastomotic channel lying dorsal and the proximal and distal channels ventral to the duodenum (Fig. 19–1). With atrophy of both the distal portion of the right vitelline vein and the ventral distal anastomotic channel, this network becomes the portal vein. This results in the duodenum lying ventral to the now sigmoid-shaped portal vein. Failure of the ventral distal channel to atrophy results in the preduodenal vein anomaly (Fig. 19–1) with resulting symptoms and radiographic signs of duodenal obstruction. The paired umbilical veins carrying oxygen anastomose with the hepatic sinusoids of the vitelline veins. The entire right umbilical vein and the proximal portion of the left vein atrophy, and a large venous tract separates from the hepatic sinusoids to form the ductus venosus which carries half of the returning oxygenated blood directly to the heart, the remaining half being distributed in the hepatic sinusoids (Fig. 19–2). The ductus venosus normally closes shortly after birth but may be probed with a catheter for 15 to 20 days, and the umbilical vein for seven to ten days. In recent years

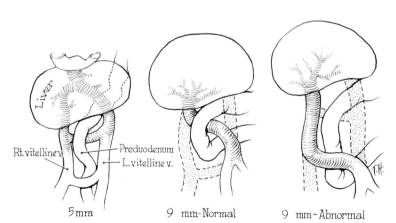

Figure 19–1. Artist's conception of vitelline veins showing the normal and abnormal development of the portal vein.

Rt. vitelline v. Preduodenum L. vitelline v.

5 mm   9 mm-Normal   9 mm-Abnormal

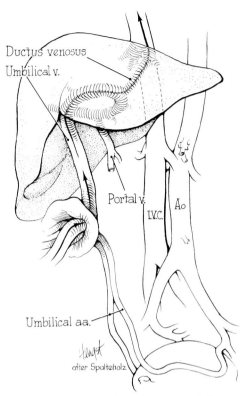

Ductus venosus

Umbilical v.

Portal v.

Ao

I.V.C.

Umbilical aa.

after Spaltzholz

Figure 19–2. Artist's conception of the neonatal umbilical vessels and ductus venosus.

these fetal channels have been used with increasing frequency for exchange transfusions, monitoring blood gases in respiratory distress, and administering various fluids, including angiographic contrast media (Figs. 19–3 and 19–4). It is important for the radiologist to know the anatomy of the umbilical artery and vein in order to determine the proper placement of catheters and to recognize the possible complications (Figs. 19–5 and 19–6, and Fig. 13–40).

Although the liver is the largest abdominal organ, its size is difficult to evaluate by conventional radiographs, manual palpation being more reliable. Sonography offers an additional method of determining the size of the liver and other solid intra-abdominal organs. Variations in position of the liver may be seen in complete situs inversus or there may be indeterminate abdominal solitus (heterotaxia) where the liver appears in a symmetrical position in the upper abdomen (see Fig. 9–2). This may in turn suggest asplenia, polysplenia, or anisosplenia associated with pulmonary

isomerism. Abnormal location of hepatic tissue may also be associated with eventration of the diaphragm, congenital defects in the abdominal wall (omphalocele, gastroschisis), and, rarely, ectopic hepatic tissue has been reported in the chest and abdomen. Various accessory lobes may be found, the most frequent of which is Riedel's lobe. These are uniformly asymptomatic and only important in that they may cast confusing abdominal densities. Isotope studies, computerized tomography, and at times diagnostic pneumoperitoneum may be helpful in delineating some of these curiosities.

Absence of the right or left lobe of the liver has been reported, both of which are rare and associated with abnormal configuration and position of the remaining liver and gallbladder. Organoaxial volvulus of the stomach has been associated with absence of the left lobe.

Congenital solitary and multiple cysts of the liver occasionally occur and may be only an incidental finding or may enlarge the liver significantly to displace the gallbladder, colon, kidney, or upper gastrointestinal tract. Approximately one half of the reported cases of multiple hepatic cysts are associated with adult polycystic disease of the kidneys.

Congenital hepatic fibrosis frequently presents clinically with abdominal enlargement, hepatomegaly, splenomegaly, and hematemesis. Bleeding due to esophageal varices associated with portal hypertension is often the first symptom. Liver function studies are characteristically normal but there may be renal disease with hypertension. Barium studies of the esophagus are helpful in showing the esophageal varices, but arterial and splenoportography may be further indicated for diagnosis and as a prerequisite to portal-to-systemic vein shunting procedures. Intravenous urography demonstrates blunted, splayed calyces, shortened infundibula, and ectatic tubules which may resemble medullary sponge kidney (Fig. 19–7). The familial incidence of congenital hepatic fibrosis is well known, and genetic transmission is considered to be autosomal recessive. Congenital hepatic fibrosis and infantile polycystic disease may be a spectrum of the same disease process.

Anomalies involving the gallbladder and

Text continued on page 396

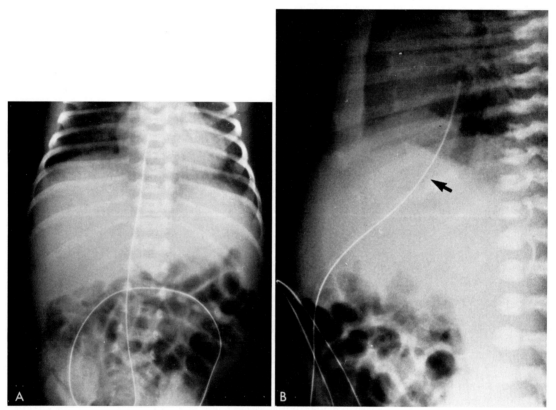

Figure 19–3. Position of umbilical vein catheter. *A,* Frontal projection shows catheter extending up the umbilical vein with the tip in the right atrium (a higher position than optimal). *B,* Lateral view illustrates the importance of identifying the position of the umbilical vein catheter extending through the ductus venosus (*arrow*) into the inferior vena cava.

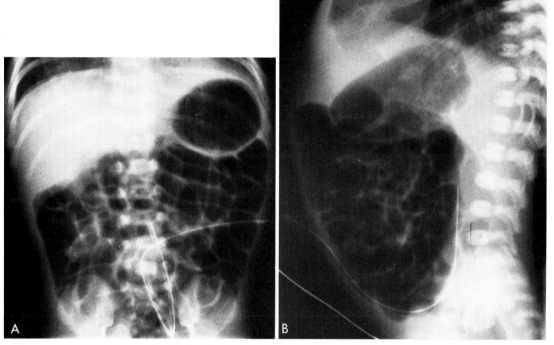

Figure 19–4. Position of umbilical artery catheter. *A,* Frontal projection shows caudal route of umbilical artery catheter passing into the iliac artery and extending into the abdominal aorta. *B,* Lateral view shows to better advantage the inferior direction of the umbilical artery.

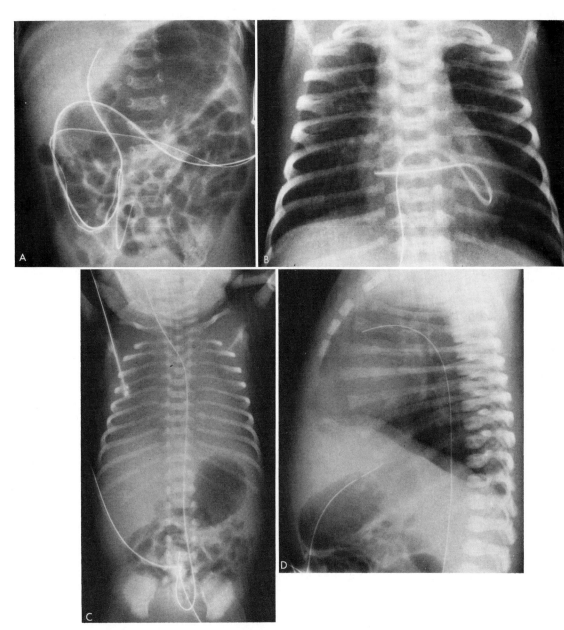

Figure 19–5. Complications of umbilical artery and vein catheterization. *A,* Umbilical vein catheter lies proximal to the ductus venosus. The air in the portal venous system has been introduced through the catheter and should not be mistaken for a complication of ischemic bowel disease. *B,* Umbilical vein catheter is passed into right atrium, through the foramen ovale into the left atrium. The tip extends into the right pulmonary vein. *C,* Umbilical artery catheter has been passed up the aorta and extends into the right common carotid artery. *D,* Umbilical artery catheter is passed up the aorta and extends into the ascending aorta, which is anteriorly positioned, suggesting transposition of the great vessels, which was subsequently proved.

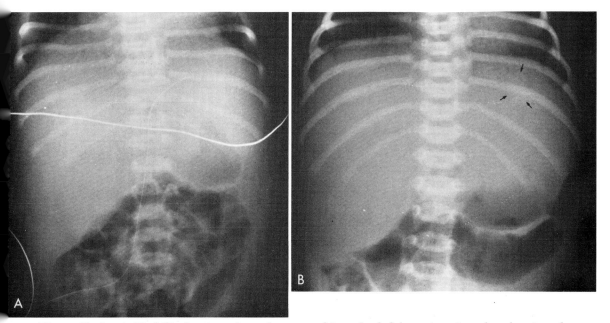

Figure 19-6. *A*, Umbilical vein catheter has passed into the left hepatic vein rather than into the inferior vena cava. *B*, Follow-up examination six weeks later shows localized area of calcification (*arrows*) in the left lobe of the liver at the site of the misdirected catheter.

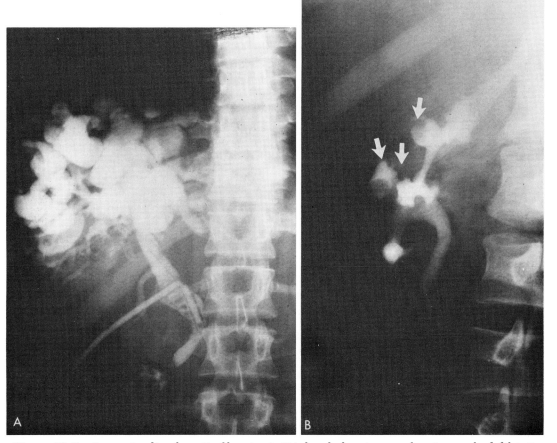

Figure 19-7. Long-standing hepatic fibrosis. *A*, T-tube cholangiogram showing marked dilatation of the biliary tree secondary to the chronic hepatic fibrosis. *B*, Alteration of minor calyces consistent with either renal tubular ectasia or medullary sponge kidney.

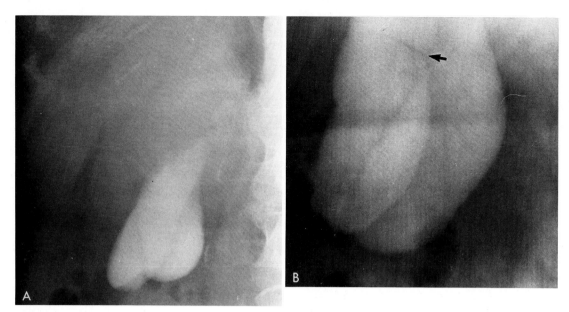

Figure 19–8. Duplication of the gallbladder. *A*, Cholecystogram shows contrast medium within two gallbladders. *B*, Duplication of the gallbladder in which a septum (*arrow*) is identified in one of the gallbladders.

biliary tract are not uncommon but many are minor, causing no symptoms. Duplications, cystic dilatations, accessory ducts, localized stenosis, and abnormal insertions may involve the hepatic, cystic, and common bile ducts. The gallbladder may be absent, duplicated, septated, or abnormal in position (Fig. 19–8). The most common abnormality is the familiar phrygian cap deformity (Fig. 19–9). Absence of the gallbladder is associated with biliary atresia and is one of the findings in polysplenia. Left-sided gallbladder is usually associated with situs inversus but may occur rarely as an isolated anomaly or with left-sided liver and situs solitus of the remaining viscera. Asplenia is suggested by a midline gallbladder associated with a symmetrical midline liver shadow. Rare fistulous communications between the biliary tract and the tracheobronchial tree should be suspected in newborns with bile-stained secretions and have been demonstrated by bronchography.

Biliary Atresia and Neonatal Hepatitis

Neonatal jaundice is usually a medical problem in which the radiologist is seldom involved. However, prolonged obstructive jaundice can be associated with various anomalies of the hepatobiliary system and the gastrointestinal tract, and in such cases the radiologist may play a vital role. Although hyperbilirubinemia may be associated with atresia of the upper small bowel, hypertrophic pyloric stenosis, or rare genetic disorders (glucuronyl transferase deficiencies, Dubin-Johnson syndrome, galactosemia), the great majority of infants with prolonged jaundice have either neonatal hepatitis or biliary atresia. No other topic in pediatrics is perhaps more controversial at this time than the differential diagnosis and management of these two conditions.

Traditionally, biliary atresia has been considered to be a congenital developmental defect. This concept has been challenged by recent investigators, and the current thinking is summarized by Landing, who proposes that neonatal hepatitis, biliary atresia, and choledochal cysts are variations of "infantile obstructive cholangiopathy" and the result of intrauterine infection. However, genetic influences cannot be excluded and may modify the basic disease process. This is a spectrum of diseases with neonatal hepatitis and biliary atresia at opposite poles, with varying degrees of involvement between these two extremes. This concept is of considerable interest from many standpoints and would explain why accurate differentiation of these diseases has not been possible with laboratory studies, including liver biopsy and operative cholangiogram.

Both biliary atresia and neonatal hepatitis present with jaundice that extends beyond 3 to 4 weeks of age in otherwise healthy-appearing infants with hepatomegaly and occasionally splenomegaly. Late in the disease malnutrition becomes evident and generalized osteoporosis and biliary rickets may develop. Esophageal varices secondary to cirrhosis and portal hypertension are also seen as late complications. With the exception of the ^{131}I rose bengal liver excretion study, laboratory studies are of little value in the differential diagnosis (Fig. 19–10). Recovery of less than 10% of the administered dose of radionuclide from the stool suggests biliary obstruction. Unfortunately the effectiveness of the test as a differential examination is limited because approximately 20% of the cases of neonatal hepatitis also fail to excrete significant amounts of the radioactive iodine in the gastrointestinal tract.

Liver biopsy may show the classic pattern of "giant cell transformation" of neonatal hepatitis as well as bile duct proliferation with periportal fibrosis typical of biliary atresia. Here again, there is considerable overlap and one frequently finds a mixed pattern of the typical pathologic findings. A clear distinction between biliary atresia and neonatal hepatitis could not be established on the basis of liver biopsy in one third of the cases studied by Hays, et al.

Until recently the clinician has had fairly definite guidelines in the management of these two conditions, following a policy of careful waiting during the first four months of life and relying on the natural history of the two diseases to make the distinction. Jaundice in infants with neonatal hepatitis usually cleared during this period, and those with biliary atresia had persistent jaundice and hepatosplenomegaly. The ra-

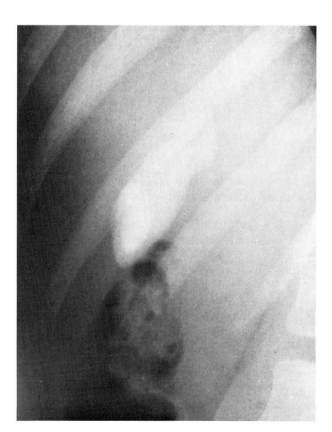

Figure 19–9. Phrygian cap in a 10 year old girl.

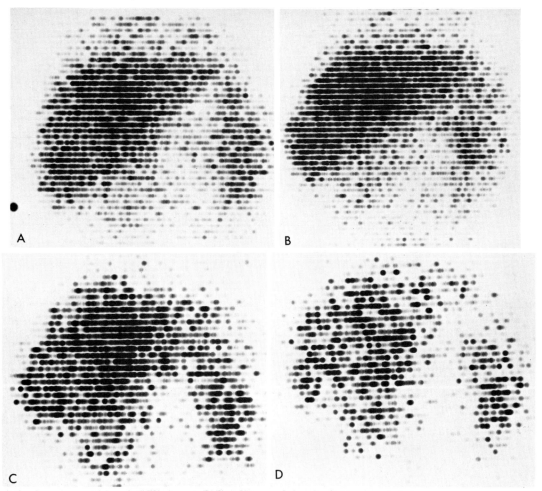

Figure 19–10. ^{131}I rose bengal excretion study in 3 month old boy with biliary atresia. *A,* Concentration of radionuclide in liver, spleen, and kidneys at 1 hour. *B,* 2-hour study. *C,* 24-hour study. *D,* 48-hour study. No excretion of the radionuclide into the gastrointestinal tract can be seen on these studies. (Courtesy of the Department of Nuclear Medicine, St. Luke's Episcopal and Texas Children's Hospitals, Houston, Texas.)

tionale of this policy has been that the salvage rate of infants with biliary atresia has been too low to justify earlier surgical exploration for the purpose of differentiating between these two conditions, since it would of necessity subject some infants with neonatal hepatitis to unnecessary surgery. However, because of improvement in surgical technics in treatment of biliary atresia and the reduced mortality of surgical investigation for making the diagnosis, many infants with jaundice, in whom neonatal hepatitis and biliary atresia are the two differential considerations, are being surgically explored prior to 2 months of age. At that time liver biopsy and operative cholangiograms are performed. The opera-

tive cholangiogram has been shown to be the most accurate method available during surgical evaluation. Even this examination, however, carries a 20% error so far as the ultimate diagnosis is concerned.

RADIOLOGIC EVALUATION. There are many radiographic patterns of involvement of the biliary tract, but three basic patterns are defined. In neonatal hepatitis the biliary system appears small in caliber and there is irregular filling of the smaller intrahepatic radicals, but there is clear communication between the liver, gallbladder, and duodenum (Fig. 19–11). Biliary atresia has been divided into correctable and noncorrectable types by Kasai. In the correctable type one sees obstruction in the com-

THE LIVER, GALLBLADDER AND PANCREAS — 399

mon bile duct or distal hepatic duct with dilated proximal channels which may be readily anastomosed to the intestinal tract (Fig. 19–12). The noncorrectable type has no extrahepatic ducts that are available for anastomosis by conventional means (Fig. 19–13). Approximately 12% of the cases explored have correctable types of atresia. If noncorrectable type biliary atresia is found some surgeons proceed with hepatoportoenterostomy or a Roux-en-Y modification. Kasai and his associates state that over 50% of noncorrectable cases may now be cured if these procedures are carried out before 10 weeks of age. Others have not had as good results and are somewhat less enthusiastic.

Choledochal Cyst

Traditionally, choledochal cyst refers to cystic dilatation of the common bile duct, but many authors have expanded this to include dilatation of any portion of the

extrahepatic biliary tree as well as intrahepatic involvement. It is a rare disease but over 600 cases have been reported in the literature, one third of which are reported by the Japanese, reflecting the Oriental prevalence. In this country one of the larger series reported from a children's hospital, spanning a 20-year period, showed an average incidence of one case every two years, or approximately one case in every 14,000 admissions. The male-to-female ratio is approximately one to three.

Most cases can be classified according to three main types described by Alonso-Lej, et al. (Fig. 19–14). Type I is the most common and consists of a rather sharply localized dilatation of the common bile duct frequently associated with distal narrowing. The dilatation is usually below the cystic duct, but dilatation extending up to and involving portions of the cystic and hepatic ducts is a modification of type I. Type II is a localized diverticulum of the common bile duct and is very rare but important in that it is the only type that is eas-

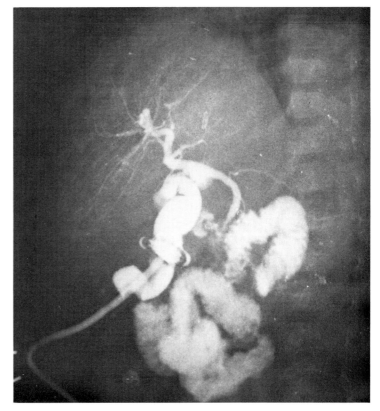

Figure 19–11. Neonatal hepatitis. Operative cholangiogram shows small compressed hepatic ducts but continuity of the ductal system with contrast media passing into the duodenum.

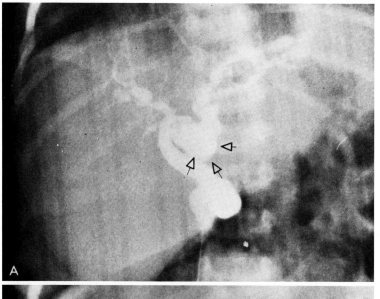

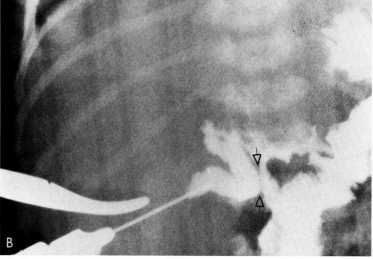

Figure 19–12. Biliary atresia in a 4 week old male infant. *A,* Atresia of the common bile duct (*arrows*) is shown by the injection of the contrast medium into the gallbladder. *B,* Repeat injection after choledochoduodenostomy shows passage of contrast medium into the duodenum. (Reprinted with permission from Taybi, H. *In* Margulis, A. R., and Burhenne, H. J., editors, *Alimentary Tract Roentgenology,* Vol. 2 (St. Louis: C. V. Mosby, 1973), p. 1506.)

ily amenable to corrective surgery. Type III is a dilatation of the intraduodenal portion of the common bile duct (and pancreatic duct) that is lined by duodenal mucosa and called a choledochocele. Some consider this a form of duodenal diverticulum. More recent authors have extended the classification to include extra- and intrahepatic biliary dilatation, as well as various types of single or multiple hepatic cysts occurring without associated disease or associated with polycystic disease or congenital hepatic fibrosis. Caroli's disease (cavernous ectasia of the intrahepatic ducts) is probably a separate disease entity.

There are many theories as to the etiology of choledochal cysts. One of the most widely accepted is that of Yotuyanagi who hypothesized excessive unequal proliferation of epithelial cells in the primitive choledochus, resulting in dilatation when canalization takes place. Dilatation of the common bile duct has been produced experimentally in puppies by curettage of the mucosa and ligation distally, indicating that the two principal factors in the development of choledochal cysts are weakening of the ductal wall and distal obstruction. The proximal insertion of the common bile duct in the pancreatic duct and reflux of pan-

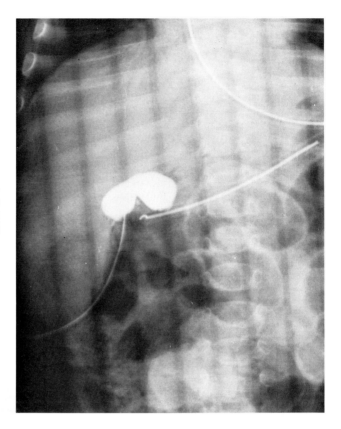

Figure 19–13. Biliary atresia. Operative cholecystogram shows no evidence of communication of the gallbladder with the bile ducts. Surgical exploration failed to demonstrate extrahepatic ducts.

creatic juice into the common bile duct leading to cholangitis, dilatation, and choledochal cyst have been offered as another cause. Landing has proposed that choledochal cysts are part of a spectrum of biliary defects (infantile obstructive cholangiopathy) which results from an acquired perinatal viral infection.

The clinical findings of choledochal cyst consist of jaundice, pain, and a palpable mass. Jaundice is the most frequent finding in infancy and pain more common in older

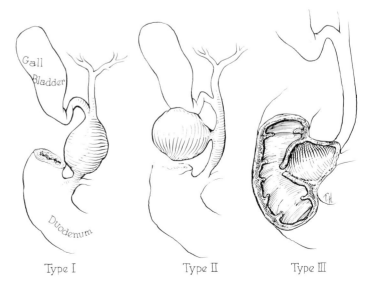

Figure 19–14. Types of choledochal cysts. Type I—cystic dilatation of the common bile duct with distal stenosis. Type II—localized diverticulum of the common bile duct. Type III—intraduodenal choledochocele.

patients. Infants frequently present with prolonged jaundice, suggesting hepatitis or biliary atresia. Older children may have hepatomegaly, vomiting, and a palpable mass. Complications include cholangitis, gallstones, cirrhosis, esophageal varices, and pancreatitis. There is also an increased frequency of malignancy, and rare instances of rupture of the gallbladder and bile peritonitis have been reported.

RADIOLOGIC EVALUATION. Although radiologic studies are helpful, they are often not specific. Abdominal radiographs may show evidence of a mass and, during intravenous pyelography, the total body opacification may demonstrate a "rim" sign surrounding an avascular cystic structure. Upper gastrointestinal tract studies are the most helpful and characteristically show displacement of the antrum and first and second portions of the duodenum anteriorly, inferiorly, and to the left (Fig. 19–15). Large cysts may displace the hepatic flexure of the colon and the right kidney inferiorly. Oral cholecystograms frequently fail to demonstrate the cyst but intravenous cholangiography may occasionally demonstrate it if the examination is done between episodes of hepatic dysfunction with normal bilirubin levels. The ^{131}I iodinated rose bengal scan frequently shows excretion into the cyst and continued use of this noninvasive technique is anticipated. Direct percutaneous puncture and opacification of the cyst has been reported but the danger of bile peritonitis is too great for popular acceptance. Operative cholangiogram is the best means to demonstrate the

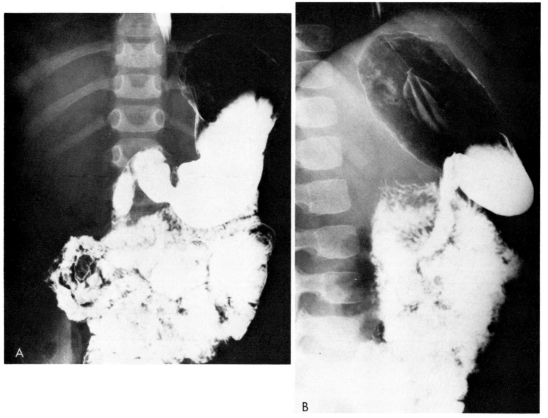

Figure 19–15. Choledochal cyst in a 4 year old girl. *A,* Upper gastrointestinal tract examination shows medial displacement of the second portion of the duodenum. *B,* Lateral view shows anterior displacement of the second portion of the duodenum.

Illustration continued on opposite page

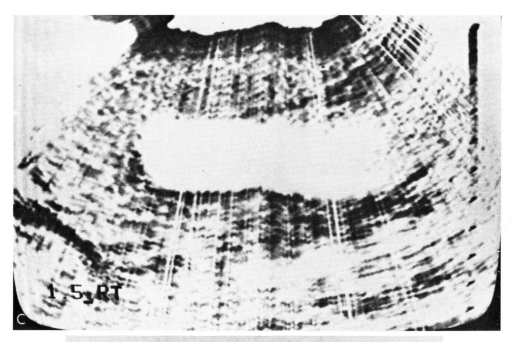

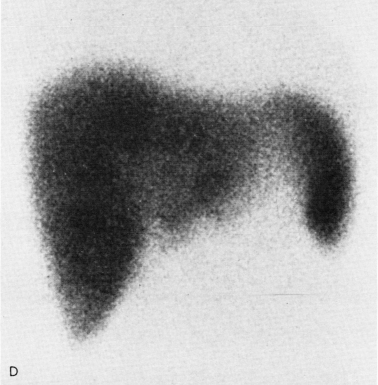

Figure 19–15 Continued. C, Longitudinal sonogram demonstrates a large, oblong sonolucent mass in the right upper abdomen. D, ^{99m}Technetium-sulfur colloid liver-spleen scan. Anterior projection shows large focal defect in area of porta hepatis compatible with choledochal cyst. (D courtesy of Department of Nuclear Medicine, St. Luke's Episcopal and Texas Children's Hospitals, Houston, Texas.)

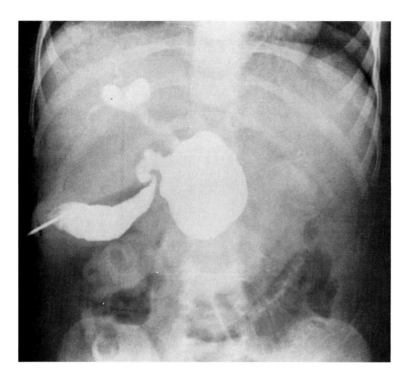

Figure 19–16. Chole-dochal cyst. Operative cho-langiogram shows cystic dilatation of the common bile duct and the branches of the hepatic duct. (Reprinted with permission from Taybi, H. *In* Margulis, A. R., and Burhenne, H. J., editors, *Alimentary Tract Roent-genology*, Vol. 2 (St. Louis: C. V. Mosby, 1973), p. 1510.)

lesion (Fig. 19–16); but the cyst frequently obscures the biliary tree, and unless multiple views are obtained or fluoroscopy is utilized to control the procedure, the true anatomic detail of the biliary tract is frequently not demonstrated. The recent addition of diagnostic abdominal ultrasound as well as computerized tomography of the viscera has been of great help in imaging solid and cystic structures. Experience is limited at this time but one can reasonably expect that future use of both these modalities, while not specific, will be of considerable value in suggesting the diagnosis of choledochal cyst. Although arteriography is not generally advocated as a primary mode of investigation in suspected cases, celiac arteriography utilized in the investigation of right upper quadrant masses will demonstrate an avascular mass with displacement of the gastroduodenal artery. Delayed films will usually demonstrate the rim sign of the choledochal cyst.

Treatment is surgical since medical management is generally ineffective. Surgical treatment consists of either wide anastomosis between the most dependent portions of the cyst and the duodenum or jejunum with a Roux-en-Y loop, or total excision of the cyst and reanastomosis of the

hepatic duct to the jejunum. The type of surgical correction utilized should be known by the radiologist in the evaluation of postoperative radiologic studies (Fig. 19–17). When the diagnosis has been established early before significant secondary liver disease has occurred, the overall prognosis in most instances is good.

INFLAMMATORY DISEASES

Cholecystitis

Cholecystitis is uncommon in children, and although acute or chronic cholecystitis may be associated with cholelithiasis, acute acalculous cholecystitis occurs as a significant separate entity and will be discussed separately.

Acute acalculous cholecystitis in children is unusual but not rare. Brenner reviewed 244 cases of biliary tract disease in childhood of which 81 cases (33%) could be classified as acute cholecystitis and in which over 70% were unassociated with stones. Similarly, about one third of 326 cases reported by Ulin were classified as acute acalculous cholecystitis. Cholecystitis has been reported in the neonate but the highest frequency is between the ages of 8 and 15 years, with an equal male-to-female ratio. The principal etiologic factors occur with almost equal frequency and include infections, hereditary constitution, metabolic factors, and unknown causes. Less than 10% of the cases in a large series were associated with hemolytic anemias. Obesity and acute systemic infections, particularly salmonella and scarlet fever, appear to be the most common predisposing factors.

Clinical symptomatology includes nausea, vomiting, fat intolerance, poorly localized abdominal pain, and right upper quadrant tenderness. Jaundice is noted in over 25% of the cases and is due to inflammatory edema of the ductal system; hence, common duct exploration is usually unnecessary. The correct preoperative diagnosis can usually be suspected from the clinical findings and adequate radiographic studies. The most common error in diagnosis is that of acute appendicitis.

RADIOLOGIC EVALUATION. Radiologic investigation may be diagnostic. If the gallbladder is distended, a discrete soft tissue mass continuous with the liver may be seen in the right upper quadrant. Invariably there is nonvisualization of the gallbladder by cholecystographic studies. Intravenous cholangiography may demonstrate the common duct but fails to opacify the gallbladder. Attempts at intravenous cholangiography in infants and young children are seldom of value because of the abundance of intestinal gas.

Cholecystectomy is recommended by nearly all surgeons, even in the neonate, and there is a reported mortality of less than 1%.

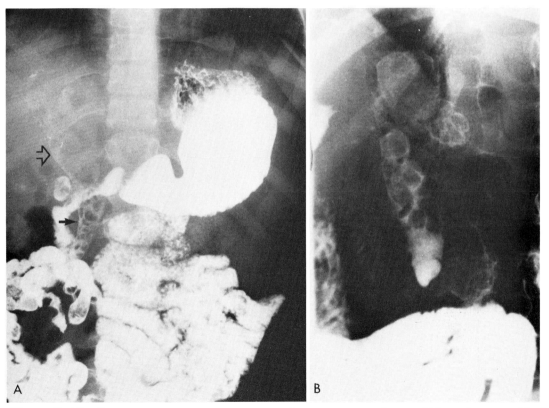

Figure 19–17. Postoperative upper gastrointestinal examination in 9 year old boy who at age 5 had anastomosis of choledochal cyst to the duodenum. *A,* Frontal view shows contrast medium in stomach and small bowel. The choledochal cyst contains barium and air (*open arrow*) and the inferior portion is filled with multiple gallstones (*closed arrow*). *B,* A delayed film shows retention of barium and air in the choledochal cyst and shows to better advantage the multiple gallstones.

Cholelithiasis

Gallstones in children are uncommon but occur slightly more often than acute cholecystitis, especially now that scarlet fever and typhoid fever have been controlled. Strauss reported an incidence of one case per 10,000 admissions. Girls are affected more often than boys, and although all ages have been reported the peak incidence is in the preadolescent and adolescent ages. Cholelithiasis is a well-known complication of chronic hemolytic anemia including sickle cell disease, spherocytosis, and thalassemia, but most reported cases are in children without chronic anemia. Overweight, previous abdominal surgery or infection, and pregnancy appear to be the most important etiologic factors. Symptoms are similar to those of adults and include recurrent episodes of nausea, vomiting, epigastric pain, and tenderness. Jaundice is noted in one third to one half the cases reported.

RADIOLOGIC EVALUATION. These studies may be diagnostic (Figs. 19–18 and 19–19). A review of gallstones in children by Harned and Babbitt indicates that opaque calculi are visualized on plain films in approximately 50% of the cases and that stones are visualized by oral cholecystogram in 70% of the cases. Nonvisualization of the gallbladder is reported in 30% of the cases. The recent use of ultrasound in the diagnosis of gallstones has been helpful in demonstrating echoes within the sonolucent gallbladder (Fig. 19–20).

Treatment is surgical, with cholecystec-

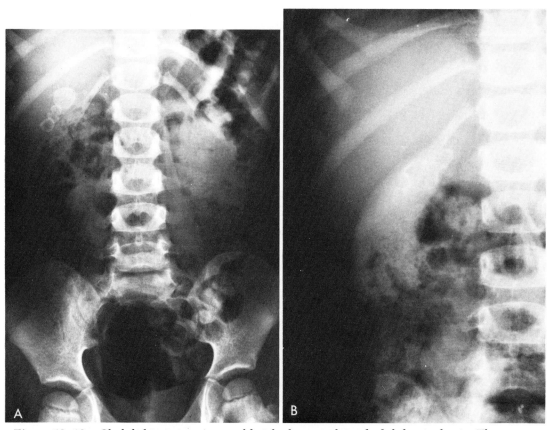

Figure 19–18. Cholelithiasis in a 4 year old girl who complained of abdominal pain. There was no history of hemolytic anemia or other known predisposing factors to cholelithiasis. *A*, Abdominal scout film shows round opaque gallstones in the right upper quadrant. *B*, Cholecystogram shows normal visualization of the gallbladder within which are the opaque calculi.

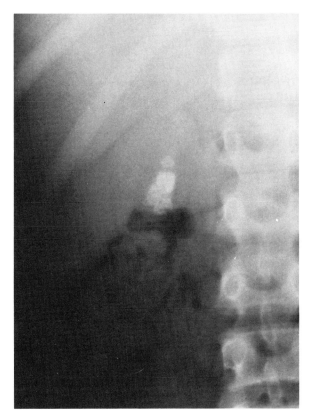

Figure 19-19. Multiple opaque gallstones in an 8 year old girl with congenital spherocytosis.

tomy the procedure of choice. Common bile duct exploration is occasionally necessary.

Liver Abscess

The most common inflammatory disease of the liver is acute viral hepatitis, which has no specific radiographic findings. Less common are the acute focal purulent inflammations which may occur in pyogenic or amoebic infections. Pyogenic liver abscesses tend to be multiple and small, although large lesions are occasionally encountered. There is slight male predominance, and most cases in children occur in patients under 5 years of age. Generally there is some underlying alteration in the immune mechanism of the body and the most frequently associated diseases are leukemia and chronic granulomatous disease of childhood. There are recent reports related to the use of indwelling umbilical vein catheters. Liver abscesses secondary

to rupture of the appendix with pylephlebitis appear to exist more in the literature than in clinical experience.

Amoebic infection arising from the terminal ileum and cecum may secondarily infect the liver, and tends to localize in the right lobe due to the streamlining of the portal venous flow. These abscesses are usually large and monolocular and consequently easier to diagnose radiographically than pyogenic infections.

RADIOLOGIC EVALUATION. The radiographic diagnosis in both situations is difficult. There may be elevation and decreased motion of the right hemidiaphragm associated with hepatic enlargement and displacement of the abdominal viscera (Fig. 19–21). Pleural effusion and even extension of the abscess into the lung may occur (Fig. 19–22). If the patient has an intravenous urogram the diagnosis may be suspected from the total body opacification (Fig. 19–23). Radionuclide liver scanning is helpful in showing a cold area of uptake (Fig. 19–23C) and ultrasound examination is helpful in demonstrating a character-

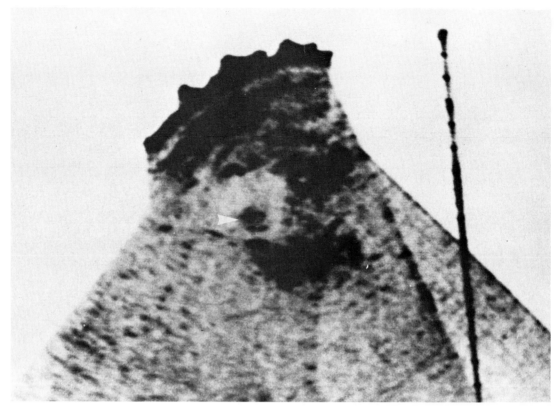

Figure 19–20. Sonogram of the gallbladder of an obese 15 year old girl whose cholecystogram had shown nonvisualization of the gallbladder. The gallstones are identified as echoes (*arrow*) within the sonolucent gallbladder.

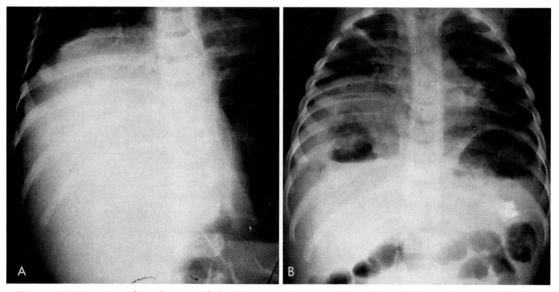

Figure 19–21. Amoebic abscess of the liver. *A,* 2½ year old child with large abscess of the liver producing elevation of the right hemidiaphragm and encroaching upon the stomach. *B,* 2 year old infant with amoebic liver abscess containing air and fluid. (Courtesy of Unidad De Pediatria, Del Hospital General De Mexico, S.S.A.)

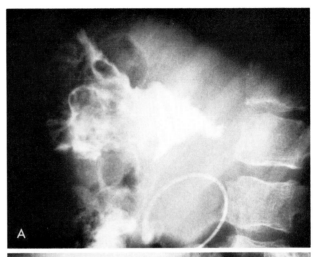
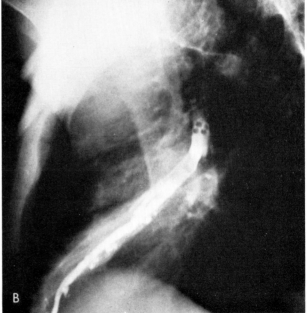

Figure 19-22. Pyogenic liver abscess in a 13 year old boy with ectodermal dysplasia. The patient had surgical exploration with drainage for a liver abscess four months prior to this examination. A chronic cough followed. *A,* Lateral view of liver following injection of water-soluble contrast medium shows large abscess cavity. *B,* Spot film shows extension of contrast medium from the liver abscess into right middle lobe bronchus.

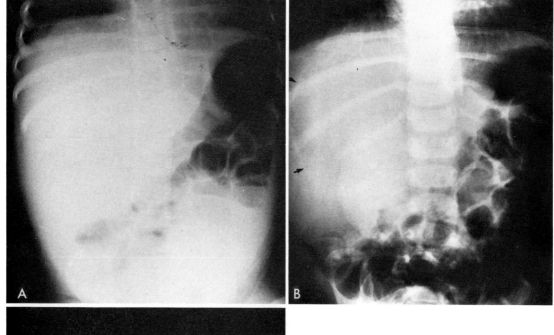

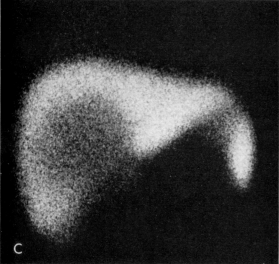

Figure 19–23. Amoebic abscess in 1 year old girl. *A*, Preliminary film shows enlargement of the liver with displacement of bowel to the left and inferiorly. *B*, Intravenous pyelography shows total body opacification with the "rim sign" (*arrows*) outlining the more radiolucent liver abscess. *C*, ^{99m}Tc-sulfur colloid liver spleen scan. Anterior projection shows large area of diminished concentration of the radionuclide in the right lobe. (*C* courtesy of the Department of Nuclear Medicine, St. Luke's Episcopal and Texas Children's Hospitals, Houston, Texas.)

istically echo-free area. Selective hepatic arteriography is confirmatory, showing hypervascularity surrounding the avascular abscess (Fig. 19–24).

Hepatic calcification in boys with recurrent infections suggests chronic granulomatous disease (Fig. 19–25). Hepatic calcifications may also occur in tuberculosis, fungal diseases, and many parasitic infections, including echinococcal disease, visceral larva migrans, and cysticercosis.

Necrotizing Angiitis

Necrotizing angiitis is a collective term applied to several pathologic conditions including periarteritis nodosa, allergic granulomatous arteritis, hypersensitivity angiitis, rheumatoid arteritis, the arteritis of collagen disease, and the necrotizing angiitis of drug abuse.

The clinical and pathologic characteristics are similar in each of these conditions

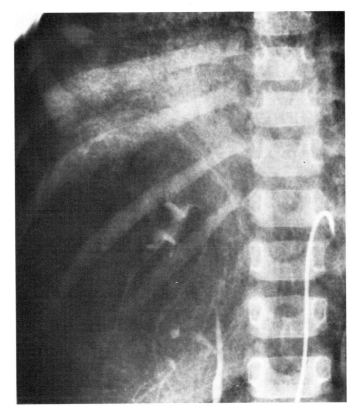

Figure 19-24. Pyogenic abscess in 5 year old child. Celiac arteriogram shows concentration of contrast medium in the hypervascular area surrounding the radiolucent abscess. (Courtesy of Dr. H. Goldstein, M. D. Anderson Hospital, Houston, Texas.)

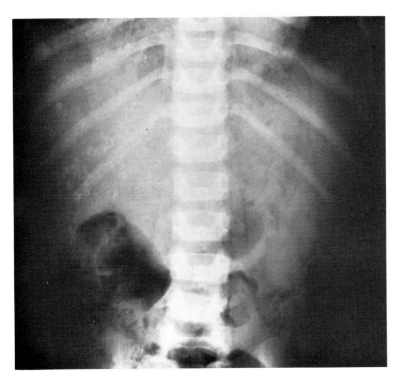

Figure 19-25. Chronic granulomatous disease in 6 year old boy. Radiograph of the abdomen shows multiple areas of calcification scattered throughout the liver.

and consist of primary inflammation and necrosis of vessels. The characteristic features of the vascular pattern of necrotizing angiitis are (1) microaneurysms which show a predilection for bifurcation sites; (2) indistinctness of vessel outlines; (3) segmental luminal irregularities; and (4) obliteration and thrombosis of vessels.

Periarteritis is an uncommon disease but is being reported more and more frequently in habitual drug users (Fig. 19–26). The drugs which are probably responsible for this type of necrotizing angiitis are difficult to identify because of the flagrant abuse of many drugs by the patient. Circumstantial evidence suggests that the amphetamine drugs are high on the list of probable offenders, but a typical drug history may also include oral or intravenous use of chlordiazepoxide HCl, diacetylmorphine, hashish, meperidine HCl, mescaline, oxycodone HCl, oxymorphone, and "STP" (2,5-dimethoxy-4-methylamphetamine).

PORTAL HYPERTENSION

Upper gastrointestinal bleeding in children is always alarming but is usually minimal in extent, without significant consequences, and frequently without a recognizable cause. However, significant bleeding is often due to esophageal varices secondary to portal hypertension. For practical purposes portal hypertension in children is secondary to intrahepatic or extrahepatic obstruction. Although the clinical presentations of both types are similar, the etiology, natural history, and prognosis are significantly different, and each type will be discussed separately. Suprahepatic obstruction of the hepatic veins or inferior vena cava is extremely rare.

Extrahepatic Obstruction

In contradistinction to adults, extrahepatic obstruction is the most common cause of

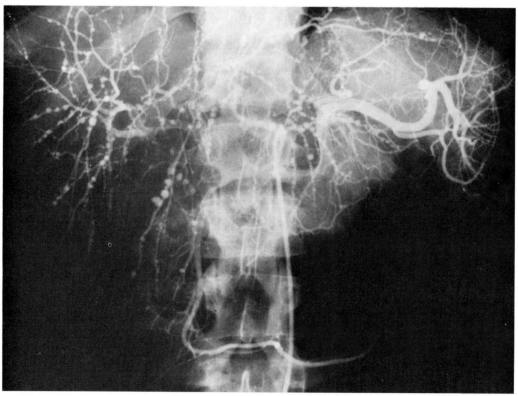

Figure 19–26. Necrotizing angiitis in 18 year old amphetamine user. Note the multiple small aneurysms of the hepatic arteries with small constricted branches. Similar changes were present in the renal and superior mesenteric arteries.

portal hypertension in children and is usually due to thrombosis of the portal vein. Most often the cause of the thrombosis is unknown, but frequently there is a history of omphalitis in the newborn or a history of sepsis and dehydration. The use of umbilical catheters for exchange transfusion in the management of respiratory distress or other acute illnesses in the newborn also has been implicated. With occlusion of the portal vein there is subsequent dilatation of all portions of the portal system and enlargement of the normal anastomotic tributaries between the portal and systemic veins, particularly around the distal esophagus and cardia of the stomach, rectum, umbilicus, mesentery, and retroperitoneal spaces. Numerous dilated tortuous channels develop in the porta hepatis between the undamaged liver and the obstructed portal vein carrying blood to the liver (hepatopetal flow), producing the angiographic appearance referred to as cavernous transformation of the portal vein. Flow of blood away from the liver (hepatofugal flow) also occurs in the normal venous channels as well as through distended collaterals, including the gastrorenal, paraumbilical, splenorenal, and splenoretroperitoneal collaterals. Many of these can be identified on appropriate vascular radiologic studies. The average age of the initial bleeding episode is 7 or 8 years but bleeding as early as 3 years of age may occur, especially if there is a history of omphalitis. A mild upper respiratory infection treated with aspirin frequently precedes the onset of hemorrhage in an otherwise healthy-appearing child. There may be evidence of melena with chronic blood loss. Splenic enlargement is always present, and there is often hematologic evidence of hypersplenism. Laboratory studies characteristically show no evidence of liver dysfunction. In the infant 6 to 8 months of age there may be splenomegaly, growth failure, and an episode of unexplained ascites which eventually clears to be followed later by bleeding from varices.

RADIOLOGIC EVALUATION. This is essential for these patients. An esophagram should be done and frequently will show evidence of varices, particularly in the older child. Follow-up studies of the stomach and duodenum are necessary to rule out other causes of upper gastrointestinal bleeding, and an excretory urogram should be performed to exclude renal tubular ectasia associated with congenital hepatic fibrosis. Angiographic demonstration of the portal system is diagnostic and may take precedence over all other studies, depending on the clinical circumstance. This may be accomplished either by splenoportography or during the venous phase of celiac, splenic, and superior mesenteric arteriography (Fig. 19–27). There are valid reasons for each examination and on occasion both may be necessary. Splenoportography has many advantages, including excellent anatomic detail and measurement of splenic pulp pressure, and is relatively easy to perform. It has the disadvantages of possible abdominal hemorrhage, usually requires a general anesthetic, and only demonstrates the venous channels. Arterial portography is more physiologic and frequently is done with local anesthesia. It demonstrates both arterial and venous structures and if properly done with high doses and delayed films will usually demonstrate the lesion with adequate anatomic detail (Fig. 19–28). It is the only method of study if there has been previous splenectomy. However, it is a more difficult and longer procedure to perform and there is more radiation exposure than with splenoportography. The details of performing either study can be found in the literature and are beyond the scope of this discussion. Typically one sees a dilated portal vein with multiple hepatopetal channels (cavernous transformation) at the hilus of the liver which supply small intrahepatic veins. Hepatofugal flow is seen filling dilated channels of the mesenteric, coronary, and short gastric veins which feed varices in the esophagus and cardia of the stomach.

Intrahepatic Obstruction

Portal hypertension due to intrahepatic obstruction is less frequent in children and is most often due to hepatic cirrhosis. It may also be associated with biliary atresia, cystic fibrosis of the pancreas, and congenital hepatic fibrosis. The latter condition has been previously discussed.

Children with intrahepatic portal hypertension are frequently ill with underlying disease, and there is often growth failure,

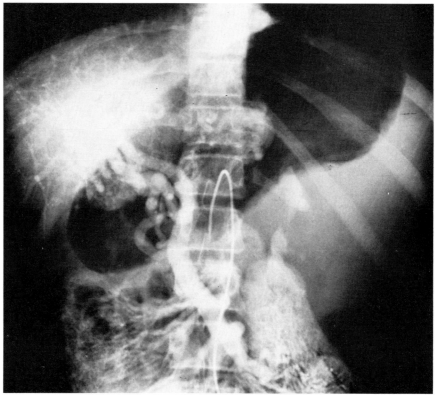

Figure 19-27. Eight year old with esophageal varices. The venous phase of the superior mesenteric angiogram shows cavernous transformation of the portal vein. (Courtesy of Dr. H. Goldstein, M.D. Anderson Hospital, Houston, Texas.)

lung disease (cystic fibrosis), encephalopathy, jaundice, ascites, and abnormal liver function studies. There is splenomegaly and the liver is usually enlarged except with advanced cirrhosis, in which case it may be shrunken. The pathophysiology of the portal vascular system in intrahepatic obstruction is very similar to that with extrahepatic obstruction except that the onset of bleeding tends to occur later and repeated bleeding episodes are not as well tolerated due to impaired coagulation mechanisms associated with diffuse liver disease.

RADIOLOGIC EVALUATION. This is much the same as outlined in the preceding section on extrahepatic obstruction. Portography is diagnostic and the radiologic findings vary with the degree of cirrhosis. In mild cases there may be only slight dilatation of the splenic and portal veins with prominent intrahepatic branches and little or no evidence of hepa-

tofugal flow. In advanced cases there is evidence of hepatofugal flow filling dilated collaterals as in extrahepatic obstruction (Fig. 19-29). The intrahepatic branches may be reduced in size and uneven, and appear straightened. Large hepatofugal collaterals may appear to drain the entire splenic bed on splenoportography and simulate extrahepatic obstruction. In this case superior mesenteric arteriography must be done to visualize the portal vein. An excretory urogram should be obtained with the angiogram. The esophagram will again usually demonstrate varices.

Surgical treatment consists of ligation of varices and a variety of surgical decompressive shunting procedures between the portal and systemic veins, including portacaval, mesocaval, and splenorenal shunts. Transposition of the spleen into the chest has also been utilized. The age, clinical course of the patient, and underlying disease process are the most important consid-

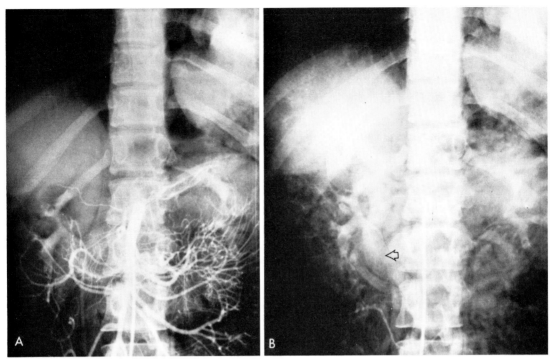

Figure 19–28. Arterioportogram with cavernous transformation of the portal vein. A, Arterial injection shows normal superior mesenteric artery. Note position of spleen in lower left hemithorax, positioned for treatment of esophageal varices. B, Delayed venous phase shows contrast medium in the superior mesenteric vein (*arrow*) and in the dilated tortuous cavernous transformation of the portal vein. (Retouched for greater clarity.)

Figure 19–29. Venous phase of arterial portography in patient with cirrhosis. Note patent portal veins with small peripheral intrahepatic branches and numerous large gastroesophageal varices (*arrows*). (Courtesy of Dr. H. Goldstein, M.D. Anderson Hospital, Houston, Texas.)

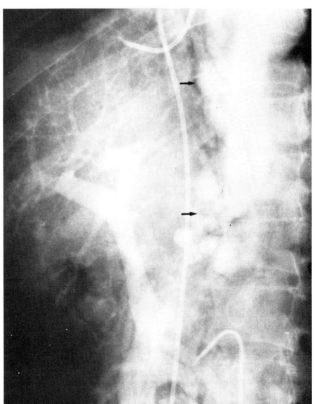

erations in corrective surgery. The angiographic demonstration of the vascular anatomy and the individual preference of the operating surgeon are also important considerations.

LIVER TUMORS

Primary liver tumors are third in frequency to Wilms' tumor and neuroblastoma among primary abdominal neoplasms. Excluding developmental and inflammatory cysts and abscesses, which are discussed elsewhere, they include benign and malignant forms. Too frequently these are relatively silent tumors which go unrecognized until there is obvious abdominal enlargement due to the large mass arising within the liver.

Benign Tumors

Excluding hemangioma, benign tumors are less common than malignant neoplasms and include hamartoma, teratoma, focal nodular hyperplasia, and adenomas. These are usually discovered by the mother or on routine physical examination and are unassociated with systemic signs and symptoms. Occasionally adenomas may develop in postinflammatory or metabolic cirrhosis. All have a good prognosis, usually resulting in cure following excision.

Hemangiomas

Most hemangiomas of the liver are benign and usually asymptomatic early in life, frequently discovered as an incidental finding during surgery or at post-mortem examination. Large hemangiomas may present as an acute emergency in the newborn with shock due to massive hemoperitoneum associated with rupture of the liver or with the classic triad of hepatomegaly, heart failure, and cutaneous hemangiomas. Hemangiomas are responsible for 10% of all liver tumors reported recently from a ten year survey, and are the most common benign tumor. Although there is considerable overlapping, two main types of hepatic hemangiomas are recognized: cavernous, which tends to be more localized, and capillary, which is usually more diffuse. Transitional forms between the two have been described and may represent different developmental stages of a single disease.

RADIOLOGIC EVALUATION. This is essential and often diagnostic. Plain films frequently suggest hepatic enlargement, and occasionally punctate calcifications are identified in the area of involvement. A properly performed intravenous urogram will often demonstrate pooling of contrast medium in the vascular spaces producing a characteristic mottled appearance (Fig. 19–30). Abdominal aortography by way of the femoral artery or by the patent umbilical artery during the first few days of life shows diagnostic increased vascularity and arteriovenous shunting. Selective celiac arteriography is frequently necessary for verification in older patients (Fig. 19–31). Radionuclide scans of the liver will usually demonstrate the lesion but are less specific than the above radiologic studies.

Treatment of symptomatic hemangioma has been surgical excision when it is confined to a resectable lobe. When the lesion is generalized in the liver, hepatic artery ligation may alleviate the symptoms of congestive heart failure. A recent report has pointed out the high risk of lobectomy, which may be up to 22%, and advocates surgical intervention only if medical measures (digitalis, steroids, etc.) fail to control the abnormal hemodynamics. Spontaneous involution has been demonstrated similar to that seen with cutaneous hemangiomas.

Malignant Tumors

Malignant liver tumors in children occur twice as frequently as benign tumors and account for two thirds of all liver tumors reported. Hepatocarcinomas affect older children, and hepatoblastomas affect infants. This subdivision is widely accepted and has meaningful significance in terms of relative prognosis. Hepatoblastoma is usually more common, although the relative incidence of the two types varies. In a recent ten-year collective survey, 51% of 252 malignant tumors were hepatoblastomas, 39% were hepatocarcinomas, and the remainder included mesenchymal

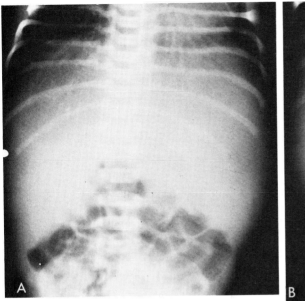
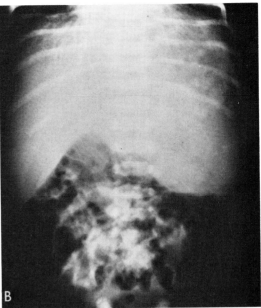
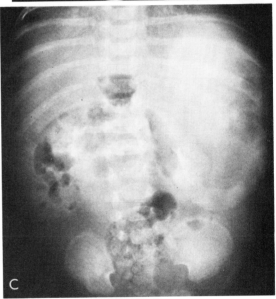

Figure 19–30. Cavernous hemangioma of left lobe of the liver. *A,* Plain film of abdomen in 1 week old child demonstrates large left upper quadrant density. *B,* Intravenous pyelogram shows collections of contrast media in dilated vascular channels in the left lobe of the liver. *C,* Film of 4 month old infant showing similar collection of contrast medium within hemangioma of the left lobe of the liver. Radiographic differentiation from splenic hemangiomas in these cases would be difficult.

tumors, various types of sarcomas, and cholangiocarcinoma. Both hepatoblastoma and hepatocellular carcinoma show male predominance. Hepatoblastoma tends to occur in the very young and is rarely seen after 3 years of age. Hepatocellular carcinoma has a peak incidence below 4 years and a second peak between 12 and 15 years. Both tumors present with abdominal enlargement, a mass, weight loss, anorexia, pain, and occasionally jaundice. Hemihypertrophy and male virilization has been re-

ported with hepatoblastoma. Spontaneous rupture of the liver is a rare complication. A large series of primary liver diseases reported by Teng, et al. included nine primary tumors. They observed significant osteoporosis, muscle atrophy, and growth failure, attributed to protein deficiency due to liver impairment (Fig. 19–32). Laboratory studies are inconsistent except for elevation of the alpha-1-fetal globulin.

RADIOLOGIC EVALUATION. These show abnormalities in over 85% of the cases

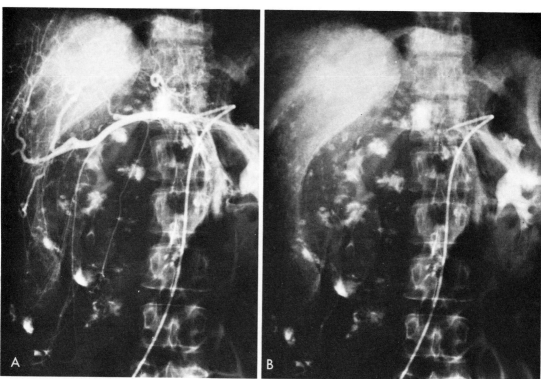

Figure 19–31. Multiple large cavernous hemangiomas of the right lobe of the liver. *A,* Selective hepatic arteriogram demonstrates deviation of the hepatic artery, presumably by a very large unopacified cyst. Multiple irregular-sized and -shaped collections of contrast material within most of the right lobe of the liver consistent with large cavernous hemangiomas. *B,* The large areas of pooled contrast material persist through the venous phase. (Courtesy of Dr. H. Goldstein, M.D. Anderson Hospital, Houston, Texas.)

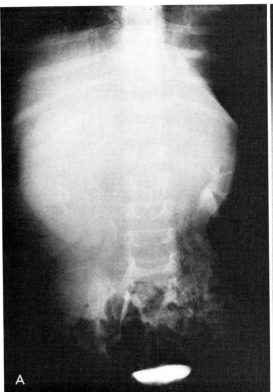

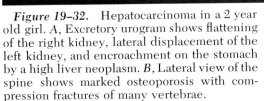

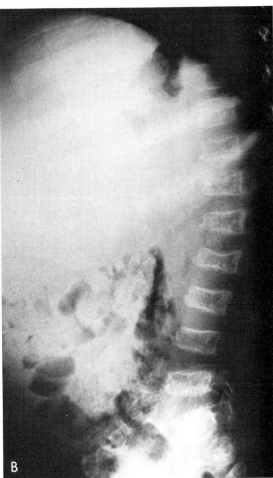

Figure 19–32. Hepatocarcinoma in a 2 year old girl. *A*, Excretory urogram shows flattening of the right kidney, lateral displacement of the left kidney, and encroachment on the stomach by a high liver neoplasm. *B*, Lateral view of the spine shows marked osteoporosis with compression fractures of many vertebrae.

with plain film evidence of hepatic and splenic enlargement. Tumor calcification is seen in 10 to 12% of the cases of hepatoblastoma, but rarely with hepatocellular carcinoma. The right hemidiaphragm is often elevated and pulmonary metastases are evident in 10% on the initial examination. Except for occasional compression of the kidney, the intravenous urogram is usually normal and is indispensable in eliminating Wilms' tumor and neuroblastoma, the most common causes of abdominal tumors in childhood. Celiac and selective hepatic arteriography are usually diagnostic of tumor involvement and also serve as a valuable guide of the vascular anatomy, not only of the tumor but also of the normal

liver parenchyma which must be preserved if partial resection is to be attempted (Fig. 19–33). The use of arteriography in the identification of metastatic disease to the liver is valuable in treatment planning (Fig. 19–34). Liver scans are also helpful noninvasive studies but are not as specific as arteriograms and cannot map the vascular anatomy.

Operative excision of malignant lesions of the liver is the only definitive treatment of significance and carries an overall survival rate of 35% for hepatoblastoma and 13% for hepatocellular carcinoma. Chemotherapy and radiation may be helpful in converting nonoperable hepatoblastoma to an operable stage.

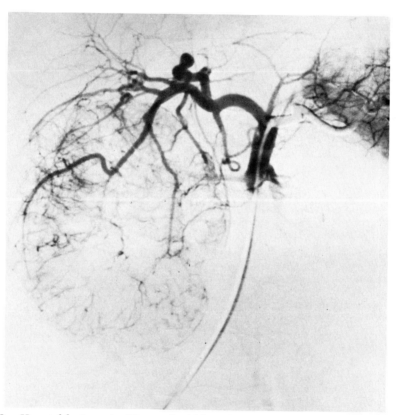

Figure 19–33. Hepatoblastoma in 22 month old boy. Subtraction film of celiac arteriogram shows large mass in the right lobe of the liver, neovascularity, and early venous shunting.

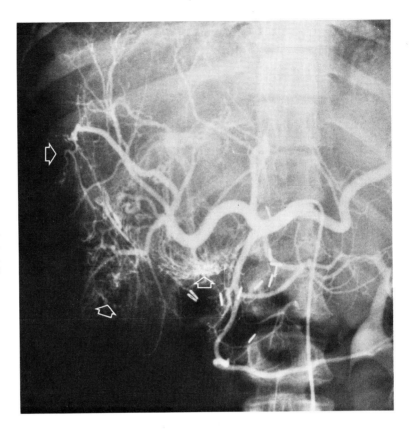

Figure 19–34. Metastatic Wilms' tumor in a 12 year old child. Selective hepatic arteriogram demonstrates multiple areas of neovascularity consistent with metastases (*arrows*). Rapid arteriovenous shunting is also demonstrated. (Courtesy of Dr. H. Goldstein, M. D. Anderson Hospital, Houston, Texas.)

THE PANCREAS

With the development of newer technics and refinement of older ones, a renewed interest in the radiologic investigation of the pancreas has emerged. This is somewhat more apparent in adults than children, largely because of the relative rarity of pancreatic abnormalities in children, with the single exception of cystic fibrosis. Except for rare calcifications, cystic fibrosis produces no demonstrable radiologic findings localized to the pancreas. The secondary changes in the lungs, paranasal sinuses, liver, and gallbladder are well known. The gastrointestinal findings may be very characteristic and have been discussed in Chapter 13.

The various radiographic modalities available to study the pancreas include routine gastrointestinal studies with hypotonic duodenography, [75Se] selenomethionine pancreatic scanning, ultrasound, and pancreatic angiography. Two more recent developments are endoscopic pancreatocholangiography and computerized body scanning. With this impressive array of procedures one should expect that abnormalities of this silent gland which have defied demonstration for so many years will become more evident. Notwithstanding this, the radiologic evaluation of the pancreas in children at the present time is often indecisive.

Congenital Lesions of the Pancreas

Although various congenital cysts and ductal anomalies have been described, they are very rare and the only two important congenital lesions of practical importance are ectopic and annular pancreas.

Ectopic pancreatic tissue may be distributed at almost any site in the gastrointestinal tract (and occasionally outside the gastrointestinal tract) but is most commonly found in the stomach and duodenum (see Fig. 9–11). With rare exceptions these are silent lesions being discovered incidentally at surgery or during radiologic examination of the gastrointestinal tract. Occasional reports suggest associated pain, vomiting, or hypertrophy of the pylorus. Barium studies characteristically show a well-defined, rounded submucosal filling defect within which is seen a central barium-filled umbilication indicating the associated ductal structure (Fig. 19–35). When this characteristic appearance is demonstrated one is able to make the diagnosis preoperatively with considerable confidence.

Annular pancreas is the most frequent and the most significant congenital lesion and is characterized by a band of pancreatic tissue which may partially or totally encircle the duodenum at or just above the ampulla. This lesion results when there is failure of the ventral pancreatic bud to rotate dorsally and fuse with the dorsal bud, which develops into the body and tail of the pancreas. A high degree of duodenal obstruction may be associated with this lesion in the newborn but many are asymptomatic and discovered incidentally later in life during radiologic examination or at surgery. An extrinsic circular defect on the outer margin of the descending duodenum is the characteristic finding seen on radiologic examination (see Fig. 12–21). When there is complete obstruction in the newborn, plain films of the abdomen will show the "double-bubble" sign of gastric and duodenal distention indistinguishable from that of duodenal atresia (see Fig. 12–19). Of interest is the combined report of the Surgical Section of the American Academy of Pediatrics, in which annular pancreas was reported in 21% of 503 patients with congenital atresia and stenosis of the duodenum. The pancreatic annulus was believed to be the obstructive factor in slightly less than one half of these cases. Consequently, annular pancreas per se may frequently be regarded as a sign of failure of normal duodenal development associated with intrinsic stenosis or atresia of the duodenum.

Pancreatitis

In contrast to adults, in whom pancreatitis is most often associated with hepatobiliary disease or alcoholism, a variety of etiologic factors may be responsible for acute pancreatitis in children.

Acute hemorrhagic pancreatitis may develop without apparent cause, but trauma, even of a trivial nature, is often responsible. Pancreatitis secondary to mumps is often suspected but difficult to prove. Fortunately it usually subsides with conservative management. Other less frequent but well known causes include steroids and immunosuppressive drugs, ascariasis, postoperative complication, annular pancreas, nutritional disturbances, hyperparathyroidism, hyperlipoproteinemia, and various atresias and stenoses involving the sphincter of Oddi and the pancreatic duct. Acute pancreatitis is occasionally associated with cystic fibrosis. Hereditary pancreatitis is transmitted as an autosomal dominant condition that affects families and should be considered in any child with recurrent episodes of acute abdominal pain. The cause of this latter condition is not known, but congenital defects of the ductal system and sphincter of Oddi may be responsible. Some cases are associated with aminoaciduria.

Regardless of the cause, the symptoms are very similar and include upper abdominal pain, vomiting, fever, leukocytosis, and occasionally jaundice. The abdomen is generally distended and tender. Shortness of breath may be associated with elevation of one or both hemidiaphragms, ascites, and pleural effusion. Delayed symptoms of polyarthritis and subcutaneous nodules associated with intramedullary fat necrosis have been reported.

RADIOLOGIC EVALUATION. Abdominal radiographs usually suggest some degree of ileus, and a distended loop of small or large bowel near the pancreas may suggest a "sentinel loop." Felson brought attention to the gasless abdomen sign (Fig. 19–36), signifying severe vomiting that occasionally is the presenting radiologic manifestation on plain films. Unexplained ascites has been reported as the presenting finding. Pancreatic calcifications are unusual but may occur in hereditary pancreatitis and in cystic fibrosis (Fig. 19–37). The abdominal fat necrosis sign of acute pancreatitis is highly specific but is not known to be reported in children. Basilar atelectasis and pleural effusion, particularly on the left, may be seen, and this observation is very significant in that amylase determinations on the pleural fluid will lead to the correct diagnosis. Contrast studies of the gastro-

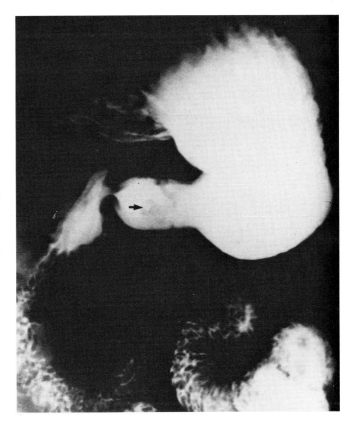

Figure 19–35. Ectopic pancreas in the antrum of the stomach. Arrow marks barium within the central umbilication. (Courtesy of Dr. H. Goldstein, M. D. Anderson Hospital, Houston, Texas.)

intestinal tract may be entirely normal and a diagnosis of pancreatitis cannot be excluded by a normal study. However, findings of mucosal edema and irritability of the stomach, duodenum, and small bowel may be highly suggestive of the proper diagnosis in the appropriate clinical setting. Extrinsic posterior indentations on the

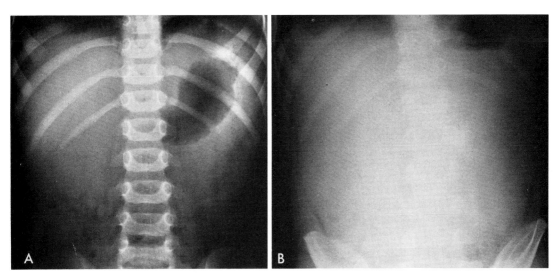

Figure 19–36. Patient with acute pancreatitis. *A,* Supine film shows gas in the stomach with little appreciable gas distal to this. *B,* Upright film shows to better advantage the deficiency of gas distal to the stomach.

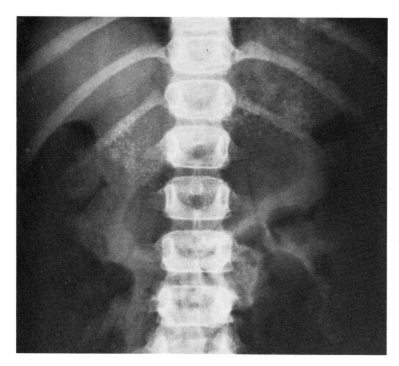

Figure 19–37. Pancreatic calcification in a child with cystic fibrosis of the pancreas and diabetes mellitus. (Courtesy of Dr. W. Berdon, Babies Hospital, New York City; reprinted from Singleton, E. B., and Gray, P. M., Jr., *Sem. Roentgenol.,* 3:267, 1968.)

stomach and widening of the duodenal loop are very helpful findings but are often not evident or very equivocal.

Further studies including radioisotope pancreatic imaging, ultrasonography, and angiography have been utilized but are often inaccurate and nonspecific and seldom performed in the pediatric age group for acute pancreatitis. Serum amylase and lipase levels are usually elevated and are highly significant but must be correlated with the clinical findings. In subacute cases the amylase may not be elevated and serum lipase determinations are more specific and reliable.

Pseudocyst of the Pancreas

Any child with a history of blunt abdominal trauma presenting with an upper abdominal mass, pain, and vomiting should suggest pseudocyst of the pancreas. The typical history is one of preceding trauma followed by a variable period of a few days to several weeks in which the acute symptoms subside, to be followed by progressive nausea, vomiting, weight loss, and development of a mass. Rarely pseudocyst may form following acute idiopathic pan-

creatitis, but trauma is believed to be responsible for at least 50% of the cases encountered in childhood. Indeed, the child under 3 years of age who presents with pseudocyst of the pancreas without obvious cause should be suspected of abuse. Pseudocyst is the commonest cause of cystic enlargement of the pancreas and is characteristically unilocular and has no epithelial lining. The body and tail are most often involved and the pseudocyst is usually localized in the upper abdomen. However, unusual locations may occur in the abdomen, and even in the chest. Serum amylase studies are elevated in about one half of the cases but pleural fluid, ascitic fluid or fluid aspirated from the cyst show more consistently diagnostic elevated amylase levels.

RADIOLOGIC EVALUATION. The findings may be very similar to those of acute pancreatitis except that there is usually more evidence of a soft tissue mass in the upper abdomen which displaces the stomach, duodenum, and at times the colon. Barium studies suggest a mass indenting and displacing the stomach when the cyst arises from the body and tail. The duodenal loop may be characteristically enlarged with mucosal effacement along the inner margin when the cyst arises in the head of the pancreas (Figs. 19–38 and 19–39). An intramural duodenal hematoma may be present and it is difficult radiologically to be certain of this associated abnormality. The splenic flexure of the colon may be depressed and intravenous urography may show indentation or depression of the left kidney. As in pancreatitis, the hemidiaphragm tends to be elevated and pleural effusion occasionally occurs, particularly on the left side.

Recent clinical experience with ultrasonography has been very rewarding, with a high degree of diagnostic accuracy reported. This is the most significant recent advance in the diagnosis of this disease and is considered by many the method of choice when pseudocyst is suspected. Characteristically a rounded sonolucent zone with a strong posterior wall is demonstrated in the area of the pancreas (Fig. 19–40). Ultrasound may be used not only in the primary diagnosis of the disease but also to follow the resolution of the lesion either after surgery or with medical management. Angiography may show changes that suggest the correct diagnosis but is seldom indicated because of the advantages of less invasive studies.

Although small cysts may occasionally resolve spontaneously, large cysts are internally drained and occasionally marsupialized.

Neutropenia – Pancreatic Insufficiency Syndrome

Shwachman et al. in 1964 described an hereditary syndrome characterized by neutropenia and pancreatic insufficiency resembling cystic fibrosis but the lungs showed no abnormality and the sweat electrolytes were normal. There is associated malabsorption, dwarfism, thrombocytopenia, and anemia. Radiographs of the long bones may show evidence of metaphyseal dysplasia and hip deformity appears to be a constant feature.

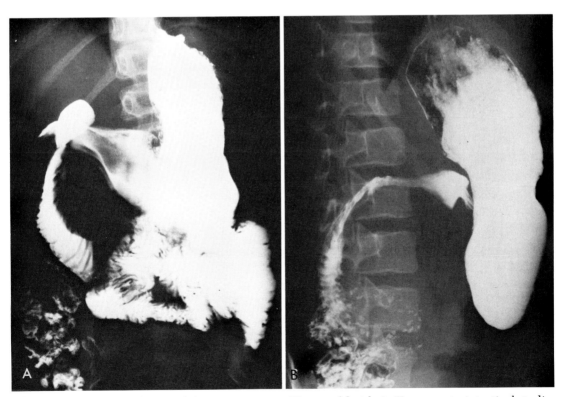

Figure 19–38. Pseudocyst of the pancreas in a 10 year old girl. *A,* Upper gastrointestinal studies show in the frontal projection indentation on the second portion of the duodenum and on the antrum of the stomach. *B,* Oblique view shows marked widening of the duodenal loop.

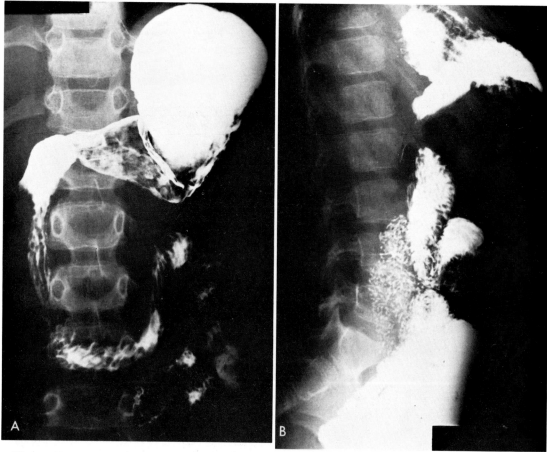

Figure 19–39. Pseudocyst of the pancreas in an 11 year old child. *A*, Frontal projection shows pressure deformity on the duodenal loop. *B*, Lateral view shows marked elevation of the antrum of the stomach.

Tumors of the Pancreas

All pancreatic tumors in children are rare and may be divided into functional and nonfunctional forms.

The nonfunctional tumors consist of various types of cysts, cystic adenomas, and carcinoma. Less than 25 cases of pancreatic carcinoma have been reported in the literature in children who range in age from 3 to 17 years. Typical symptoms consist of pain, anorexia, vomiting, weight loss, and a palpable abdominal mass. Jaundice may be present but is less common than in adults. The tumor is often far advanced at the time of diagnosis and metastases to the regional lymph nodes, liver, and lungs are already present. The diagnosis is usually suggested by upper gastrointestinal examination, showing enlargement of the head of the pancreas impinging on the duodenal loop (Fig. 19–41). Hypotonic duodenography has greatly improved the diagnostic accuracy of the upper gastrointestinal examination. Celiac and subselective arteriographic studies usually suggest an avascular mass with arterial encasement and venous stenosis or occlusion.

The functional tumors include the beta and nonbeta pancreatic islet cell tumors. Pancreatic cholera and glucagon-secreting islet cell tumors have been recognized recently but are extremely rare.

The beta-cell insulinoma results in profound hypoglycemia and has been reported in the neonate but is usually manifest later in life. Repeated convulsions and loss of consciousness associated with hypoglyce-

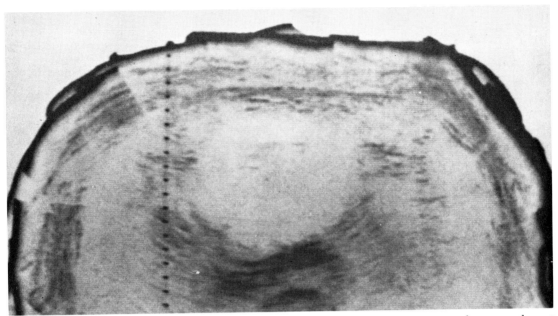

Figure 19–40. Pseudocyst of the pancreas in a young adult. The transverse scan shows sonolucent area, indicating the location of the pseudocyst.

Figure 19–41. Carcinoma of the head of the pancreas in an 18 month old boy with right upper quadrant mass and jaundice. There is widening of the duodenal loop with constriction of the postbulbar portion of the duodenum. The inferior vena cava showed invasion on a venogram. (Courtesy of Dr. H. Grossman, Duke University Medical Center, Durham, N.C.; reprinted from Singleton, E. B., and Gray, P. M., Jr., *Sem. Roentgenol.*, 3:267, 1968.)

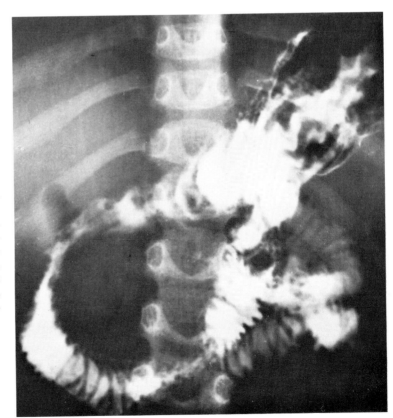

mia early in life may result in brain damage. Fatigue, nausea, anxiety, and sweating are frequently seen in older children. The most important laboratory study is the determination of the level of fasting blood sugar, which is usually under 50 mg per 100 ml. Serum insulin levels as well as the intravenous tolbutamide insulin stimulating test may be helpful in diagnosis but both have limitations and require careful interpretation.

The insulin-producing tumors are usually single, but may be multiple and can only be demonstrated radiographically by pancreatic angiography. Characteristically one sees a small dense stain during the capillary and venous phase of the angiogram, usually in the body and tail of the pancreas (Fig. 19–42). Ten per cent are estimated to be malignant and liver metastases frequently occur. As with the Zollinger-Ellison syndrome these tumors may be a part of a more generalized endocrine adenomatosis. Tumors less than 1 cm in size are not usually visualized, but the overall angiographic accuracy is estimated variously from 60 to 90%.

Treatment is surgical excision and the preoperative angiogram may be of great assistance in localizing the lesion.

Nonbeta islet cell tumors (Zollinger-Ellison syndrome) are characterized by recurrent intractable peptic ulcer disease, gastric hypersecretion, and profuse diarrhea in one third to one half the cases. The disease is rare in children, with less than 25 cases reported in children under 16 years, and has not been reported in infancy. It may be a manifestation of familial multiple endocrine adenomatosis (Wermer's syndrome) with tumoral hyperplasia of the parathyroid, pituitary, adrenal, thyroid, and pancreatic islets.

The radiologic manifestations include (1) large gastric folds with excessive gastric fluid even on fasting and without evidence of obstruction; (2) intractable peptic ulcers, which may be single or multiple and which

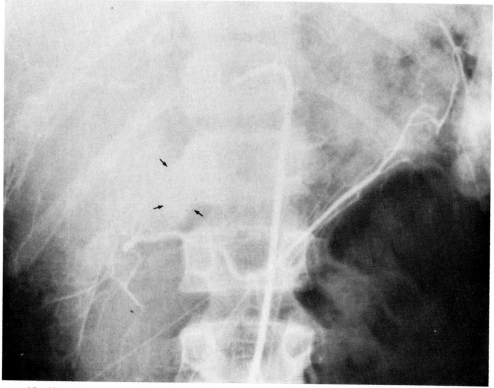

Figure 19–42. Nine year old male with seizures and episodes of hypoglycemia. Parenchymal phase of celiac arteriogram demonstrates a discrete oval-shaped stain (*arrows*) in the region of the head of the pancreas. At surgery this was proven to be an insulinoma.

are diagnostically atypical in location (post-bulbar, jejunal) in 25% of the cases; (3) dilatation and edema of the second portion of the duodenum (megaduodenum; (see Fig. 13–17); and (4) edema, increased secretions, and altered motility of the small bowel. Gastric analysis reveals a marked increase in volume and acidity and radioimmune assay of the serum shows elevated serum gastrin levels.

Celiac and superior mesenteric arteriography may demonstrate the lesion but radiographic localization is usually more difficult than in insulinomas. The incidence of malignancy is approximately 60%, and metastases to the regional lymph nodes and liver often occur. Treatment consists of surgical resection.

REFERENCES

Introduction

Baker, D. H., Berdon, W. E., and James, L. S. Proper localization of umbilical arterial and venous catheters by lateral roentgenograms, *Pediatrics, 43*:34, 1969.

Boles, E. T., Jr., and Smith, B. Preduodenal portal vein, *Pediatrics, 28*:805, 1961.

Campbell, R. E. Roentgenologic features of umbilical vascular catheterization in newborns, *Am. J. Roentgenol., 112*:68, 1971.

Diamond, L. K., Allen, F. H., Jr., and Thomas, W. O., Jr. Erythroblastosis fetalis: Treatment with exchange transfusion, *N. Engl. J. Med., 244*:39, 1951.

Emmanouilides, G. C., and Hoy, R. C. Transumbilical aortography and selective arteriography in newborn infant, *Pediatrics, 39*:337, 1967.

James, L. S. Complications arising from catheterization of the umbilical vessels. Problems of Neonatal Intensive Care Units. Report of the 59th Ross Conference on Pediatric Research, Columbus, 1969, pp. 36–43.

Johnson, G. F. Congenital preduodenal portal vein, *Am. J. Roentgenol., 112*:93, 1971.

Meyer, W. W., and Lind, J. The ductus venosus and mechanism of its closure, *Arch. Dis. Child., 41*:597, 1966.

Rosen, M. S., and Reich, S. B. Umbilical venous catheterization in the newborn: Identification of correct positioning, *Radiology, 95*:335, 1970.

Scott, J. M. Iatrogenic lesions in babies following umbilical vein catheterization, *Arch. Dis. Child., 40*:426, 1965.

Siggard-Anderson, O., and Engel, K. A new acid-base monogram, *Scand. J. Clin. Lab. Invest., 12*:177, 1960.

Congenital Anomalies of the Liver and Gallbladder

Avnet, N. L. Roentgenologic features of congenital bilateral anterior diaphragmatic eventration, *Am. J. Roentgenol., 88*:743, 1962.

Baker, D. H., and Harris, R. C. Congenital absence of the intrahepatic bile ducts, *Am. J. Roentgenol., 91*:875, 1964.

Bartone, N. F., and Grieco, R. V. Absent gallbladder and cystic duct, *Am. J. Roentgenol., 110*:252, 1970.

Blyth, H., and Ockenden, B. G. Polycystic disease of kidneys and liver presenting in childhood, *J. Med. Genet., 8*:257, 1971.

Boyden, E. A. Phrygian cap in cholecystography; a congenital anomaly of the gallbladder, *Am. J. Roentgenol., 33*:589, 1935.

Deligeorgis, D., Yannakos, D., and Doxiadis, S. Normal size of liver in infancy and childhood; x-ray study, *Arch. Dis. Child., 48*:790, 1973.

Etter, L. E. Left-sided gallbladder; necessity for films of entire abdomen in cholecystography, *Am. J. Roentgenol., 70*:987, 1953.

Feldman, M. Polycystic disease of the liver, *Am. J. Gastroenterol., 29*:83, 1958.

Firestone, F. N., and Taybi, H. Bilateral diaphragmatic eventration: Demonstrated by pneumoperitonography, *Surgery, 62*:954, 1967.

Gross, R. E. *The Surgery of Infancy and Childhood* (Philadelphia: W. B. Saunders, 1953) pp. 525–541.

Grossman, H., and Seed, W. Congenital hepatic fibrosis, bile duct dilatation, and renal lesions resembling medullary sponge kidney (congenital "cystic" disease of the liver and kidneys), *Radiology, 87*:46, 1966.

Hays, D. M., Woolley, M. M., Snyder, W. H., Jr., Reed, G. B., Gwinn, J. L., and Landing, B. J. Diagnosis of biliary atresia: Relative accuracy of percutaneous liver biopsy, open liver biopsy, and operative cholangiography, *J. Pediatr., 71*:598, 1967.

Hess, W., *Surgery of the Biliary Passages and the Pancreas* (Princeton, N.J.: D. Van Nostrand, 1965).

Kasai, M. Treatment of biliary atresia with special reference to hepatic porto-enterostomy and its modifications, *Progr. Pediatr. Surg., 6*:5, 1974.

Kerr, D. N. S., Warrick, C. K., and Hart-Mercer, J. A lesion resembling medullary sponge kidney in patients with congenital hepatic fibrosis, *Clin. Radiol., 13*:85, 1962.

Landing, B. H. Considerations of the pathogenesis of neonatal hepatitis, biliary atresia and choledochal cyst—the concept of infantile obstructive cholangiopathy, *Progr. Pediatr. Surg., 6*:113, 1974.

LeRoux, B. T. Heterotrophic intrathoracic liver. *Thorax, 16*:68, 1961.

Lieberman, E., Salinas-Madrigal, L., Gwinn, J. L., Brennan, L. P., Fine, R. N., and Landing, B. H. Infantile polycytic disease of the kidneys and liver: Clinical, pathologic, and radiologic correlation and comparison with congenital hepatic fibrosis, *Medicine, 50*:277, 1971.

Lindner, H. H., and Green, R. B. Embryology and surgical anatomy of the extra-hepatic biliary tract, *Surg. Clin. North Am., 44*:1273, 1964.

Meyers, H. I., and Jacobson, G. Displacement of stomach and duodenum by anomalous lobes of the liver, *Am. J. Roentgenol., 79*:789, 1958.

Moller, J. H., Nakib, A., Anderson, R. C., and Edwards, J. E. Congenital cardiac disease associated with polysplenia, *Circulation, 36*:789, 1967.

Nahum, H., Poree, C., and Sauvegrain, J. The study of the gallbladder and biliary ducts, *Progr. Pediatr. Radiol., 2*:65, 1969.

Neuhauser, E. B. D., Elkin, M., and Landing, B. H.

Congenital direct communication between the biliary system and the respiratory tract, *Am. J. Dis. Child.*, 83:654, 1952.

Reilly, J. E., and Neuhauser, E. B. D. Renal tubular ectasia in cystic disease of the kidney and liver, *Am. J. Roentgenol.*, 84:546, 1960.

Rosenfield, N., and Treven, S. Liver-spleen scanning in pediatrics, *Pediatrics*, 53:692, 1974.

Shehadi, W. H., and Jacox, H. W. *Clinical Radiology of the Biliary Tract* (New York: McGraw-Hill, 1963).

Singleton, E. B., Dutton, R. V., and Wagner, M. L. Radiographic evaluation of lung abnormalities, *Radiol. Clin. North Am.*, 10:333, 1972.

Waggett, J., Stool, S., Bishop, H. C., and Kirtz, M. B. Congenital bronchobiliary fistula, *J. Pediatr. Surg.*, 5:566, 1970.

Williams, C., and Williams, A. M. Abnormalities of the bile duct, *Ann. Surg.*, 141:598, 1955.

Choledochal Cyst

Alonso-Lej, F., Rever, W. R., and Pissagno, D. J. Congenital choledochal cysts, with a report of 2, and an analysis of 94, cases, *Int. Abstr. Surg.*, 108:1, 1959.

Babbitt, D. P., Starshak, R. J., and Clemett, A. R. Choledochal cyst: A concept of etiology, *Am. J. Roentgenol.*, 119:57, 1973.

Blythe, H., and Ockenden, B. G. Polycystic disease of the kidney and liver presenting in childhood, *J. Med. Genet.*, 8:257, 1971.

Chem, W. J., Chang, C. H., and Hung, W. T. Congenital choledochal cyst: With observations on rupture of the cyst and intrahepatic ductal dilatation, *J. Pediatr. Surg.*, 8:529, 1973.

Dickinson, J. Acute cholecystitis due to scarlet fever, *Am. J. Dis. Child.*, 121:331, 1971.

Duckett, J., Angelo, J. E., and Longino, L. Surgical treatment of idiopathic dilatation of the common bile duct (choledochal cyst) in 14 children, *J. Pediatr. Surg.*, 6:421, 1971.

Gilday, D. L., Brown, R., and Macpherson, R. I. Choledochal cyst—a case diagnosed by radiographic and ultrasound collaboration, *J. Can. Assoc. Radiol.*, 20:25, 1969.

Gorwitz, J. T., and Kimmeeling, R. Perforated choledochal cyst with bile peritonitis in an infant: Case report and surgical management, *Surgery*, 59:878, 1966.

Han, S. Y., Collins, L. C., and Wright, R. M. Choledochal cyst: Report of five cases, *Clin. Radiol.*, 20:332, 1969.

Hays, D. M., Goodman, G. N., Snyder, W. H., and Wooley, M. M. Congenital cystic dilatation of the common bile duct, *Arch. Surg.*, 98:457, 1969.

Holder, T. M., Stuber, J. L., and Templeton, A. W. Sonography as a diagnostic aid in the evaluation of abdominal masses in infants and children. *J. Pediatr. Surg.*, 7:532, 1972.

Ishida, M., Tsuchida, Y., Saito, S., and Hori, T. Primary excision of choledochal cysts, *Surgery*, 68:884, 1970.

Jones, P. G., Smith, E. D., Clarke, A. M., and Kent, M. Choledochal cysts: Experiences with radical excision. *J. Pediatr. Surg.*, 6:112, 1971.

Klotz, D., Cohn, B. D., and Kottmeier, P. K., Choledochal cysts: Diagnostic and therapeutic problems, *J. Pediatr. Surg.*, 8:271, 1973.

Landing, B. H. Considerations of the pathogenesis of neonatal hepatitis, biliary atresia and choledochal cyst—the concept of infantile obstructive cholangiopathy, *Progr. Pediatr. Surg.*, 6:113, 1974.

Lieberman, E., Salinas-Madrigal, L., Gwinn, J. C., Brennan, C. P., Fine, R. N., and Landing, B. H. Infantile polycystic disease of the kidney and liver, *Medicine*, 50:277, 1971.

Mujahed, Z., Glenn, F., and Evans, J. Communicating cavernous ectasia of the intrahepatic ducts (Caroli's disease), *Am. J. Roentgenol.*, 113:21, 1971.

O'Neill, J. A., Jr., and Clatworthy, H. W. Jr., Management of choledochal cysts: A fourteen-year follow-up, *Am. Surg.*, 37:230, 1971.

Rabinowitz, J. G., Kinkhabwala, M. N., and Rose, J. S. Rim sign in choledochal cyst: Additional diagnostic feature, *J. Can. Assoc. Radiol.*, 24:226, 1973.

Rosenfield, N., and Griscom, N. T. Choledochal cysts: Roentgenographic techniques, *Radiology*, 114:113, 1973.

Rosenfield, N., and Treves, S. Liver-spleen scanning in pediatrics, *Pediatrics*, 53:692, 1974.

Saito, S., and Ishida, M. Congenital choledochal cyst (cystic dilatation of the common bile duct), *Progr. Pediatr. Radiol.*, 6:63, 1974.

Silberman, E. L., and Glaessner, T. S. Roentgen features of congenital cystic dilatation of the common bile duct: A report of two cases, *Am. J. Roentgenol.*, 82:470, 1964.

Steinbach, H. L., Crane, J. T., and Bruyn, H. B. The roentgen demonstration of cirrhosis of the liver with fatty metamorphosis: Report of a case due to congenital fibrocystic disease, *Radiology*, 62:858, 1954.

Tada, S., Yasukochi, H., Shida, H., Motegi, F., and Fukuda, A. Choledochal cyst demonstrated by ^{131}I rose bengal scanning, *Am. J. Roentgenol.*, 116:587, 1972.

Yotuyanagi, S. Contributions to aetiology and pathology of idiopathic cystic dilatation of common bile duct, with report of three cases, *Gann J. (Tokyo)*, 30:601, 1936.

Cholecystitis and Cholelithiasis

Bloom, R. A., and Swain, V. A. J. Non-calculous distention of the gallbladder in children, *Arch. Dis. Child.*, 41:503, 1966.

Brenner, R. W., and Stewart, C. F. Cholecystitis in children, *Rev. Surg.*, 21:327, 1964.

Crystal, R. F., and Fink, R. L. Acute acalculous cholecystitis in childhood: A report of 2 cases, *Clin. Pediatr.*, 10:423, 1971.

Dickinson, S. J., Corley, G., and Santulli, T. V. Acute cholecystitis as a sequel to scarlet fever, *Am. J. Dis. Child.*, 121:331, 1971.

Hanson, B. A., Mahour, G. H., and Woolley, M. M. Diseases of the gallbladder in infancy and childhood, *J. Pediatr. Surg.*, 6:277, 1971.

Harned, R. K., and Babbitt, D. P. Cholelithiasis in children, *Radiology*, 117:391, 1975.

Kiesewetter, W. B. Cholecystitis and cholelithiasis. *In* Mustard, W. T., Ravitch, M. M., Snyder, W. H., Jr., Welch, K. J., and Benson, C. D., editors, *Pediatric Surgery* (2nd ed.; Chicago: Year Book Medical Publishers, 1969), pp. 745–747.

Marks, C., Espinosa, J., and Hyman, L. J. Acute acalculous cholecystitis in childhood, *J. Pediatr. Surg.*, 3:608, 1968.

Mintz, A. A., Church, G., and Adams, E. D. Cholelithiasis in sickle cell anemia, *J. Pediatr.*, 47:171, 1955.

Morales, L., Taboada, E., Toledo, L., and Radrigan, W. Cholecystitis and cholelithiasis in children, *J. Pediatr. Surg.*, 2:565, 1967.

Munster, A. M., and Brown, J. R. Acalculous cholecystitis, *Am. J. Surg.*, 113:730, 1967.

Newman, D. E. Gallstones in children, *Pediatr. Radiol.*, 1:100, 1973.

Phillips, J. C., and Gerald, B. E. The incidence of cholelithiasis in sickle cell disease, *Am. J. Roentgenol.*, 113:27, 1971.

Strauss, R. G. Scarlet fever with hydrops of the gallbladder, *Pediatrics*, 44:741, 1969.

Strauss, R. G. Cholelithiasis in childhood, *Am. J. Dis. Child.*, 117:689, 1969.

Ulin, A. W., Nosal, J. L., and Martin, W. L. Cholecystitis in childhood: Associated obstructive jaundice, *Surgery*, 31:312, 1952.

Liver Abscess

Caldicott, W. J. H., and Baehner, R. L. Chronic granulomatous disease of childhood, *Am. J. Roentgenol.*, 103:133, 1968.

Dehner, L. P., and Kissane, J. M. Pyogenic hepatic abscesses in infancy and childhood, *J. Pediatr.*, 74:763, 1969.

McCarty, E., Pathmanand, C., Sunakorn, P., and Scherz, R. G. Amoebic abscess in childhood: A case study of a 21 month old Thai child and a literature review, *Am. J. Dis. Child.*, 126:67, 1973.

Nebesar, R. A., Tefft, M., and Colodny, A. H. Angiography of liver abscess in granulomatous disease of childhood, *Am. J. Roentgenol.*, 108:628, 1970.

Novy, S. B., Wallace, S., Goldman, A. M., and Ben-Menachem, Y. Pyogenic liver abscess: Angiographic diagnosis and treatment by closed aspiration, *Am. J. Roentgenol.*, 121:388, 1974.

Preimesberger, K. F., and Goldberg, M. E. Acute liver abscess in chronic granulomatous disease of childhood, *Radiology*, 110:147, 1974.

Sutcliffe, J., and Chrispin, A. R. Chronic granulomatous disease, *Br. J. Radiol.*, 43:110, 1970.

Williams, J. W., Rittenberry, A., Dillard, R., and Allen, R. G. Liver abscess in newborn: Complication of umbilical vein catheterization, *Am. J. Dis. Child.*, 125:111, 1973.

Wolfson, J. J., Quie, P. G., Laxdal, S. D., and Good, R. A. Roentgenologic manifestations in children with a genetic defect of polymorphonuclear leukocyte function (chronic granulomatous disease of childhood), *Radiology*, 91:37, 1968.

Necrotizing Angiitis

Citron, B. P., Halpern, M., McCarron, M., Lundbert, G. D., McCormick, R., Pincus, I. J., Tatter, D., and Haverback, B. J. Necrotizing angiitis associated with drug abuse, *N. Engl. J. Med.*, 283:1003, 1970.

Halpern, M., and Citron, B. P. Necrotizing angiitis associated with drug abuse, *Am. J. Roentgenol.*, 111:663, 1971.

Lang, E. K. Arteriographic diagnosis of periarteritis nodosa, *J. Indiana State Med. Assoc.*, 60:928, 1967.

Portal Hypertension

Auvert, J., Michel, J. R., and Farge, C. The radiological approach to the diagnosis of portal hypertension, *Progr. Pediatr. Radiol.*, 2:99, 1969.

Bookstein, J. J., and Whitehouse, W. M. Splenoportography, *Radiol. Clin. North Am.*, 2:447, 1964.

Buonocore, E., Collmann, I. R., Kerley, H. E., and Lester, T. L. Massive upper gastrointestinal hemorrhage in children, *Am. J. Roentgenol.*, 115:289, 1972.

Ehrlich, F., Pipatanagul, S., Sieber, W. K., and Kiesewetter, W. B. Portal hypertension: Surgical management in infants and children, *J. Pediatr. Surg.*, 9:283, 1974.

Fellows, K. E., Jr., and Nebesar, R. A. Abdominal, hepatic and visceral angiography. *In* Gypes, M. T., editor, *Angiography in Infants and Children* (New York: Grune & Stratton, 1974), Chapter 6, pp. 193–232.

Hsia, D. Y., and Gellis, S. S. Portal hypertension in infants and children, *Am. J. Dis. Child.*, 90:290, 1955.

Kerr, D. N., Warrick, C. K., and Hart-Mercer, J. A lesion resembling medullary sponge kidney in patients with congenital hepatic fibrosis, *Clin. Radiol.*, 13:85, 1962.

Martin, L. W. Changing concepts of management of portal hypertension in children, *J. Pediatr. Surg.*, 7:559, 1972.

Myers, N. A., and Robinson, M. M. Extrahepatic portal hypertension in children, *J. Pediatr. Surg.*, 8:467, 1973.

Oski, F. A., Allen, D. M., and Diamond, L. K. Portal hypertension—a complication of umbilical vein catheterization, *Pediatrics*, 31:297, 1963.

Pinkerton, J. A., Holcomb, G. W., Jr., and Foster, J. H. Portal hypertension in childhood, *Ann. Surg.*, 175:870, 1972.

Reilly, B. J., and Neuhauser, E. B. D. Renal tubular ectasia in cystic disease of the kidney and liver, *Am. J. Roentgenol.*, 84:546, 1960.

Rosch, J., and Dotter, C. T. Extrahepatic portal obstruction in children and its angiographic diagnosis, *Am. J. Roentgenol.*, 112:143, 1971.

Sherman, N. J., and Clatworthy, H. W., Jr. Gastrointestinal bleeding in neonates; A study of 94 cases, *Surgery*, 62:614, 1967.

Spencer, R. Gastrointestinal hemorrhage in infancy and childhood: 476 cases, *Surgery*, 55:718, 1964.

Turunen, M., and Laitinen, H. Collateral circulation between a spleen transposited into the thoracic cavity and the V. cava superior, *Ann. Surg.*, 149:443, 1959.

Viamonte, M., Warren, W. D., Formon, J. J., and Martinez, L. O. Angiographic investigation in portal hypertension, *Surg. Gynecol. Obstet.*, 130:37, 1970.

Voorhees, A. B., Jr., Harris, R. C., Britton, R. C., Price, J. B., and Santulli, T. V. Portal hypertension in children: 98 cases, *Surgery*, 58:540, 1965.

Voorhees, A. B., Jr., and Price, J. B., Jr. Extrahepatic portal hypertension: A retrospective analysis of 127 cases and associated clinical implications, *Arch. Surg.*, 108:338, 1974.

Liver Tumors

Clatworthy, H. W., Jr., Boles, E. T., Jr., and Kottmier, E. K. Liver tumors in infancy and childhood, *Ann. Surg.*, 154:475, 1971.

Exelby, P. R., Ali, E. -D., Huvos, A. G., and Beattie, E. J., Jr. Primary malignant tumors in children, *J. Pediatr. Surg.*, 6:272, 1971.

Exelby, P. R., Filler, R. M., and Grosfeld, J. L. Liver tumors in the particular reference to hepatoblastoma and hepatocellular carcinoma: American Academy of Pediatrics Surgical Section Survey—1974, *J. Pediatr. Surg.*, 10:329, 1975.

Ishak, K. G., and Glunz, P. R. Hepatoblastoma and hepatocarcinoma in infancy and childhood: Report of 47 cases, *Cancer*, 20:396, 1967.

Margulis, A., Nice, C., and Rigler, L. Roentgen findings in primary hepatoma in infants and children, *Radiology*, 66:809, 1956.

Martin, L. W., and Woodman, K. S. Hepatic lobectomy for hepatoblastoma in infants and children, *Arch. Surg.*, 98:1, 1969.

McBride, C., and Wallace, S. Cancer of the right lobe of the liver, *Arch. Surg.*, 105:289, 1972.

McCarthy, C. S., Davies, E. R., Wells, P. N. T., Rose, S. G. M., Follett, D. H., Muir, K. M., and Read, A. E. A comparison of ultrasonic and isotope scanning in the diagnosis of liver disease, *Br. J. Radiol.*, 43:100, 1970.

McDonald, P. Hepatic tumors in childhood, *Clin. Radiol.*, 18:74, 1967.

Moss, A. A., Clark, R. E., Palubinskas, A. J., and de Lorimier, A. A. Angiographic appearance of benign and malignant hepatic tumors in children, *Am. J. Roentgenol.*, 113:61, 1971.

Nebesar, R. A., Tefft, M., and Filler, R. M. Correlation of angiography and isotope scanning in abdominal diseases of children, *Am. J. Roentgenol.*, 109:323, 1970.

Nikaldoh, H., Boggs, J., and Swenson, O. Liver tumors in infants and children: Clinical and pathologic analysis of 22 cases, *Arch. Surg.*, 101:245, 1970.

Novy, S., Wallace, S., Medellin, H., and McBride, C. Angiographic evaluation of primary malignant hepatocellular tumors in children, *Am. J. Roentgenol.*, 120:353, 1974.

Sorsdahl, O. A., and Gay, B. B., Jr. Roentgenologic features of a primary carcinoma of the liver in infants and children, *Am. J. Roentgenol.*, 100:117, 1967.

Taylor, K. J. W., Carpenter, D. A., and McCready, V. R. Gray-scale echography in the diagnosis of intrahepatic disease, *J. Clin. Ultrasound*, 1:284, 1973.

Tefft, M. More common radionuclide examinations in children: Indications for use with a discussion of radiation dose received, *J. Pediatr.*, 48:802, 1956.

Teng, C. T., Dachsner, C. W., Singleton, E. B., Rosenberg, H. S., Cole, V. W., Hill, L. L., and Brennan, J. C. Liver disease and osteoporosis in children, *J. Pediatr.*, 59:684, 1961.

Hemangiomas

Berdon, W. E., and Baker, D. H. Giant hepatic hemangioma with cardiac failure in the newborn infant: Value of high-dosage intravenous urography and umbilical angiography, *Radiology*, 92:1523, 1969.

de Lorimier, A. A., Simpson, E. B., Baum, R. S., and Carlsson, E. Hepatic-artery ligation for hepatic hemangiomatosis, *N. Engl. J. Med.*, 277:333, 1967.

Golberg, S. J., and Fonkalsrud, E. Successful treatment of hepatic hemangioma with corticosteroids, *J.A.M.A.*, 208:2473, 1969.

Graivier, L., Votteler, T. P., and Dorman, G. W. Hepatic hemangiomas in newborn infants, *J. Pediatr. Surg.*, 2:299, 1967.

Leonidas, J. C., Strauss, L., and Beck, R. Vascular tumors of liver in newborns: Pediatric emergency, *Am. J. Dis. Child.*, 125:507, 1973.

Matolo, N. M., and Johnson, D. G. Surgical treatment of hepatic hemangioma in the newborn, *Arch. Surg.*, 106:725, 1973.

O'Connor, J. F., and Neuhauser, E. B. D. Total body opacification in conventional and high-dose intravenous urography in infancy, *Am. J. Roentgenol.*, 90:63, 1963.

Selke, A. C., and Cornell, S. H. Infantile hepatic hemangioendothelioma, *Am. J. Roentgenol.*, 106:200, 1969.

Slovis, T. L., Berdon, W. E., Haller, J. O., Casarella, W. J., and Baker, D. H. Hemangiomas of the liver in infants: Review of diagnosis, treatment and course, *Am. J. Roentgenol.*, 123:791, 1975.

Touloukian, R. J. Hepatic hemangioendothelioma during infancy: Pathology, diagnosis and treatment with predisone, *Pediatrics*, 45:71, 1970.

The Pancreas—Introduction

Andersen, D. H. Cystic fibrosis of the pancreas and its relation to celiac disease: A clinical and pathologic study, *Am. J. Dis. Child.*, 56:344, 1938.

di Sant'Agnese, P. A., and Talamo, R. C. Pathogenesis and pathophysiology of cystic fibrosis of the pancreas, *N. Engl. J. Med.*, 277:1287, 1344, 1399, 1967.

Eaton, S. B., Jr., and Ferrucci, J. T., Jr. *Radiology of the Pancreas and Duodenum* (Philadelphia: W. B. Saunders, 1973).

Esterly, J. R., and Oppenheimer, E. H. Observations in cystic fibrosis of the pancreas. I. The gallbladder, *Bull. Johns Hopkins Hosp.*, 110:247, 1962.

Grossman, H., Berdon, W. E., and Baker, D. H. Gastrointestinal findings in cystic fibrosis, *Am. J. Roentgenol.*, 97:227, 1955.

Reeves, R. J., and Moran, F. T. Diffuse pancreatic calcifications. An analysis of 6 cases, *Radiology*, 51:219, 1948.

Singleton, E. B., and Gray, P. M., Jr. Radiologic evaluation of pancreatic disease in children, *Sem. Roentgenol.*, 3:267, 1968.

Congenital Lesions of the Pancreas

Atallah, M. K., and Melhem, R. E. Annular pancreas in infancy: Report of 3 Cases, *Am. J. Roentgenol.*, 90:740, 1963.

Barbosa, J. J., de Castro, J., Dockerty, M. B., and Waugh, J. M. Pancreatic heterotopia: Review of recent literature and report of 41 authenticated surgical cases of which 25 were clinically significant, *Surg. Gynecol. Obstet.*, 82:527, 1946.

Besemann, E. F., Auerbach, S. H., and Wolfe, W. W., The importance of roentgenologic diagnosis of aberrant pancreatic tissue in the gastrointestinal tract, *Am. J. Roentgenol.*, 107:71, 1969.

Boyden, E. A., Cope, J. G., and Bill, A. H., Jr. Anatomy and embryology of congenital intrinsic obstruction of the duodenum, *Am. J. Surg.*, 114:190, 1967.

Eklof, O., Lassrich, A., Stanley, P., and Chrispin, A. R. Ectopic pancreas, *Pediatr. Radiol.*, 1:24, 1973.

Elliot, C. B., Kliman, M. R., and Elliot, K. A. Pancreatic annulus: A sign or a cause of duodenal obstruction? *Can. J. Surg.*, 11:357, 1968.

Fonkalsrud, E. W., de Lorimier, A. A., and Hays, D. M. Congenital atresia and stenosis of the duodenum: A review compiled from the members of the Surgical Section of the America Academy of Pediatrics, *Pediatrics*, 43:79, 1969.

Free, E. A., and Gerald, B. Duodenal obstruction in the newborn due to annular pancreas, *Am. J. Roentgenol.*, 103:321, 1968.

Hope, J. W., and Gibbons, J. F. Duodenal obstruction due to annular pancreas, *Radiology*, 63:473, 1954.

Lucaya, J., and Ochoa, J. B. Ectopic pancreas in the stomach, *J. Pediatr. Surg.*, 11:101, 1976.

Pancreatitis

Berenson, J. E., Spitz, H. B., and Felson, B. The abdominal fat necrosis sign, *Radiology*, 100:567, 1971.

Blumenthal, H. T., and Probstein, J. G. Acute pancreatitis in the newborn, in infancy and in childhood, *Am. Surg.*, 27:533, 1961.

Farrell, G. E., and Prillaman, P. E. Pleural effusions in acute pancreatitis, *South Med. J.*, 57:505, 1964.

Felson, B. Letter from the editor, *Sem. Roentgenol.*, 3:215, 1968.

Frey, C., and Redo, S. F. Inflammatory lesions of the pancreas in infancy and childhood, *Pediatrics*, 32:93, 1963.

Gilbert, M. G., and Carbonnell, M. L. Pancreatitis in childhood associated with ascariasis, *Pediatrics*, 33:589, 1964.

Grosfeld, J. L., and Cooney, D. R. Pancreatic and gastrointestinal trauma in children, *Pediatr. Clin. North Am.*, 22:2, 365, 1975.

Gross, J. B., Gambill, E. E., and Ulrich, J. A. Hereditary pancreatitis. Description of a fifth kindred and summary of clinical features, *Am. J. Med.*, 33:358, 1962.

Hartley, R. C. Pancreatitis under the age of 5 years: A report of 3 cases, *J. Pediatr. Surg.*, 2:419, 1967.

Hendren, W. H., Greep, J. M., and Patton, A. S. Pancreatitis in childhood: Experience with 15 cases, *Arch. Dis. Child.*, 40:132, 1965.

Immelman, E. J., Bank, S., Krige, H., and Marks, I. N. Roentgenologic and clinical features of intramedullary fat necrosis in bones in acute and chronic pancreatitis, *Am. J. Med.*, 36:96, 1964.

Kalwinsky, D., Fritelli, G., and Oski, F. A. Pancreatitis presenting as unexplained ascites, *Am. J. Dis. Child.*, 128:734, 1974.

Kattwinkel, J., Lapey, A., di Sant'Agnese, P. A., and Edwards, W. A. Hereditary pancreatitis: 3 kindreds and a critical review of the literature, *Pediatrics*, 51:55, 1973.

Keating, J. P., Shackelford, G. D., Shackelford, P. G., and Ternberg, J. L. Pancreatitis and osteolytic lesions, *J. Pediatr.*, 81:350, 1972.

Moossa, A. R. Acute pancreatitis in childhood: A study of 16 cases and review of the literature, *Progr. Pediatr. Surg.*, 4:111, 1972.

Poppel, M. H. The roentgen manifestations of pancreatitis, *Sem. Roentgenol.*, 3:227, 1968.

Riemenschneider, T. A., Wilson, J. F., and Vernier, R. L. Glucocorticoid-induced pancreatitis in children, *Pediatrics*, 41:428, 1968.

Roseman, D. M., Kowlessar, O. D., and Sleisenger, M. H. Pulmonary manifestations of pancreatitis, *N. Engl. J. Med.*, 263:294, 1960.

Shwachman, H., Lebenthal, E., and Khaw, K. T. Recurrent acute pancreatitis in patients with cystic fibrosis with normal pancreatic enzymes, *Pediatrics*, 55:86, 1975.

Sibert, J. R. Hereditary pancreatitis in a Newcastle family, *Arch. Dis. Child.*, 48:618, 1973.

Singleton, E. B., and Gray, P. M., Jr. Radiologic evaluation of pancreatic disease in children, *Sem. Roentgenol.*, 3:267, 1968.

Sperling, M. A. Bone lesions in pancreatitis, *Australas. Ann. Med.*, 17:334, 1968.

Spjut, H. J., and Anderson, M. S. Pathology of the pancreas. *Sem. Roentgenol.*, 3:217, 1968.

Weens, H. S., and Walker, L. A. The radiologic diagnosis of acute cholecystitis and pancreatitis, *Radiol. Clin. North Am.*, 2:89, 1964.

Whitten, D. M., Feingold, M., and Eisenklam, E. J. Hereditary pancreatitis, *Am. J. Dis. Child.*, 116:426, 1968.

Williams, W. H., and Hendren, W. H. Intrapancreatic duodenal duplication causing pancreatitis in a child, *Surgery*, 69:708, 1971.

Witte, C. L., and Schanzer, B. Pancreatitis due to mumps, *J.A.M.A.*, 203:1068, 1968.

Pseudocyst of the Pancreas

Bongiovi, J. J., and Logosso, R. D. Pancreatic pseudocyst occurring in the battered child syndrome, *J. Pediatr. Surg.*, 4:220, 1969.

Caravati, C. M., Ashworth, J. S., and Frederick, P. Pancreatic pseudocysts. A medical evaluation, *J.A.M.A.*, 197:572, 1966.

Filly, R. A., and Freimanis, A. K. Echographic diagnosis of pancreatic lesions: Ultrasound scanning techniques and diagnostic findings, *Radiology*, 96:575, 1970.

Fu, W. R., and Stanton, L. W. Angiographic study of pseudocysts of the pancreas, *J. Can. Assoc. Radiol.*, 20:176, 1969.

Galligan, J. J., and Williams, H. J. Pancreatic pseudocysts in childhood: Unusual case with mediastinal extension, *Am. J. Dis. Child.*, 112:479, 1966.

Kilman, J. W., Kaiser, G. C., King, R. D., and Shumacker, H. B. Pancreatic pseudocysts in infancy and childhood, *Surgery*, 55:455, 1964.

Leopold, G. R. Pancreatic echography: A new dimension in the diagnosis of pseudocyst, *Radiology*, 104:365, 1972.

Pena, S. D. J., and Medovy, H. Child abuse and pancreatic pseudocysts of the pancreas, *J. Pediatr.*, 83:1026, 1973.

Reuter, S. R., and Redman, H. C. *Gastrointestinal Angiography* (Philadelphia: W. B. Saunders, 1972).

Shockman, A. T., and Marasco, J. A. Pseudocysts of the pancreas, *Am. J. Roentgenol.*, 101:628, 1967.

Thomford, N. R., and Jesseph, J. E. Pseudocysts of the pancreas. A review of 50 cases, *Am. J. Surg.*, 118:86, 1969.

Wool, G., and Goldring, D. Pseudocysts of the pancreas: Report of 5 cases and review of the literature, *J. Pediatr.*, 70:586, 1967.

Neutropenia—Pancreatic Insufficiency Syndrome

Bodian, M., Sheldon, W., and Lightwood, R. Congenital hypoplasia of the exocrine pancreas, *Acta Paediatr.*, 53:282, 1964.

Fellman, K., Kozlowski, K., Senger, A. Unusual bone changes in exocrine pancreas insufficiency with cyclic neutropenia, *Acta Radiol.*, 12:428, 1972.

Shwachman, H., Diamond, L. K., Oski, F. A., and Khaw, K. T. The syndrome of pancreatic insufficiency and bone marrow dysfunction, *J. Pediatr.*, 65:645, 1964.

Stanley, P., and Sutcliffe, J. Metaphyseal chondrodysplasia with dwarfism, pancreatic insufficiency and neutropenia, *Pediatr. Radiol.*, 1:119, 1973.

Taybi, H., Mitchell, A. D., and Friedman, G. D. Metaphyseal dysostosis and the associated syndrome of pancreatic insufficiency and blood disorders, *Radiology*, 93:563, 1969.

Tumors of the Pancreas

Boijsen, E., and Samuelsson, L. Angiographic diagnosis of tumors arising from the pancreatic islets, *Acta Radiol. (Stockholm).*, 10:161, 1970.

Buchta, R. M., and Kaplan, J. M. Zollinger-Ellison syndrome in a 9 year old: A case report and review of this entity in childhood, *Pediatrics*, 47:594, 1971.

Christoforidis, A. J., and Nelson, S. W. Radiological manifestations of ulcerogenic tumors of the pancreas, *J.A.M.A.*, 198:511, 1966.

Friesen, S. R. Effect of total gastrectomy on the Zollinger-Ellison tumor: Observation by second look procedure, *Surgery*, 62:609, 1967.

Fulton, R. E., Sheddy, P. F., McIlrath, D. C., and Ferris, D. O. Preoperative angiographic localization of insulin-producing tumors of the pancreas, *Am. J. Roentgenol.*, 123:367, 1975.

Gray, R. K., Rosch, J., and Grollman, J. H., Jr. Arteriography in the diagnosis of islet-cell tumors, *Radiology*, 97:39, 1970.

Korobkin, M. T., Palubinskas, A. J., and Glickman, M. G. Pitfalls in arteriography of islet-cell tumors of the pancreas, *Radiology*, 100:319, 1971.

Mah, P. T., Loo, D. C., and Tock, E. P. C. Pancreatic acinar cell carcinoma in childhood. *Am. J. Dis. Child.*, 128:101, 1974.

McGuigan, J. E., and Trudeau, W. L. Immunochemical measurement of elevated level of gastrin in the serum of patients with pancreatic tumors of the Zollinger-Ellison variety, *N. Engl. J. Med.*, 278:1308, 1968.

Moynan, R. W., Neerhout, R. C., and Johnson, T. S.

Pancreatic carcinoma in childhood: Case report and review, *J. Pediatr.*, 65:711, 1964.

Nelson, S. W., and Christoforidis, A. J. Roentgenologic features of the Zollinger-Ellisone syndrome—ulcerogenic tumor of the pancreas, *Sem. Roentgenol.*, 3:254, 1968.

Passaro, E., Basso, N., and Walsh, J. H. Calcium challenge in the Zollinger-Ellison snydrome, *Surgery*, 72:60, 1972.

Reuter, S. R., and Redman, H. C. *Gastrointestinal Angiography* (Philadelphia: W. B. Saunders, 1972).

Rickham, P. P. Islet-cell tumors in childhood, *J. Pediatr. Surg.*, 10:83, 1975.

Robinson, M. J., Clarke, A. M., Gold, H., and Connelly, J. F. Islet-cell adenoma in the newborn: Report of 2 patients, *Pediatrics*, 48:232, 1971.

Rosenlund, M. L., Crean, G. P., Johnson, D. G., Holtzapple, P. G., and Brooks, F. P. The Zollinger-Ellison syndrome in a ten year old boy, *J. Pediatr.*, 75:443, 1969.

Schotland, M. G., Kaplan, S. L., and Grumbach, M. M. The tolbutamide tolerance test in the evaluation of childhood hypoglycemia, *Pediatrics*, 39:838, 1967.

Schwartz, D. L.: White, J. J., Saulsbury, F., and Haller, J. A., Jr. Gastrin response to calcium infusion: An aide in the improved diagnosis of Zollinger-Ellison syndrome in children, *Pediatrics*, 54:599, 1974.

Tuttle, R. J., Strasberg, Z., and Cole, F. M. Angiographic diagnosis of insulinoma in a 6 year old boy, *Radiology*, 104:355, 1972.

Wermer, P. Genetic aspects of adenomatosis of endocrine glands, *Am. J. Med.*, 16:363, 1954.

Zboralske, F. F., and Amberg, J. R. Detection of the Zollinger-Ellison syndrome: The radiologist's responsibility, *Am. J. Roentgenol.*, 104:529, 1968.

Zollinger, R. M. Islet cell tumors and the alimentary tract, *Am. J. Roentgenol.*, 126:933, 1976.

Zollinger, R. M., and Ellison, E. H. Primary peptic ulceration of jejunum associated with islet cell tumors of pancreas, *Ann. Surg.*, 142:709, 1955.

INDEX

Illustrations are indicated by italic numerals;
tables are indicated by an italic "t" following
page number.

435